The Healthy Italian

COOKING FOR THE LOVE OF FOOD AND FAMILY

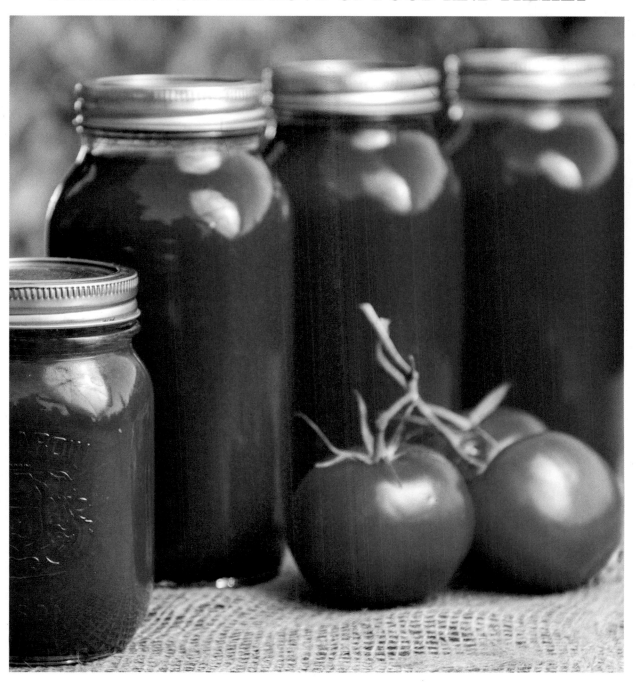

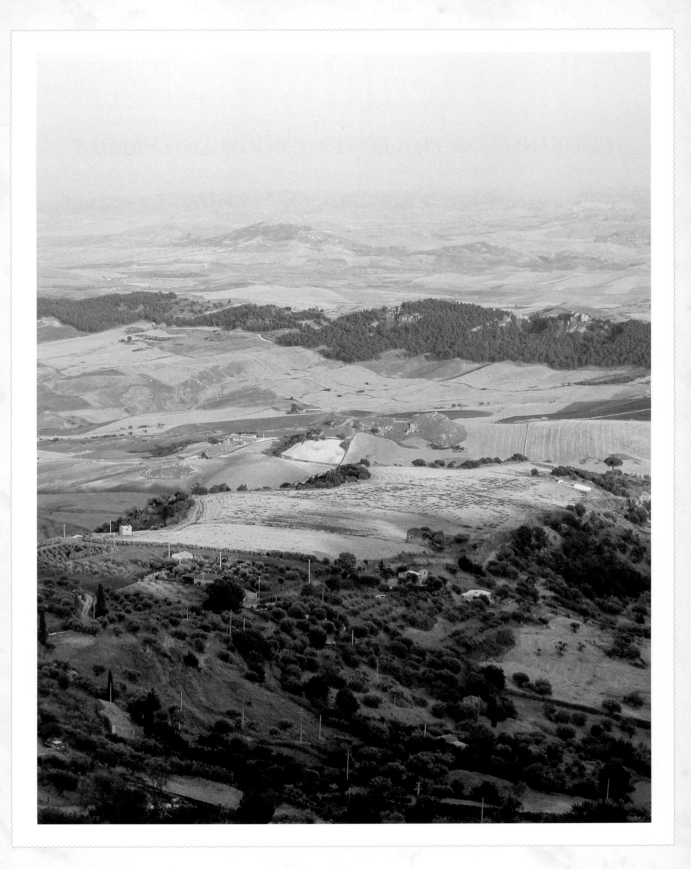

The Healthy Italian

COOKING FOR THE LOVE OF FOOD AND FAMILY

FINA SCROPPO

PHOTOGRAPHY BY MICHAEL RAO

DANVID & COMPANY INC.

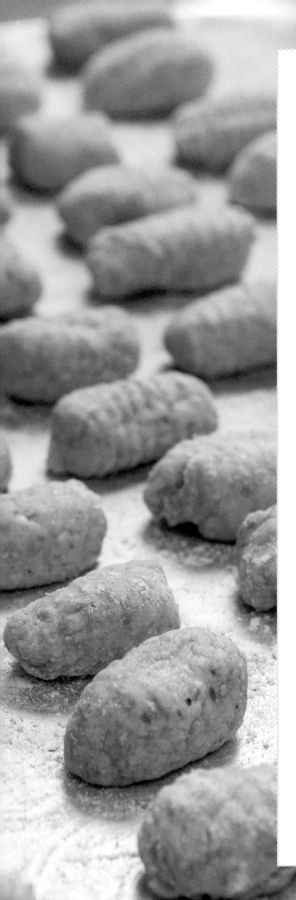

Library and Archives Canada Cataloguing in Publication

Scroppo, Fina, author
          The healthy Italian : cooking for the love of food and family / by Fina Scroppo ; photography by Michael Rao.

Includes index.
ISBN 978-0-9920075-0-8 (pbk.)

          1. Cooking, Italian. I. Title.

TX723.S37 2013   641.5945   C2013-906119-3

Art director: Stephanie White
Food photography: Michael Rao
Editor: Suzanne Moutis
Contributing editor: Liza Finlay
Nutrition consultant: Emily Kennedy, MSc, RHN, registered nutritionist
Publisher: Danvid & Company Inc.

Printed in Canada by Transcontinental Printing

For all inquiries, please contact us at **www.thehealthyitalian.ca**

If you're interested in bulk purchases of **The Healthy Italian**, we offer an aggressive discount. Please contact us at **www.thehealthyitalian.ca**

Recipe analysis calculated using NutriBase Nutrition and Fitness Software (CyberSoft, Inc.) www.nutribase.com

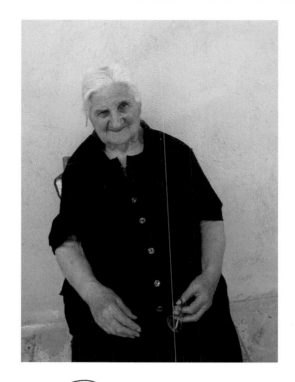

Dedication

....

For my late grandmother,
Nonna Maria Grazia,
and all those grandmothers
who influence our cooking,
shape our lives and
inspire our futures.

....

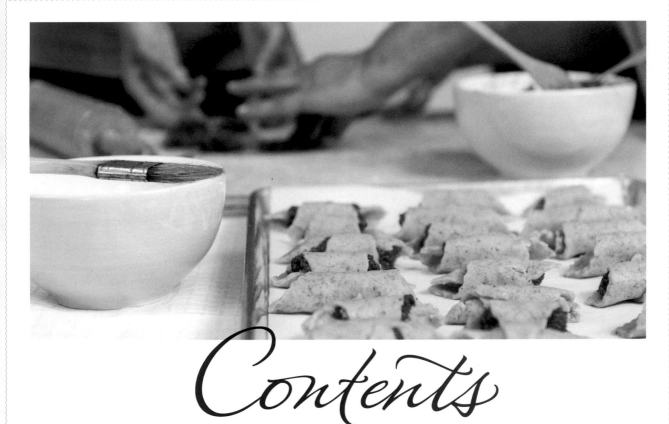

Contents

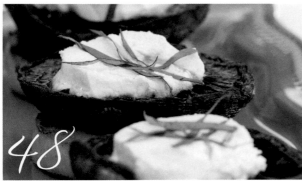

48

SALADS

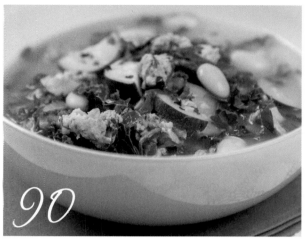

90

SOUPS & STEWS

THE RITUAL

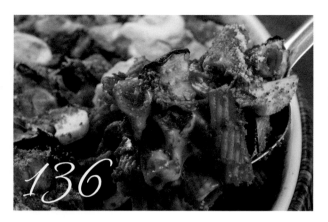

136

260

TRADITIONS

246

PIZZAS & FRITTATAS

DESSERTS

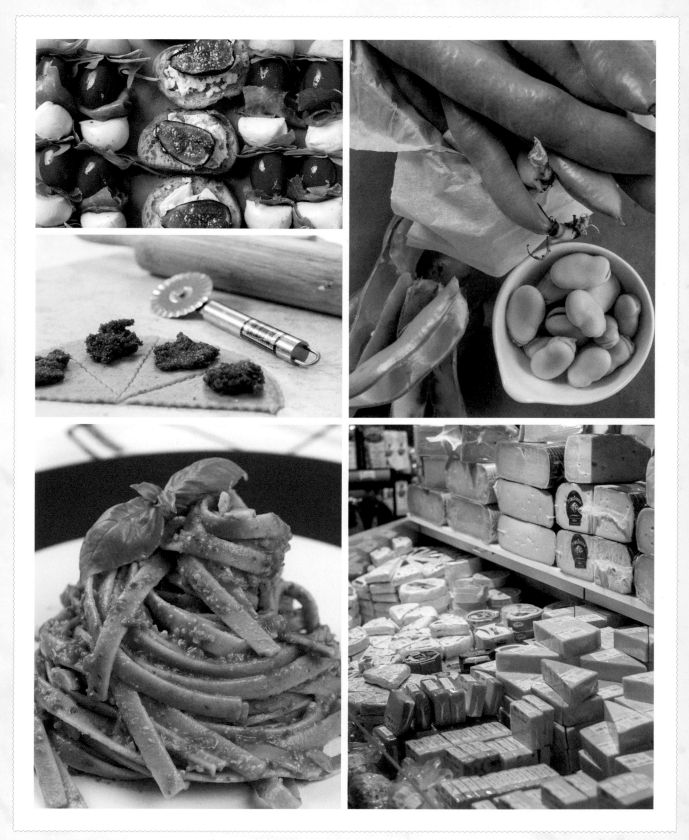

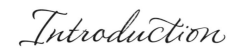

Introduction

I'M THRILLED TO SHARE *THE HEALTHY ITALIAN* WITH YOU. After more than two decades working as an editor and writer, I was determined to produce this book. Finally, I was ready to take this opportunity to marry my journalism experience with my love of Italian food and cooking. But this cookbook is so much more than that. What makes it extra special — besides the fact that it's packed with delicious authentic Italian recipes made healthy, pages and pages of mouth-watering photography and tons of tips to get meals on the table easier — is that this project is a personal passion of mine. Growing up Italian, food has always been at the epicenter of my life. Today, as a busy mom and passionate home cook, I lean on what I know best — Italian food. But the challenge there has been to cook Italian healthfully without compromising taste, fit it into my day and feel good about serving those meals to my family. That was the seed for *The Healthy Italian.* Throughout the cookbook, you'll see glimpses of the personal connections I make to this incredibly versatile cuisine through stories that I hope will entertain as well as inspire you not only to lead a healthier lifestyle but also to sit down and enjoy a delicious homemade meal with the people that matter most to you.

There were many factors that played a role in why I produced this cookbook now, but one of the biggest reasons is that it has never been easier to cook healthy meals. While it's true that packaged foods entice us away from the kitchen, it's also a fact that grocery stores continue to stock produce aisles and shelves with more and more nutritious options to create delectable, healthy meals with convenience. And applying those options to Italian cuisine is no exception. *The Healthy Italian* makes it even easier with a section on helping you stock the essential pantry staples. In every recipe, you'll find at-a-glance icons so the home cook has instant information on preparing meals, such as labels like gluten-free, meatless, 30 minutes or less and make ahead (with the number of days you can prepare a recipe ahead of time). I've paid particular attention to convenience in every recipe but, more importantly, I've focused on great taste — my family wouldn't have it any other way!

If you're passionate about good food and nutritious eating, I hope you'll make *The Healthy Italian* a favorite family resource. After all, it's about cooking for the love of food and family.

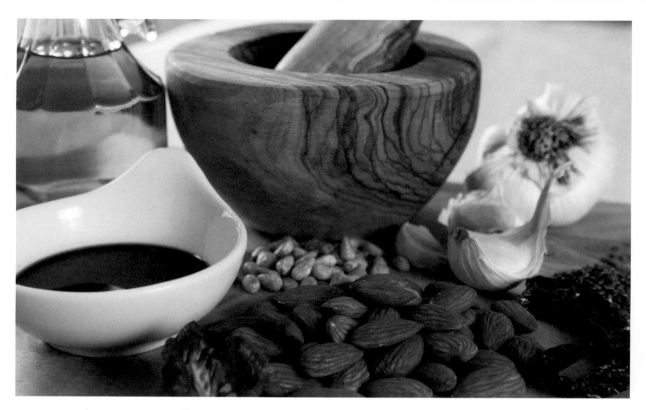

The Healthy Italian Pantry

MY PANTRY HAS ALWAYS BEEN AN ESSENTIAL RESOURCE FOR COOKING DELICIOUS FAMILY RECIPES. In our house, the *cantina* (also known as the cold cellar) becomes the prime storage for a host of homemade basics that we devote weekends to prepare — tomato sauce, canned whole tomatoes, roasted red peppers, olives, marinated vegetables and more. Olive oil, balsamic vinegar, dried beans, pasta, grains, flours, spices and nuts fill the kitchen pantry. Together with fresh produce, nutrient-rich pantry ingredients form the foundation for so many delicious Italian dishes that are both good for you and brimming with flavor. And when a pantry is stocked with wholesome ingredients, whipping up a healthy Italian meal is so much easier. Here are some healthy pantry basics to get you started.

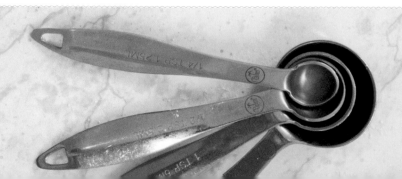

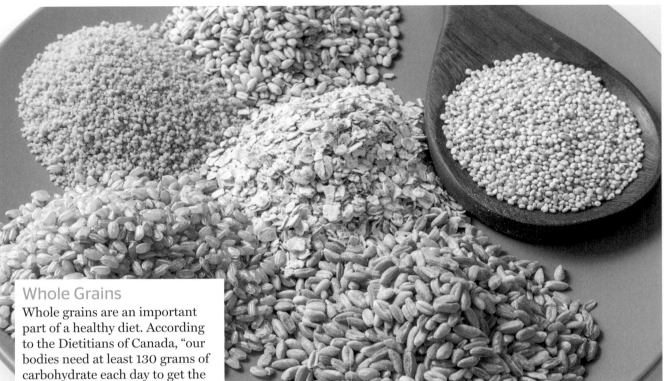

Whole Grains

Whole grains are an important part of a healthy diet. According to the Dietitians of Canada, "our bodies need at least 130 grams of carbohydrate each day to get the glucose or sugar that fuels our brains." Use a wide range of whole grains both in traditional meals that use them and in dishes where you wouldn't normally expect to find them — toss them into salads, substitute them for pasta in soups and rice in risottos, mix them into stuffing or season them simply to create a savory side dish. Experiment with these different grains, which are great sources of fiber and other important vitamins and minerals, for a variation in texture and taste.

➤ Short-grain brown rice/brown Arborio rice
➤ Farro
➤ Barley
➤ Cornmeal (polenta)
➤ Oats (rolled or quick oats, oat bran)
➤ Quinoa: although technically an edible seed, it's used like a grain

Whole-Grain Flours

Where once refined flours ruled the Italian pantry, there's now a

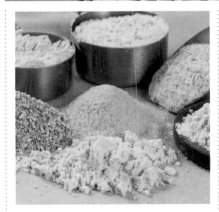

host of better-for-you flours made from healthy grains and seeds that offer greater benefits, such as fiber and protein. What's best, they're widely available at your local grocery store so you don't need to make a special trip to the bulk-food store.

➤ Whole-grain flour
➤ Oat flour
➤ Brown rice flour
➤ Quinoa flour
➤ Spelt flour

➤ Whole wheat flour: while not a whole-grain flour, it can be a better alternative to all-purpose or other refined flours, especially when combined with whole-grain flours. Look for whole-grain whole wheat flour, which uses the entire kernel of grain
➤ Whole durum semolina: while not a whole-grain flour, durum and semolina flours (usually sold as a combined flour) can offer other benefits, such as a little more protein and elasticity in pizza dough (for more information, see page 236)
Note: enriched wheat flour is not a whole-grain flour
➤ Gluten-free flours: potato flour (and starch), rice flour, chickpea flour (check labels to make sure there isn't cross-contamination with other flours), oats (if you have Celiac disease or eat a gluten-free diet, look for certified gluten-free oat flour or oats to mill as flour)

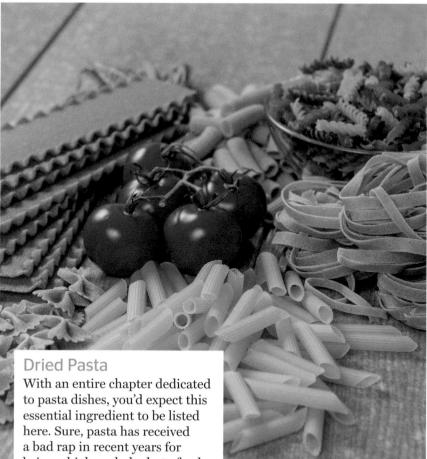

Dried Pasta

With an entire chapter dedicated to pasta dishes, you'd expect this essential ingredient to be listed here. Sure, pasta has received a bad rap in recent years for being a high-carbohydrate food, but some newer pasta varieties made with good-for-you grains improve its nutritional profile. They're also better tasting than the first generation of whole wheat/whole-grain pastas, and that's a big bonus when pasta is the star of any dish. Stock up on a variety of long and short pastas in various shapes — some are better suited to certain recipes and accompanying sauces. Different shapes are also a great way to make an "old" pasta recipe "new" again. Here are some of the pasta varieties readily available:

- ➤ Whole-grain
- ➤ Spelt
- ➤ Durum-semolina pastas using whole durum flour (see note in "Whole-Grain Flours")

- ➤ Mixed grain varieties that use a combination of whole grains, such as kamut and quinoa, or a combination of these with other whole grains)
- ➤ Gluten-free: brown rice or corn pasta

Breadcrumbs/Coating

There's been much debate about which breadcrumbs make the healthiest coating for meats, vegetables and appetizer dishes. There are a few basics I keep in mind when choosing my breadcrumbs: avoid seasoned breadcrumbs, which are loaded with sodium and preservatives; chose a whole-grain breadcrumb if it's available; or make my own.

- ➤ Whole wheat/whole-grain breadcrumbs: If you can't find them in your grocery store, try this simple method. Toast whole-grain bread. Let dry, uncovered, for two days. Whirl in the food processor until it becomes crumbs. Store in an airtight container for up to two weeks or in your freezer for up to one month
- ➤ Spelt breadcrumbs: these are a great substitute for chunkier coatings. The larger crumbs add a light, crispy coating to dishes
- ➤ Quinoa: Whirl the dry seeds in a food processor for a chunkier coating or pulse in a mill or a coffee grinder to achieve a finer consistency

Canned Fish

Canned seafood is a terrific source of selenium, omega-3 fatty acids, vitamin D and calcium (when bones are included). Look for fish packed in water, but if you prefer a fish packed in oil for more flavor, choose a brand packed in olive oil. Drain the excess oil and limit the amount of additional oil you use in the salad or pasta sauce you're adding it to.

- ➤ Tuna: Choose a canned light tuna that contains these tuna species: skipjack, yellowfin or tongol, which are relatively low in mercury. Avoid albacore (white) tuna, which can have higher levels of mercury
- ➤ Anchovies: Find them in the refrigerated section next to the fish counter. Packed in salt, they'll need to be rinsed well before using
- ➤ Sardines: Choose unseasoned varieties packed in water

Beans/Legumes

These great providers of iron, fiber and magnesium, among other nutrients, add bulk and

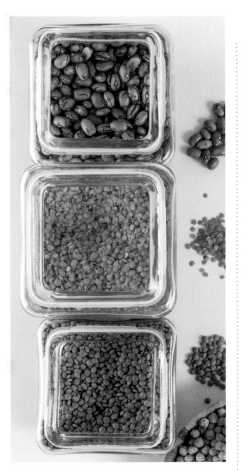

GLUTEN-FREE OPTIONS

The following pantry products may contain gluten. Check labels in these ingredients:
➤ Baking powder
➤ Broths: chicken, beef or vegetable — check

for wheat, fillers, hydrolyzed plant protein and other gluten additives
➤ Chickpea flour
➤ Oat bran; rolled oats — the label should say

"non-contaminated gluten-free oats"
➤ Italian herb seasoning
➤ Rice crackers
➤ Store-bought pesto
➤ Store-bought tomato sauce

vacuum-packed, there's a host of vegetables that add wonderful flavor to dishes. Because salt is used to preserve some of these pantry ingredients, they'll require a soaking in warm water or a good rinse.

➤ Whole peeled tomatoes: Canned or jarred, choose no-salt-added or low-salt brands. San Marzano or Roma tomatoes provide the best flavor
➤ Tomato purée (passata): See "whole peeled tomatoes," above
➤ Sun-dried tomatoes: Choose dry-

packed sun-dried tomatoes, not ones packed in oil. Reconstitute in warm water and rinse
➤ Dried mushrooms, such as porcini or cremini: Reconstitute in warm water and rinse
➤ Roasted red peppers: Choose brands packed with no oil or salt
➤ Artichokes: Packed in water in cans or packed in brine in jars
➤ Capers: Packed in brine in jars
➤ Olives: Vacuum-sealed or packed in brine

creaminess to so many dishes. Canned beans and legumes are easy to sprinkle into dishes; choose brands labeled "no salt added." While dried beans require an overnight soak, they can give more flavor to recipes. Delicate legumes can be added directly into dishes while cooking.

➤ Beans (Romano, cannellini, white kidney, navy): canned or dried. Dried varieties need to be soaked in water for at least 12 hours
➤ Chickpeas: canned or dried
➤ Red and brown lentils: Canned or dried. Because dried lentils cook so quickly and they're so tasty, I add them to many of my soups

Vegetables (Canned/ Preserved/Dried)

From dried to canned to

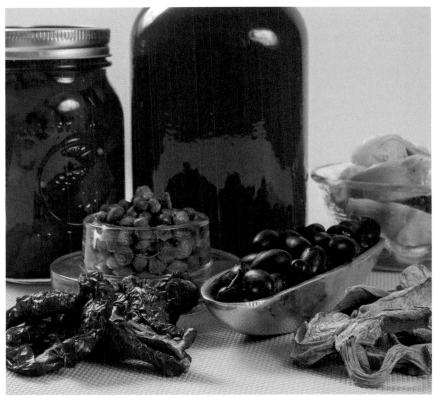

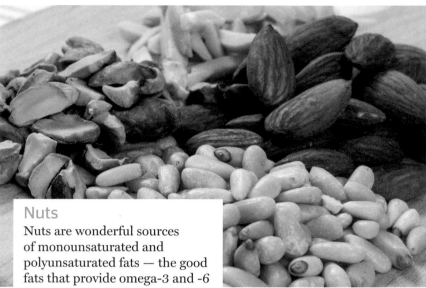

Nuts

Nuts are wonderful sources of monounsaturated and polyunsaturated fats — the good fats that provide omega-3 and -6 fatty acids. Sprinkle these nuts in small quantities on salads, pasta, stuffing or appetizers as part of a balanced diet.

➤ Almonds, pine nuts, pistachios, walnuts: Choose natural or dry-roasted, unsalted nuts

Extra-Virgin Olive Oil

Not only does extra-virgin olive oil taste great, but it also has many health benefits as a monounsaturated fat. Look for extra-virgin olive oil, which means it has been produced from the first pressing of olives without the aid of heat or chemicals. Best used over salads or for moderate heating.

Balsamic Vinegar

Look for aged balsamic for a sweeter, more full-bodied taste. Some of the finest balsamic vinegar comes from Modena in the Emilia-Romagna region of Italy.

Seasoning, Dried Herbs and Spices

Cooking with fresh seasoning and spices not only provides enormous taste but also sensory-awakening aromas. Just a pinch of dried herbs and spices can intensify the flavor of dishes and limit the amount of salt or sugar in recipes. Dried herbs and spices can retain their intense flavor for up to a year when sealed properly.

➤ Sea salt: While there's no difference in the amount of sodium in sea salt versus table salt, sea salt has a more full-bodied flavor
➤ Freshly ground black pepper (peppercorns)
➤ Garlic and onions
➤ Oregano
➤ Fennel seeds
➤ Bay leaves
➤ Rosemary
➤ Saffron
➤ Paprika
➤ Crushed red pepper chili flakes (peperoncini)
➤ Italian herb seasoning
➤ Cinnamon
➤ Cloves

Sugars

Raw sugars, honey, agave nectar/syrup, coconut palm

Sodium-Reduced Broths

There are a multitude of broths now on the market that give you a choice between salt content — from traditional high-sodium to reduced-sodium to no-salt-added broths. Don't be confused with the words "reduced" or "low" — "reduced" means less than the original and is not necessarily a low-sodium product. Check labels for sodium content and adjust seasoning in dishes where it's being used if necessary. Make your own vegetable broth by boiling six to eight cups of water with carrots, potatoes, leeks, celery, parsley, bay leaf and basil for an hour. Strain vegetables and store in refrigerator for two to three weeks.

FRIDGE BASICS

Aside from the pantry, keep these ingredients on hand in your refrigerator:
➤ Fresh produce: fresh is best and holds the greatest amount of nutrients when consumed within days. In particular, stock the fridge with onions, carrot and celery — they form the base for so many dishes known as "soffitto" in Italian.
➤ Fresh herbs: Today's grocery stores are stocked with herbs all year-round. Choose from parsley, basil, rosemary, mint and oregano — some of the most common herbs used in Italian cooking. Experiment with different leafy greens, from spinach to kale to Swiss chard to rapini (broccoli rabe).
➤ Low-fat cheeses or bold, flavorful cheeses that require only a little bit for a big taste. Parmesan cheese is not the same as Parmigiano-Reggiano cheese, which is made using a specific, regulated recipe and production method. Parmesan is often an imitation cheese.

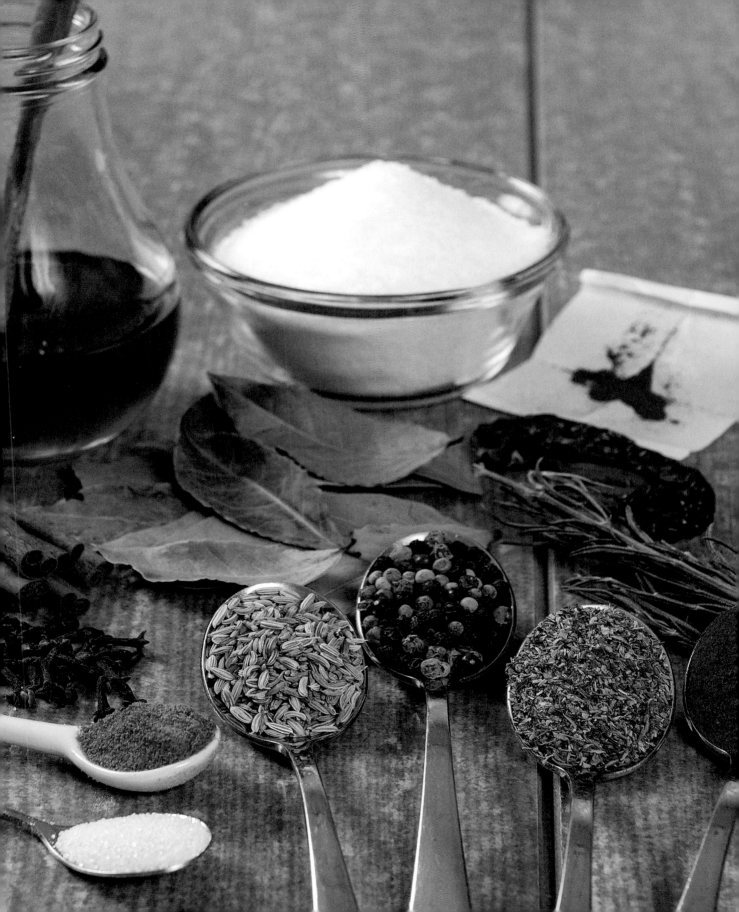

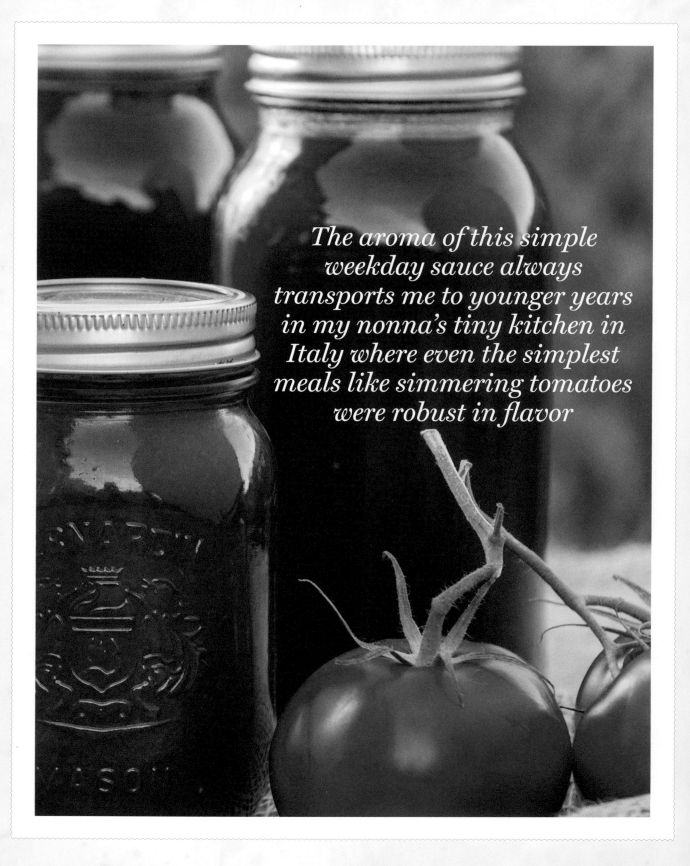

The aroma of this simple weekday sauce always transports me to younger years in my nonna's tiny kitchen in Italy where even the simplest meals like simmering tomatoes were robust in flavor

The Basics

Salse e condimenti basilari

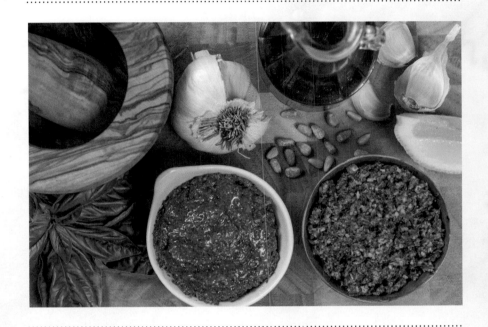

I remember the day he came home and announced that he had learned the "secret" to making the best basil pesto

Basic Pasta Tomato Sauce
Salsa di pomodoro

IF THERE IS ONE RECIPE THAT DEFINES AUTHENTIC ITALIAN COOKING, it's this one — the quintessential pasta tomato sauce. And it is the foundation for so many extraordinary dishes. We woke up to this version, my mom's signature sauce, every Sunday morning. If it wasn't the sizzle of the garlic and onions that roused us, it was the wafting aroma of tomatoes and herbs making its way into our bedrooms. It was the signal that today was *the* day when our family could look forward to spending time together, if only over a plate of fresh pasta with delicious homemade tomato sauce.

1 tbsp	extra-virgin olive oil
1	onion, minced
2	cloves garlic, minced
4 tbsp	no-salt-added tomato paste
1 cup	water
4 cups	no-salt-added tomato purée (passata)
1	small carrot, grated (about ¼ cup)
2 to 3	bay leaves
2 tbsp	chopped fresh basil
1 tbsp	chopped fresh parsley
1 tsp	Italian herb seasoning
¼ tsp	sea salt

Freshly ground black pepper to taste

➤ In a large pot, heat olive oil over medium-high heat. Add onion and garlic and cook until onions are softened, about 2 minutes. Add tomato paste and stir in water to dissolve. Stir in tomato purée, grated carrot, herbs, salt and pepper.

➤ Reduce heat to low, cover and bring to a gentle simmer. Cook for 1 hour, stirring occasionally. Remove and discard bay leaves before serving tossed with pasta. Sauce will keep in the refrigerator for up to one week and freezes for up to one month.

⇄ VARIATIONS Some like it hot! If you do, you can easily dial up the heat in this sauce to make it *arrabbiata* (meaning "angry" in Italian). Simply add 2 tsp minced fresh chili pepper (*peperoncini*) or 1 tsp dried crushed red pepper flakes when adding the onion and garlic to the oil. If you're using the fresh chili, don't forget to wear gloves when slicing it.

➤ Make a meat sauce by adding 10.5 ounces/300 grams lean ground turkey or extra-lean ground beef; cook with onion and garlic, breaking up large pieces, until no longer pink before adding remaining ingredients.

⌂ HIGH IN...VITAMINS A AND C

Go ahead and smother your favorite pasta with this tomato sauce. Just ½ cup delivers almost equal amounts of vitamins A and C at roughly one-third of their daily value, thanks to the richly pigmented tomato purée and carrot added to this simple sauce.

 4 CUPS   GLUTEN-FREE   MEATLESS

PER CUP 161 CALORIES | 4 G TOTAL FAT (1 G SATURATED FAT) | 0 MG CHOLESTEROL | 255 MG SODIUM | 31 G CARBOHYDRATE | 7 G FIBER | 5 G PROTEIN

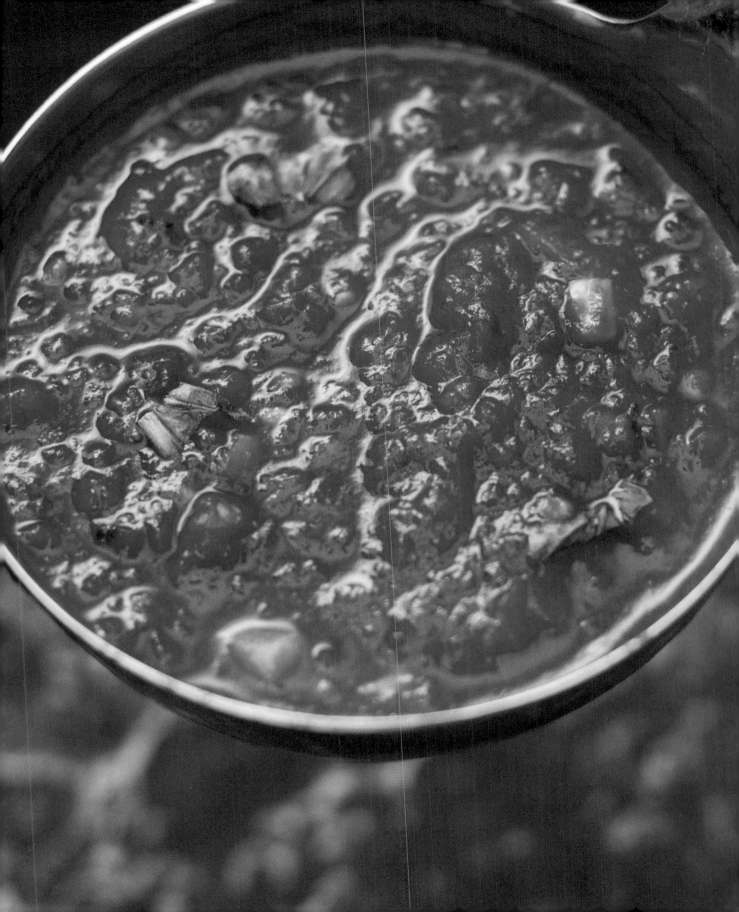

Sunday (Lean) Meatballs

Polpette di carne magra della Domenica

WE DON'T LIMIT OUR MEATBALLS to "on top of spaghetti." We drop them into soups, smash them in between crusty buns or eat them just the way they are. After learning to make tomato sauce, this was the next recipe I mastered, thanks to my mom, who not only makes the most incredibly moist and mouth-smacking meatballs but also shapes them as skillfully as the famous Italian Renaissance sculptors carved their iconic works of art.

Meatballs

½ cup	oat bran or ¾ cup quick-cooking oats (not instant)*
⅓ cup	1% milk
1 lb	(454 g) extra-lean ground beef
1 lb	(454 g) lean ground turkey or chicken
1	egg, beaten
1	egg white
2	cloves garlic, minced
½ cup	minced onion
¼ cup	minced fresh parsley
3 tbsp	freshly grated Parmigiano-Reggiano cheese
2 tbsp	minced fresh basil
½ tsp	sea salt
Pinch	freshly ground black pepper

Tomato Sauce (prepared al sugo)

1 tsp	extra-virgin olive oil
1 tbsp	chopped onion
1	clove garlic, minced
1 can	(5.5 oz/156 mL) no-salt-added tomato paste
3 cups	water
4 cups	no-salt-added tomato purée (passata)
1 tbsp	chopped fresh basil
½ tsp	sea salt
2	bay leaves

➤ In a large bowl, combine oat bran with milk and let soak until fully absorbed. Add the meat to bowl, breaking it up as you go, and stir in egg and egg white.

➤ Add remaining ingredients and mix well until combined. (Go ahead, use your hands!) Wet hands and using 2 tbsp at a time shape mixture into balls.

➤ **To cook them in tomato sauce, prepare the sauce.** In a medium pot, heat olive oil over medium-high heat. Add onion and garlic and cook until onions are softened, about 1 minute. Add tomato paste, stirring with water until fully dissolved. Add tomato purée and seasonings; bring to a boil. Drop in meatballs slowly, one at a time. Cover and bring to a boil. Reduce heat to medium-low and let simmer for 1 to 1½ hours, stirring periodically after 10 minutes of cooking. Remove and discard bay leaves. Serve meatballs and sauce over pasta or on their own with a side of salad.

➤ **If cooking without sauce:** Preheat oven to 375°F. Coat a shallow baking pan with cooking spray, place meatballs on pan and lightly spray them. Place pan in preheated oven and cook for 25 minutes, turning halfway through cooking, or until meatballs are cooked through and no longer pink in the center.

➤ **To freeze meatballs:** Place meatballs on a greased baking pan and freeze for about two to three hours. Transfer and store meatballs in a freezer bag or container for up to a month.

⇆VARIATION Give this recipe an iron boost by adding a handful or two of shredded baby spinach into the meat mix before shaping into meatballs.

↻LOW IN...FAT

Using extra-lean ground meats instead of the traditional trio of pork, beef and veal slashes both the amount of fat and saturated fats by half, yet they still have the same succulent texture as the ones Mom used to make.

32-34 MEDIUM MEATBALLS OR
42-45 COCKTAIL SIZE MEATBALLS

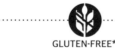

GLUTEN-FREE*
CHECK LABEL

MAKE AHEAD

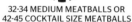

PER 4 MEATBALLS 216 CALORIES | 9 G TOTAL FAT (3 G SATURATED FAT) | 86 MG CHOLESTEROL | 253 MG SODIUM | 3 G CARBOHYDRATE | 0 G FIBER | 29 G PROTEIN

Quick Marinara Sauce
Sugo alla marinara

THE AROMA OF THIS SIMPLE weekday sauce always transports me to younger years in my nonna's tiny kitchen in Italy where even the simplest meals like simmering tomatoes were robust in flavor. Use it to top pasta, grilled meats or fish, or a multigrain pizza crust.

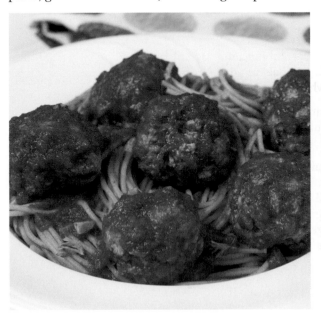
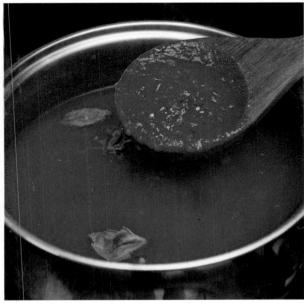

2 cans	(28 oz/796 mL each) no-salt-added San Marzano whole peeled tomatoes with purée or juice, or 5 cups fresh very ripe tomatoes, chopped
1½ tbsp	extra-virgin olive oil
1	onion, chopped
3	cloves garlic, minced
Pinch	granulated sugar
3 tbsp	chopped fresh basil
½ tsp	Italian herb seasoning
½ tsp	dried oregano
½ tsp	sea salt
Freshly ground black pepper to taste	

➤ In the bowl of a food processor or blender, pulse tomatoes with liquid until smooth and set aside. In a large pot, heat olive oil over medium-high heat. Add onion and garlic and cook until onions are softened, about 2 minutes. Add sugar, basil and remaining seasonings and spices.

➤ Reduce heat to low, cover and simmer. Stir occasionally while cooking for 20 minutes.

⇆VARIATION For a fresh-tasting pizza sauce à la Margherita, add 2 tbsp of tomato paste to the ingredients at the same time you're adding in the puréed tomatoes into the pot. Add an additional 1 tbsp chopped fresh basil just before placing on pizza crust.

5 CUPS   30 MIN OR LESS   GLUTEN-FREE   MEATLESS

PER CUP 84 CALORIES | 4 G TOTAL FAT (1 G SATURATED FAT) | 0 MG CHOLESTEROL | 246 MG SODIUM | 11 G CARBOHYDRATE | 3 G FIBER | 2 G PROTEIN

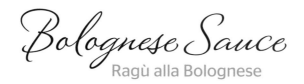

Bolognese Sauce
Ragù alla Bolognese

LIKE MOST NORTH AMERICANS, I always thought that Bolognese sauce was just a basic tomato sauce simmered with ground meat. That is, until my aunt corrected me. She takes pride in the cuisine of Emilia-Romagna, which is where she lives and it's believed the sauce was first named after its capital city of Bologna. It has so much more character by blending meats (lean, in this case) with few, if any, tomatoes simmered slowly with the most fragrant of ingredients.

9 oz	(250 g) lean ground turkey
9 oz	(250 g) extra-lean ground beef
3	slices reduced-sodium extra-lean deli-style prosciutto cotto or ham, chopped (2 oz/56 g)
1	onion, chopped
2	cloves garlic, chopped
1 cup	finely diced carrots
1 cup	finely diced celery hearts
½ cup	red wine
1½ cups	canned good-quality no-salt-added diced tomatoes, drained
2 tbsp	no-salt-added tomato paste
½ to 1 cup reduced-sodium beef or chicken broth	
2 to 3	bay leaves
2 tbsp	chopped fresh basil
1 tbsp	chopped fresh parsley
1 tsp	Italian herb seasoning
¼ tsp	sea salt
Pinch	ground nutmeg
Freshly ground black pepper to taste	
½ cup	1% milk

➤ Coat a large pot with cooking spray and heat over medium-high heat. Add ground turkey, beef and prosciutto cotto, breaking up the large pieces and stirring continuously until almost no longer pink. Stir in onion, garlic, carrots and celery. Cook until vegetables have softened, about 2 to 3 minutes. Pour in wine and scrape any bits at the bottom of the pot as you stir for 2 more minutes.

➤ Add diced tomatoes, tomato paste and ½ cup of beef broth. Stir in bay leaves, basil, parsley, Italian herb seasoning, salt, nutmeg and pepper. Reduce heat to low, cover and bring to a gentle simmer. Stir occasionally while cooking for 30 minutes. Add milk and simmer for 1 hour, stirring occasionally and adding in remaining beef broth if sauce is drying up. Remove bay leaves and discard.

➤ Toss sauce with whole-grain torn fresh pasta or with dried egg noodles like tagliatelle or fettuccine, or over Sweet Potato Polenta (*see recipe, page 22*).

⇄ **VARIATION** Italian ragù doesn't traditionally add diced tomatoes, but I like mine a little more tomatoey. You could stick to a more authentic version by replacing the tomatoes for more broth — about 1 cup will do.

MAKE AHEAD Prepare and refrigerate the sauce two to three days ahead of using it.

↻ LOW IN...SATURATED FAT

All meats have some level of saturated fat but this recipe reduces that amount by a whopping 54 percent from the original "classico" Bolognese sauce.

6 CUPS GLUTEN-FREE MAKE AHEAD

PER CUP 171 CALORIES | 9 G TOTAL FAT (3 G SATURATED FAT) | 62 MG CHOLESTEROL | 213 MG SODIUM | 3 G CARBOHYDRATE | 0 G FIBER | 19 G PROTEIN

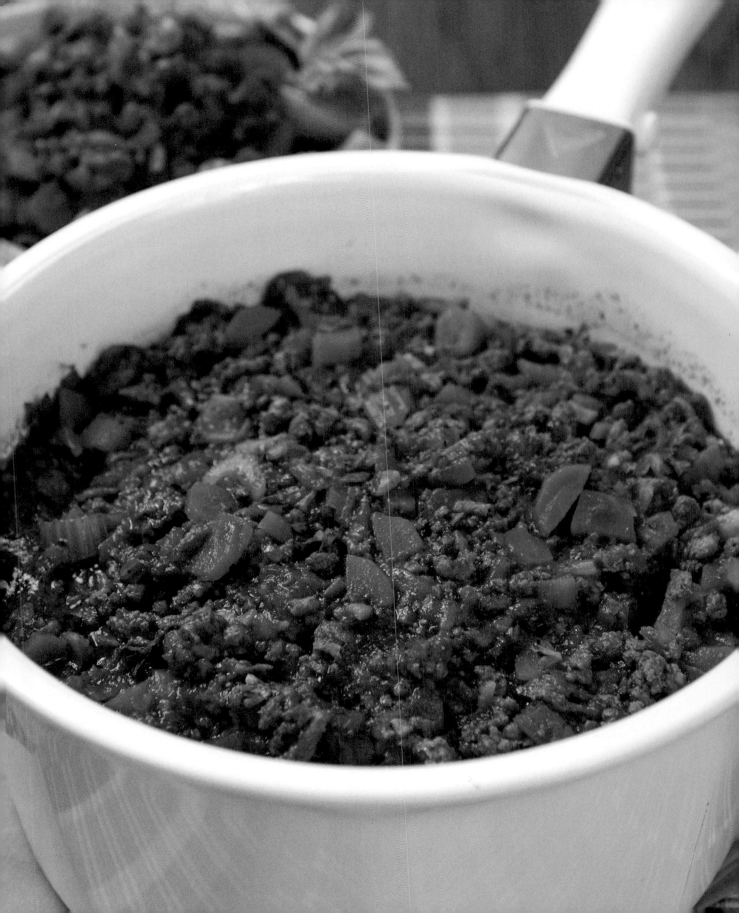

Béchamel Sauce

Besciamella

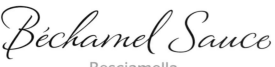

THERE WAS HARDLY A SUNDAY THAT WENT BY when we didn't have the Italian channel on TV in the background while preparing a traditional big lunch. The cooking show by TV chef and operatic singer Pasquale Carpino was always a favorite, as we enjoyed catching glimpses of him whipping up delicious dishes while he sang. During one episode, it wasn't his singing that caught my attention; it was his *besciamella* sauce that he substituted for tomato sauce. That was the beginning of my love affair with this white sauce from northern Italy, which some say has been borrowed from its French neighbors. Because it's so easy to make and offers so much versatility, I toss it in my homemade macaroni and cheese, in between lasagna layers or in basil pesto for even more creamy goodness.

2 tbsp	light butter
2 tbsp	corn flour* or all-purpose flour
1½ cups	1% milk
½ cup	reduced-sodium vegetable or chicken broth
¼ tsp	Dijon mustard
Pinch	ground nutmeg
½ tsp	sea salt
Freshly ground black pepper to taste	
1 tsp	freshly grated Parmigiano-Reggiano cheese

➤ In a medium pot, melt butter over medium-high heat and whisk in flour until it forms a paste. Add in milk a little at a time as mixture thickens. Whisk in broth, Dijon mustard, nutmeg, salt and pepper. Bring sauce to a gentle boil and reduce heat to low. Whisk occasionally as it simmers for 5 more minutes. Remove from stove, stir in cheese and toss with pasta.

⍫LOW IN...SATURATED FAT

This creamy sauce is a great alternative to a typical cheesy sauce like Alfredo, which is loaded with butter, heavy cream and cheese and dumps three-quarters of the daily value of fat in just one serving. While this béchamel has just seven percent of the daily value of fat per serving, it's still big on taste.

2 CUPS

30 MIN OR LESS

GLUTEN-FREE*

MEATLESS

PER ½ CUP 84 CALORIES | 4 G TOTAL FAT (2 G SATURATED FAT) | 14 MG CHOLESTEROL | 174 MG SODIUM | 9 G CARBOHYDRATE | 0 G FIBER | 3 G PROTEIN

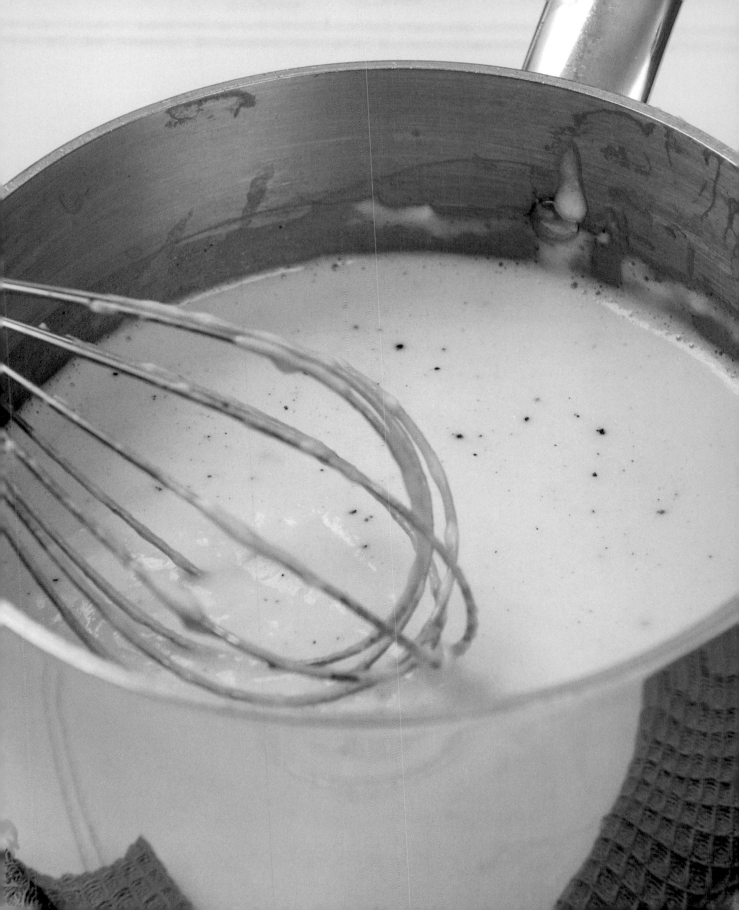

Basil Pesto Genovese
Pesto alla Genovese

MY DAD LOVED LEARNING NEW WAYS TO ENJOY VEGETABLES so he'd often ask customers at the grocery store where he worked for their family recipes. I remember when he came home one day and announced that he had learned the "secret" to making the best basil pesto, as revealed by a customer from Genova — the birthplace of basil pesto and explorer Christopher Columbus. It was a boiled potato, thrown into the mix for an irresistibly creamy consistency. We've been making it like that ever since. We use it as a pasta sauce, as a dip on our appetizer platters, and even as a salad dressing for extra flavor.

1	small white potato, peeled
2 cups	packed fresh basil (2 oz/60 g)
½ cup	packed fresh curly parsley sprigs (0.5 oz/20 g)
2	cloves garlic, coarsely chopped
2 tsp	roasted pine nuts
3 tbsp	freshly grated Pecorino Romano cheese
Pinch	sea salt
Freshly ground black pepper to taste	
3 tbsp	extra-virgin olive oil

⇄ VARIATION For a nutritional boost to this pesto, replace half the basil with baby arugula or baby kale leaves.

➤ In a small pot filled with water, boil potato until center is tender when pierced with a fork. Cut into cubes and reserve ¼ cup. Save the rest of the potato for another use.

➤ Place all ingredients, except potato and oil, in the bowl of a food processor or blender and pulse until combined. Add potato and stream in olive oil and whirl until smooth, scraping down sides and bottom halfway through.

➤ Toss with pasta, spread over polenta or top an appetizer. Keep pesto in refrigerator for two to three weeks with a small amount of oil on top or store in a freezer-safe container (hold back on the cheese until thawed and ready to use).

MAKE AHEAD Boil the potato up to a few hours or one day ahead.

TIP Parsley mellows out the slightly bitter taste of the basil. Make sure both herbs are patted dry before adding them into the food processor.

♫ HIGH IN...FLAVONOIDS

Basil, the main ingredient in this pesto, has an impressive amount of flavonoids, which are plant-based compounds found in richly pigmented herbs, fruits and vegetables that function as powerful antioxidants in the body. The flavonoids found in basil offer protection against the damage of cells and chromosomes from free-radical activity and radiation. Adding basil to foods has also found to inhibit the growth of bacteria. This pesto is also high in vitamins C and K.

 1 CUP
 30 MIN OR LESS
 GLUTEN-FREE
 MEATLESS
 MAKE AHEAD

PER 2 TBSP 69 CALORIES | 7 G TOTAL FAT (1 G SATURATED FAT) | 3 MG CHOLESTEROL | 85 MG SODIUM | 2 G CARBOHYDRATE | 0 G FIBER | 2 G PROTEIN

Almond-Gremolata Pesto
Pesto di gremolata e mandorle

I LIKE PAIRING GRILLED CHICKEN OR SHRIMP WITH GREMOLATA, a typical Milanese condiment made with lemon zest, parsley and garlic. But, here, it gets a twist for a more robust accompaniment that combines basil and almonds to make this zesty chunky pesto.

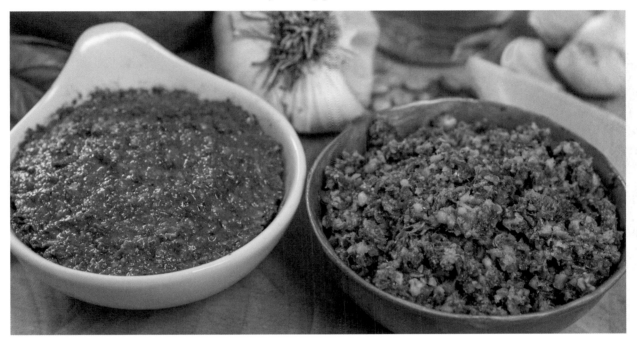

1 cup	packed fresh parsley sprigs
¼ cup	packed fresh basil
¼ cup	toasted slivered almonds
2	cloves garlic
1 tbsp	freshly grated Parmigiano-Reggiano cheese

Zest of 1 lemon

2 tbsp	freshly squeezed lemon juice
¼ tsp	sea salt

Freshly ground black pepper to taste

2 tbsp	extra-virgin olive oil

➤ Combine all ingredients, except oil, in the bowl of a food processor or blender and pulse until finely chopped. Stream in olive oil and whirl until chunky, scraping down sides and bottom in between.

MAKE AHEAD This pesto can be stored for up to one week in the refrigerator before using.

¾ CUP   30 MIN OR LESS   GLUTEN-FREE   MEATLESS   MAKE AHEAD

PER 2 TBSP 72 CALORIES | 7 G TOTAL FAT (1 G SATURATED FAT) | 1 MG CHOLESTEROL | 151 MG SODIUM | 2 G CARBOHYDRATE | 1 G FIBER | 2 G PROTEIN

Balsamic Reduction Sauce

Riduzione di aceto balsamico

THE REGION KNOWN FOR CULINARY CONTRIBUTIONS like Parma prosciutto, Bolognese sauce and hand-crafted pastas, such as tortellini, also came up with this gastronomic delight, so you know it demands attention. Its sharp, tear-jerking scent fills my house when I make it — a sort of proclamation that just a drizzle will make a big impact. My family loves to spoon this tangy, syrupy sauce over grilled meats like pork loin, grilled vegetables and bocconcini and tomato salad.

2 cups	balsamic vinegar
1 tbsp	maple syrup
1	clove garlic, minced
1	sprig fresh rosemary

➤ In a small pot, combine vinegar, maple syrup, garlic and rosemary. Bring to a gentle boil, then reduce heat to medium-low.

➤ Simmer for 40 minutes, stirring occasionally, until mixture is reduced by half and mixture turns syrupy.

➤ Remove garlic and rosemary and drizzle sauce lightly over roasted meats, grilled vegetables or salad. Stores for two to three weeks in the refrigerator.

TIP As this sauce slowly simmers, the fumes of the vinegar can be a real eye stinger, so let in some fresh air. Just think, your house will smell very clean without you even picking up a mop!

⇆ VARIATION Try this reduction over fruit, such as fresh strawberries, ripe cantaloupe or glazed figs.

1 CUP   GLUTEN-FREE   MEATLESS

PER 2 TBSP 63 CALORIES | 0 G TOTAL FAT (0 G SATURATED FAT) | 0 MG CHOLESTEROL | 15 MG SODIUM | 13 G CARBOHYDRATE | 0 G FIBER | 0 G PROTEIN

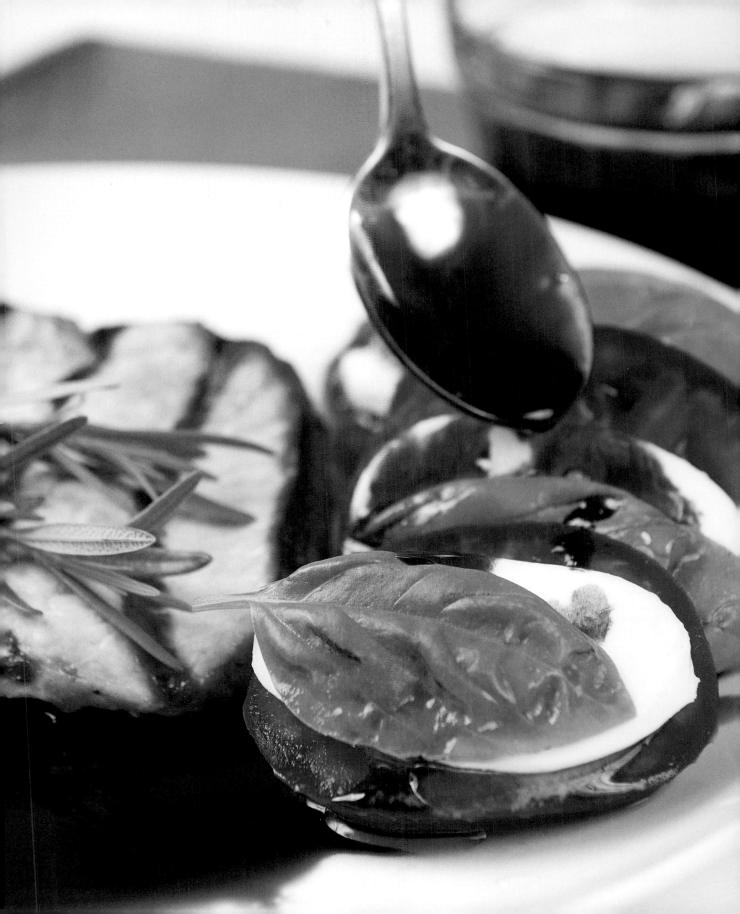

Sweet Potato Polenta

Polenta di patate dolci

MY SISTER-IN-LAW NADIA IS A HUGE FAN OF POLENTA. Hot from the pot, grilled with portobellos or mixed into a cake batter, she can't resist it. In fact, her family makes a ritual of eating it like so many other Italian families do — poured directly from the stove and onto a wooden board at the center of the table and topped with a heaping mound of homemade Italian sausages simmered in a savory sauce. Both young and old take a seat at the table and dig in to the extra-large sharing plate that doesn't need to be passed around. Naturally, I couldn't include this polenta recipe unless it met with her approval.

3 cups	cubed sweet potatoes (about 2 medium sweet potatoes)
2 tsp	chopped fresh rosemary
½ tsp	sea salt
7 cups	water
1½ cups	fine yellow cornmeal (see tip)
1 tbsp	extra-virgin olive oil
1 tbsp	freshly grated Parmigiano-Reggiano cheese
	Bolognese Sauce or Basic Pasta Tomato Sauce for serving (*see recipes in this chapter*)

TIP There are different textures of cornmeal — from coarse to medium types. Although package labels don't always note the type, compare brands and choose a finer grain if you prefer a smoother, less gritty polenta. Products labelled instant polenta include cornmeal that has been precooked to reduce cooking time — it tends to be smoother but more refined. Cornmeal is not the same as corn flour, which has a finer, powdery consistency and should not be used here.

⇆ VARIATION Depending on your topping, you may want to flavor the polenta by cooking it in different broths, for example, chicken, vegetable or even a wild mushroom. Some polenta aficionados prefer to add some milk during the last few minutes of cooking for a creamier porridge.

➤ Add sweet potatoes, rosemary and salt to a large pot with the water and bring to a boil. Cook potatoes for 15 minutes, until soft. Remove from heat and break up sweet potato with a hand masher.

➤ Return pot to burner and bring mixture to a gentle simmer; slowly pour in cornmeal in a fine stream. Whisk continuously, making sure to smooth out the lumps. Once all cornmeal has been added, reduce heat to low and use a wooden spoon to stir continuously for about 25 to 30 minutes, until mixture is creamy (less gritty) and comes away from the sides of the pot. Wear oven mitts while stirring to protect your hands from hot bubbling splatters! Stirring the polenta often breaks down the starches and results in a creamier texture. Stir in olive oil and cheese just before serving. Serve hot in individual bowls. Drizzle extra olive oil or top with your favourite sauce.

➤ Alternatively, pour hot polenta into a large serving dish (a 9 x 13-inch works well) and flatten out evenly with the back of a greased spoon. Polenta will set quickly so you need to move fast. Drizzle olive oil on top and let cool. When firm, cut into slices and serve. Serve polenta with sauces, stews, fish, cheeses or grilled vegetables.

➤ **If using as an appetizer**, cut firm polenta into slices, coat a baking pan with cooking spray and bake in an oven at 350°F for 15 minutes. Top with your favorite toppings, such as goat's cheese or pesto (*see Basil Pesto Genovese, page 18, and Grilled Portobello Mushrooms & Polenta, page 48*).

⋂ HIGH IN...BETA-CAROTENE

The addition of sweet potato to this polenta boosts not only its vibrant color but also its source of alpha- and beta-carotene, both of which are converted into vitamin A. And it comes in extraordinary amounts here, with almost double the amount of vitamin A recommended in a day's worth.

6 SERVINGS
12 AS APPETIZER

GLUTEN-FREE

MEATLESS

MAKE AHEAD
AS AN APPETIZER

PER MEAL SERVING 191 CALORIES | 4 G TOTAL FAT (1 G SATURATED FAT) | 1 MG CHOLESTEROL | 231 MG SODIUM | 36 G CARBOHYDRATE | 7 G FIBER | 3 G PROTEIN

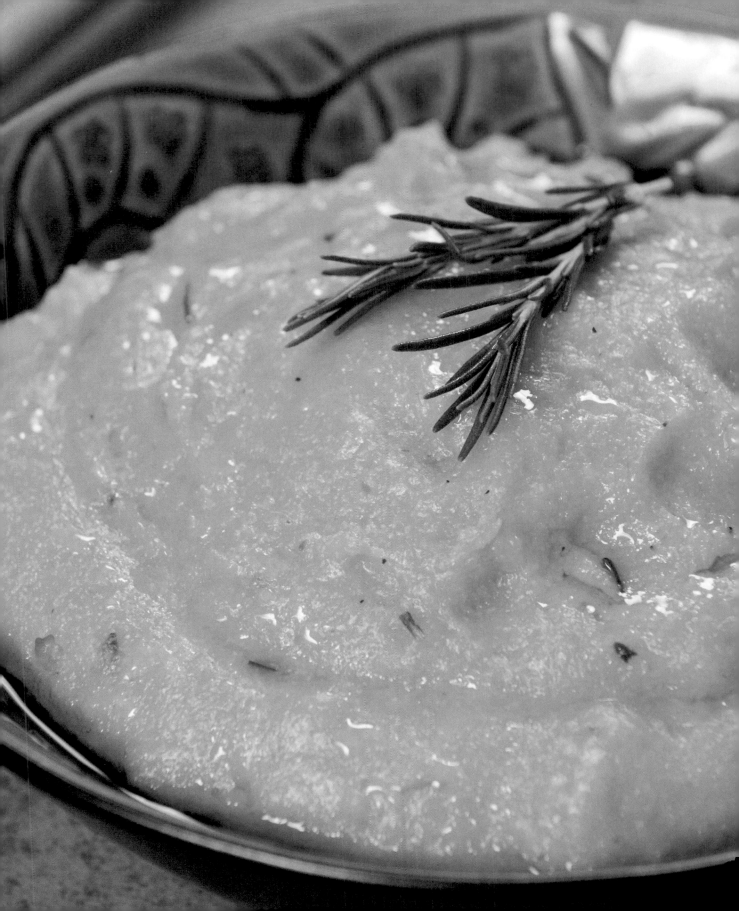

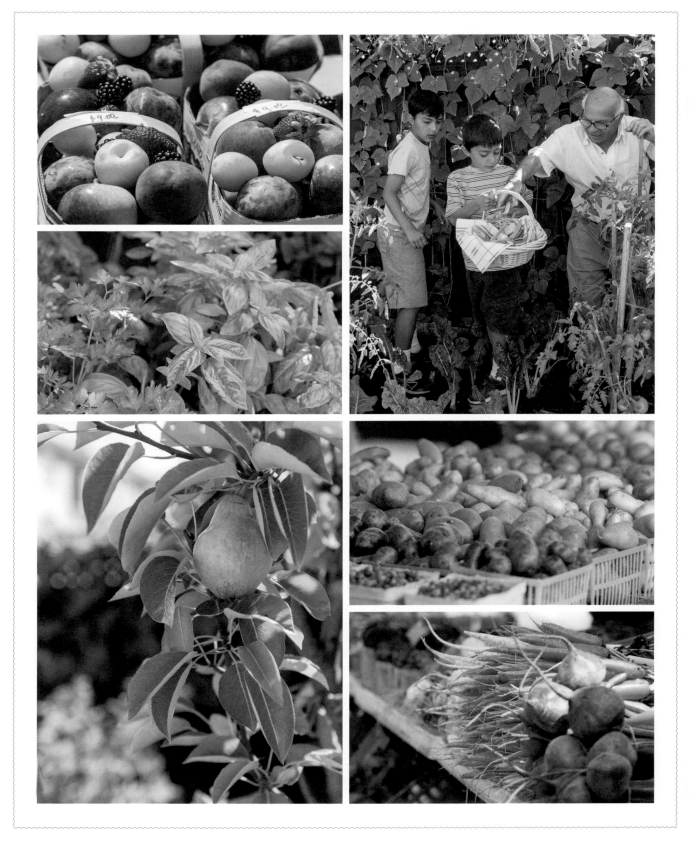

Beginnings
Fresh Ingredients

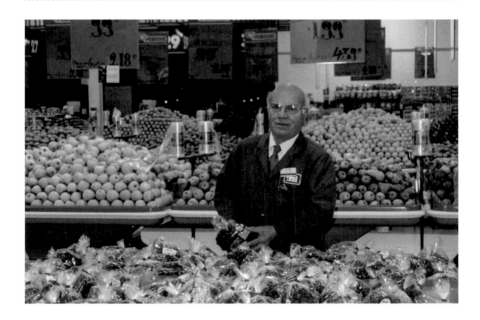

It's no secret that healthy cooking always starts with an assortment of freshly picked vegetables, fruits and herbs. I was fortunate enough to learn that lesson early in my life, and it became entrenched in my family's cooking repertoire. Our family's love affair with food began with my dad's immersion into the grocery business, which had a huge influence on what we cooked and ate at home. Dad landed his first job at the Ontario Food Terminal when he emigrated from Italy to Canada in 1957; later he managed grocery stores, many of which carried produce catered to the Italian community. Dad's love of fresh produce extended beyond business and into our home, where he nurtured his own garden for months at a time, proud of what he could grow on a little plot of land, from tomatoes and green beans to Swiss chard and vegetable marrow to eggplants and herbs. Whether these "raw materials" came from the garden or the grocery store, it meant we were exposed to a whole new universe of food, sometimes even unusual produce we'd never tasted before. Of course, the real mastery took place in the kitchen, where Mom was always clever at combining what she had been taught by generations before her and new techniques she had picked up along the way. Together, they fostered a lifelong appreciation for good-quality, nutritious ingredients and a passion for cooking them to perfection.

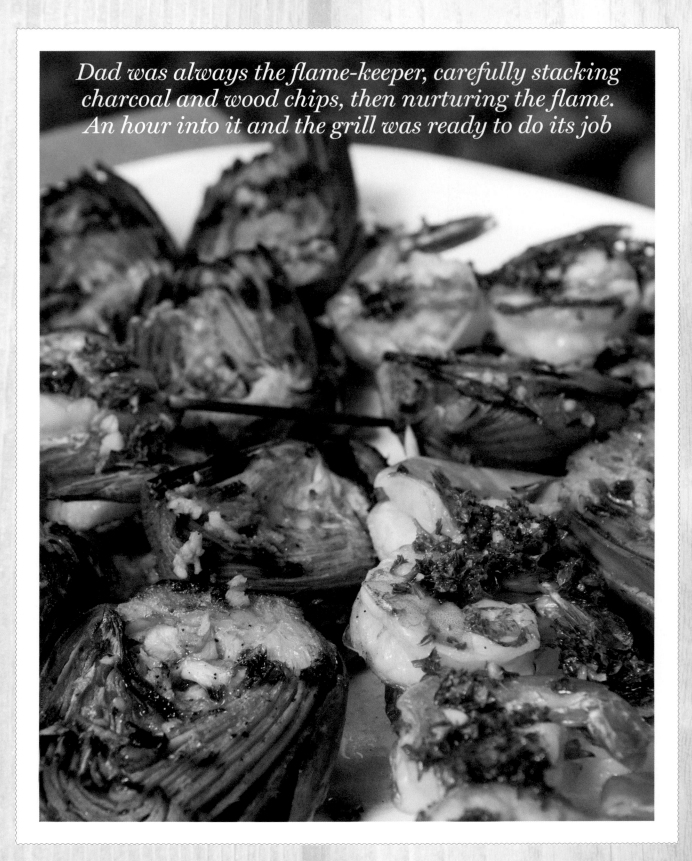

Dad was always the flame-keeper, carefully stacking charcoal and wood chips, then nurturing the flame. An hour into it and the grill was ready to do its job

Appetizers

Antipasti

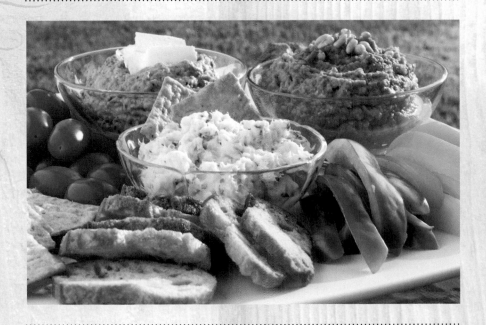

*I was quite content to skip dinner that night
and indulge in a smorgasbord of tapenades and
dips, much like these regional favorites,
along with a little Chianti*

Mussels Marinara
Cozze alla marinara

WHEN WE ACCOMPANIED MOM TO THE FISH MARKET during the winter holidays, we'd pinch our noses and hold our breaths. My kids do the same today when the fishy odor greets us at the entrance. But soon after, they become mesmerized by the quantity and quality of seafood and the familiar anthem is played out: "Mom, can we get this...can we get that?" They become swept away by the energetic vibe of the overwhelming crowd — not the smell — that shuffles from aisle to aisle to fill their carts with specialties for Christmas Eve dinner. This is one of them in our family. My kids roll up their sleeves when they see this bowl of seafood goodness come to the table...and there are no pinched noses in sight.

2 lbs	(1 kg) mussels, cleaned
1½ tbsp	extra-virgin olive oil
4	cloves garlic, minced
1 cup	thinly sliced red onions
½ cup	white wine
1½ cups	canned no-salt-added diced tomatoes
1 cup	no-salt-added tomato purée (passata)
½ cup	finely grated carrots
¼ cup	thinly sliced fennel
¼ cup	chopped fresh parsley
½ tsp	dried oregano
½ tsp	crushed red pepper flakes
½ tsp	sea salt
Freshly ground black pepper to taste	

➤ Make sure the mussels are on ice and refrigerated until you're ready to use them. Run mussels under cold water to remove any grit and debeard them (you'll want to remove the little threads that are attached to them if they aren't already removed). Discard any open mussels. Set aside.

➤ In a large pot, heat olive oil over medium-high heat. Add garlic and red onions and cook until onions are softened, about 2 minutes. Stir in wine, tomatoes, tomato purée, carrots and fennel. Cook for 2 minutes, then add remaining ingredients, except mussels. Reduce heat to medium-low and cook for 20 minutes.

➤ Add mussels, stir well and cook for 10 more minutes, or until mussels have opened. Ladle hot mussels and broth into bowls and serve with multigrain bread for dunking.

⌂ HIGH IN...PROTEIN

Mussel meat is an excellent source of protein similar to red meat — here a serving has more than 50 percent of the daily value. What sets it apart is that it's low in calories and fats, too, especially saturated fats. Mussels also help flex muscles, boasting one of the highest concentrations of vitamin B12 in food — the daily recommendation is 2.4 micrograms yet just 3 ounces of mussels contain a whopping 20.40 micrograms.

 8 SERVINGS   40 MIN OR LESS   GLUTEN-FREE   MEATLESS

PER SERVING 114 CALORIES | 4 G TOTAL FAT (1 G SATURATED FAT) | 16 MG CHOLESTEROL | 450 MG SODIUM | 10 G CARBOHYDRATE | 2 G FIBER | 8 G PROTEIN

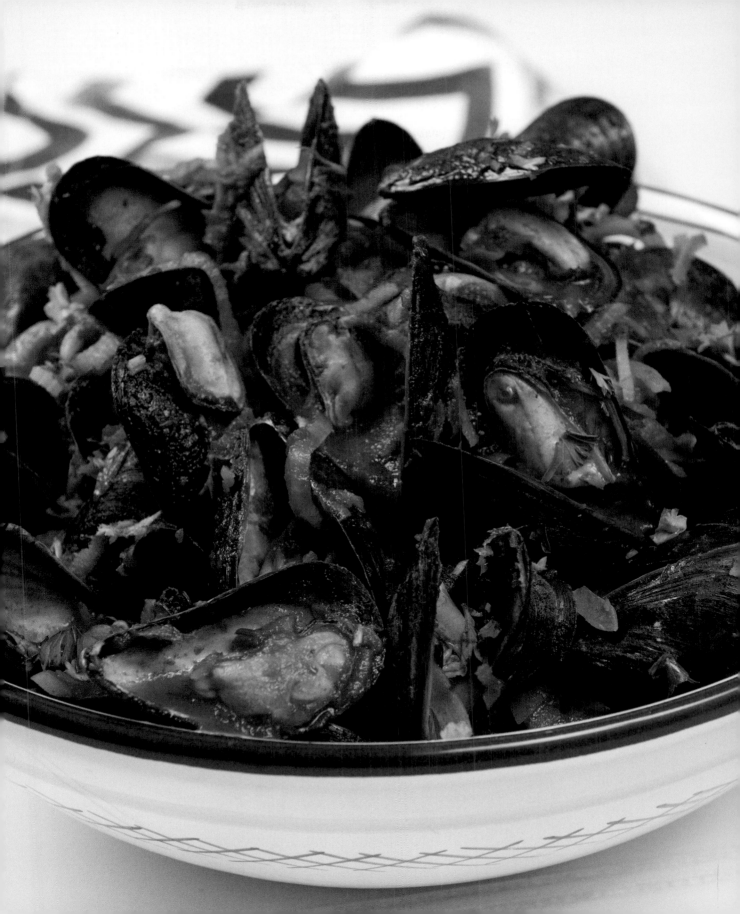

Zucchini & Herb Patties
Frittatine di zucchine e erbe

"IF YOU LOVE SOMETHING, LET IT GO; if it comes back to you, it was truly never to be." I've used the popular phrase with some literary doctoring to best describe how I feel about serving zucchini to my family. I love it; they don't, so it usually comes back to me. But, when I serve this recipe, all I get back is the empty plate. Besides taste, my respect for this tender vegetable stems from watching the plant's sprawling growth in our veggie patch, from a sunny yellow blossom to an elongated vegetable ripe for the picking. Shredded in a batter of eggs and flour — here we swap regular flour for chickpea flour for more taste and protein — and mixed with a wallop of fresh herbs, zucchini can't grow fast enough.

Patties

2	eggs, beaten
1	egg white
½ cup	chopped green onions or finely minced onion
1 tbsp	extra-virgin olive oil
3 tbsp	1% reduced-sodium cottage cheese
¼ cup	freshly grated Parmigiano-Reggiano cheese
3 tbsp	chopped fresh parsley
2 tbsp	minced fresh mint
½ tsp	dried oregano
¼ tsp	sea salt
Pinch	freshly ground black pepper
½ cup	chickpea flour (*see page 34 for more info*)
2 tsp	baking powder
2 cups	finely grated zucchini (see tip)

Serving Sauce (optional)

½ cup	low-fat plain Greek yogurt
1 tbsp	chopped fresh mint
1 tbsp	freshly squeezed lime juice
1	clove garlic, crushed or minced
Pinch	sea salt

➤ Combine all patty ingredients except chickpea flour, baking powder and zucchini in a large bowl. Mix well.

➤ Stir chickpea flour and baking powder into bowl with wet ingredients until well blended. Fold in zucchini until completely coated into mixture. Mixture will seem thick at first but will quickly soften to a paste.

➤ Coat a medium non-stick skillet with cooking spray and set to medium-low heat (no hotter or patties will brown too quickly). Working in batches, drop zucchini batter by the scant tablespoon, about four at a time in the skillet and cook about 1½ minutes per side or until golden brown. Repeat with remaining batter, coating skillet with cooking spray each time. Keep warm and serve immediately. Enjoy on their own or serve with sauce, if using.

TIP Trim the ends of zucchini, but don't peel skin to get the most of its nutritional impact. Use a box grater to shred zucchini so it cooks more evenly.

⇆ VARIATION When in season, try substituting an equal amount of finely chopped zucchini blossoms for 1 cup of the grated zucchini.

⌂ HIGH IN...VITAMIN C

Every ¼ cup of raw zucchini has about 10 percent of the daily value of vitamin C. While it has less than half of the vitamin C found in an orange, zucchini also has less than half the calories. The green onions and fresh herbs in this recipe further boost the amount of vitamin C. The skin of zucchini is also a terrific source of vitamin A. Both vitamins are a powerful pair for protecting against skin ailments, osteoarthritis, asthma, atherosclerosis, age-related macular degeneration and reducing the duration and severity of some viruses like the common cold.

 18-20 PATTIES   30 MIN OR LESS   GLUTEN-FREE   MEATLESS

PER PATTY(20) 23 CALORIES | 1 G TOTAL FAT (0 G SATURATED FAT) | 1 MG CHOLESTEROL | 110 MG SODIUM | 2 G CARBOHYDRATE | 1 G FIBER | 2 G PROTEIN

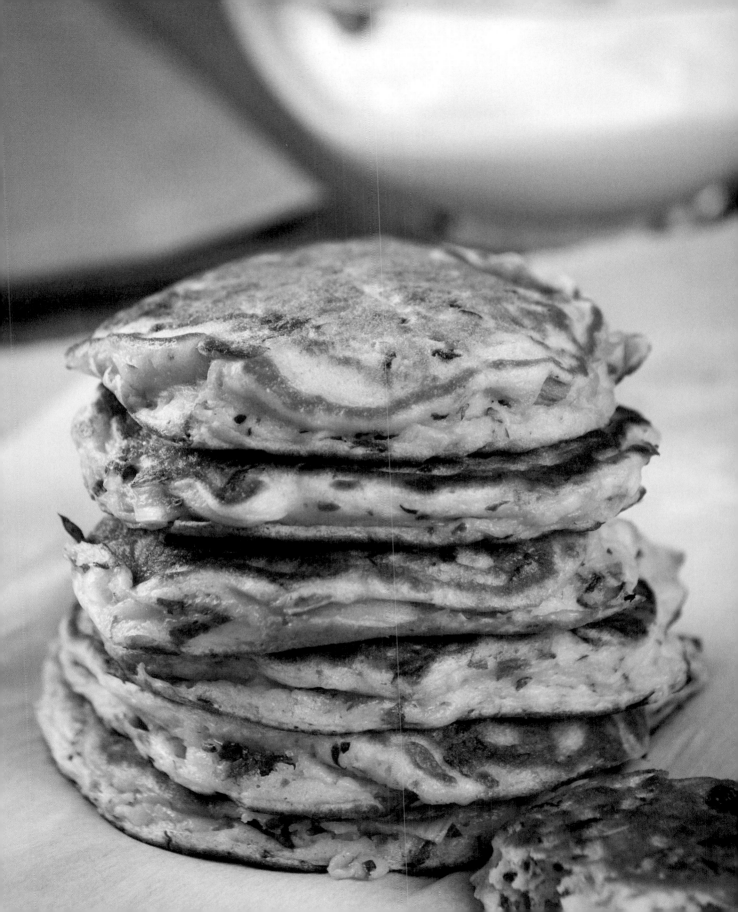

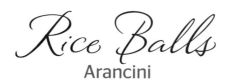

Rice Balls
Arancini

I'LL NEVER FORGET THE MANY TRAIN TRIPS we took in Italy, in particular the crossing of the Mediterranean from mainland Sila, Calabria, to Messina, Sicily. As soon as the train pulled into the ferry and we scurried up to the top deck, it was an awakening of the senses — a mystic volcanic mountain in the distance, the sweltering heat of the sun penetrating the piercing blue sky, the crashing sea waves. But the wafting aroma of arancini (rice balls), perfectly shaped into cones like the approaching Mount Etna, was what really held our attention. We were definitely all aboard!

2 tsp	extra-virgin olive oil
1 tsp	light butter
¼ cup	minced onion
3 cups	brown arborio or brown short-grain rice
5 cups	reduced-sodium vegetable or chicken broth
1 cup	packed shredded part-skim mozzarella (4 oz/113 g)
1 cup	prepared tomato sauce (*see Basic Pasta Tomato Sauce recipe, page 10*), divided
1 cup	whole wheat dry breadcrumbs
½ cup	cornmeal
Sea salt and freshly ground black pepper to taste	
4	egg whites, beaten
¼ cup	frozen small green peas, thawed
2 oz	(56 g) part-skim mozzarella, cut into 20 ½-inch (1-cm) cubes
Extra prepared tomato sauce for serving	

MAKE AHEAD While rice balls require a few steps, you'll actually benefit from dividing them up. Cook the rice and sauce a day or two before baking.

➤ In a large pot, heat olive oil and butter on medium-high heat. Add onion and cook until softened, about 1 to 2 minutes. Add rice and stir until well coated. Add a ladle of broth at a time to the pot to allow liquid to be absorbed before adding more, stirring continuously. When all liquid is absorbed, reduce heat to medium-low, cover and cook for another 40 minutes. Add more broth if rice dries out and is not well cooked. Remove from heat.

➤ Mix in shredded mozzarella and ¾ cup prepared tomato sauce until fully and evenly incorporated. Let cool and refrigerate for at least 2 hours or preferably overnight.

➤ Preheat oven to 425°F. To assemble: Fill one bowl with breadcrumbs; fill another bowl with cornmeal, salt and pepper. In a small bowl, add egg whites. In a fourth bowl, combine ¼ cup tomato sauce and peas. Have your mozzarella cubes ready, too.

➤ Wet your hands, portion out a scant ½ cup of rice mixture and shape into a ball. Make a well in center of ball, add about 1 tsp of tomato sauce with 4 to 5 peas and push in a piece of cheese. Close up hole and reshape ball. Roll it in cornmeal, dredge in egg white, then finish rolling in breadcrumbs. Place on a baking sheet lined with parchment paper. Repeat with remaining balls. Lightly coat them with cooking spray. Cook for 15 to 20 minutes in preheated oven, transferring pan to upper rack during the last 5 minutes of cooking time, until rice balls are lightly browned. Serve with tomato sauce.

⌂ HIGH IN...FIBER

White starchy rice is replaced with brown short-grain rice, which bolsters the fiber in these golden nuggets. Giving them a crispy shell without deep-frying also avoids at least triple the amount of fat.

20 MEDIUM RICE BALLS   MEATLESS   MAKE AHEAD

PER RICE BALL(20) 148 CALORIES | 4 G TOTAL FAT (1 G SATURATED FAT) | 5 MG CHOLESTEROL | 247 MG SODIUM | 36 G CARBOHYDRATE | 3 G FIBER | 7 G PROTEIN

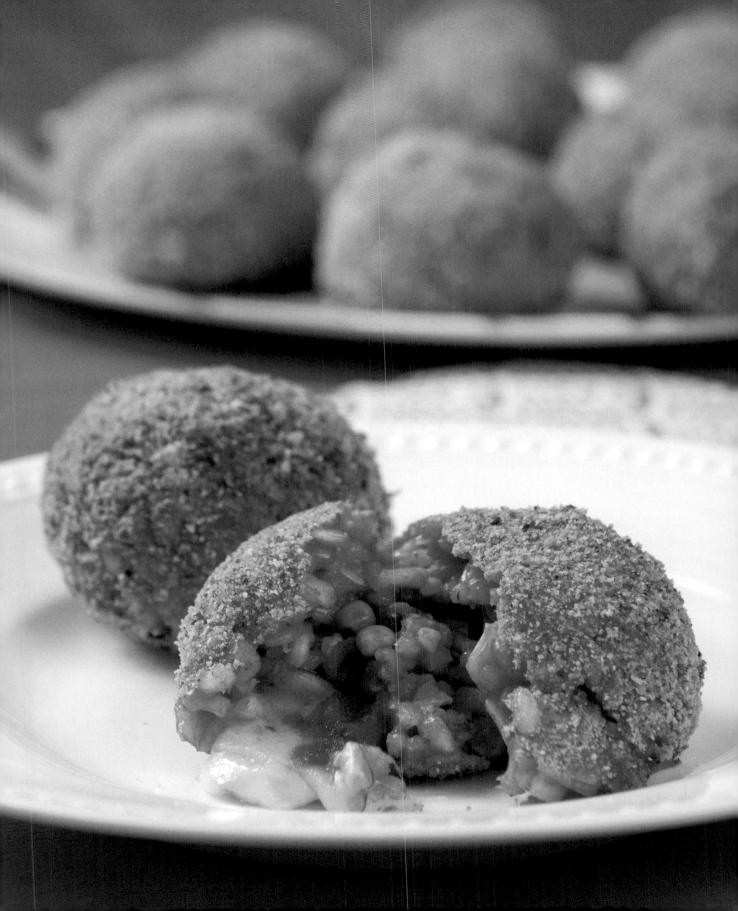

Chickpea Polenta "Fritters"
Panelle

STREET FOOD IN ITALY ISN'T YOUR CLASSIC NORTH AMERICAN FARE of hotdogs and ice cream. A trip down memory lane walking the streets with Italian cousins conjures up the intoxicating aromas of roasted sugared almonds, pizza *al taglio* (by the slice), rice balls and grilled paninos with fresh bocconcini and prosciutto. It's a gastronomical explosion of the senses. So, too, is this street food particular to Sicily's capital city of Palermo, which takes a batter of chickpea flour and deep fries it before stuffing it in between bread slices. Here, *panelle* are seasoned for even more flavor and skip the deep fryer to either be enjoyed on their own, as a platform for dips or paired with a simple giardiniera or seared cheese.

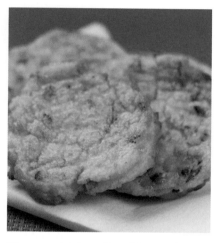

1½ cups	chickpea flour* (see tip)
1 tsp	sea salt
1 tbsp	chopped fresh rosemary, or 1 tsp dried rosemary
¼ tsp	freshly ground black pepper
2 cups	cold water
2 tbsp	whole flaxseeds

MAKE AHEAD Pop mixture out of muffin tins, then refrigerate for one to two days. Broil just before serving.

TIP You can find chickpea flour in the specialty food or East Indian food aisle of your grocery store. This flour is gluten-free but check the label to ensure wheat fillers haven't been added.

➤ Lightly grease two 12-cup muffin tins with cooking spray. Set aside.

➤ Combine chickpea flour, salt, rosemary and pepper in a bowl.

➤ In a medium pot, add water and slowly whisk in the chickpea flour mixture until fully dissolved (do this while the water is cold!). Bring the pot to the burner over medium heat and whisk continuously until mixture thickens to resemble porridge. Reduce heat to low and continue to whisk for another 4 to 5 minutes, until mixture pulls away from the sides and bottom of the pot. Stir in seeds. Allow mixture to cool slightly.

➤ Portion out about 1 heaping tablespoon of mixture into each muffin cup using a wet spoon and your hands to evenly fill bottom of cup to a thickness of about ¾ inch (2 cm). Let cool for about 30 minutes.

➤ Preheat oven to broil setting. Carefully transfer each patty onto a baking sheet lined with parchment paper. Lightly spray each side of panelle pieces with cooking spray and place in oven, about 6 inches from broil element, to cook for 7 to 8 minutes on each side, until they're golden brown.

⌒ HIGH IN...PROTEIN

Chickpea flour, also known as gram or besan flour, is a great substitute for other flours because it's higher in protein (½ cup offers 11 g of protein compared to 8 g of protein in the same amount of whole wheat flour or 6 g in all-purpose flour). The body breaks down this vegetarian-friendly protein into amino acids, which help build and repair muscles and tissues. Consuming legumes such as chickpea flour along with a source of vitamin C (tomatoes, citrus) can help absorb the type of iron contained.

20-24 PIECES

GLUTEN-FREE*
CHECK LABEL

MEATLESS

MAKE AHEAD

PER 4 PIECES 118 CALORIES | 3 G TOTAL FAT (0 G SATURATED FAT) | 0 MG CHOLESTEROL | 370 MG SODIUM | 14 G CARBOHYDRATE | 3 G FIBER | 6 G PROTEIN

Same-Day Fresh Giardiniera
Giardiniera fresca

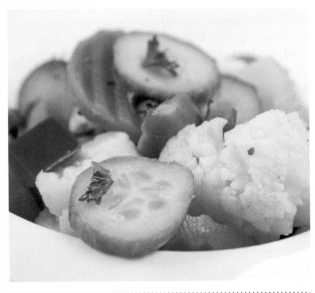

2 cups	good-quality store-bought giardiniera with brine (choose one with cauliflower and carrots)
1 cup	thinly sliced mini cucumbers
½ cup	sliced celery
½ cup	cubed red bell peppers
1 tbsp	green olives in brine, rinsed
1 tbsp	thinly sliced red onions
1 tbsp	each: chopped fresh parsley, peppercorns and extra-virgin olive oil

Freshly ground black pepper to taste

➤ Drain giardiniera (reserving liquid) and place in a large bowl. Add remaining ingredients and toss well with 2 tbsp of reserved brine. Season with pepper. Serve at room temperature or chill for 2 hours to let flavors settle in.

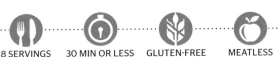

8 SERVINGS   **30 MIN OR LESS**   **GLUTEN-FREE**   **MEATLESS**

PER SERVING 11 CALORIES | 0 G TOTAL FAT (0 G SATURATED FAT) | 0 MG CHOLESTEROL | 413 MG SODIUM | 2 G CARBOHYDRATE | 1 G FIBER | 1 G PROTEIN

Pan-Seared Tuma with Red Peppers
Tuma fritta con peperoni rossi

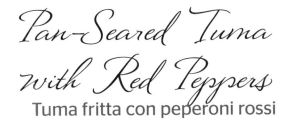

¼ cup	uncooked quinoa
Pinch	sea salt
¼ cup	egg white, beaten
12 oz	(340 g) tuma cheese (see tip)
¼ cup	roasted red peppers, or store-bought roasted red peppers (*see recipe tip, page 140*)

➤ Add quinoa into the bowl of a mill or coffee grinder and whirl until it reaches a near flour consistency (alternatively, you can use quinoa flour). Combine milled quinoa with salt in a shallow bowl or pie plate. Pour egg white in another small bowl.

➤ Cut tuma thinly into ½-inch (1-cm) strips, about 2 x 3 inches (5 x 7.5 cm) in size — you'll get about 10 strips. Dip strips into egg white, then press into quinoa flour until well coated.

➤ Heat a medium non-stick skillet on high heat; coat with cooking spray. Add tuma and sear until lightly golden, about 2 minutes on each side. Serve hot topped with strips of roasted red peppers.

TIP Tuma is a mild-tasting, firm soft cheese much like pressed ricotta that is very low in salt. If you can't find tuma, substitute large bocconcini or mozzarella.

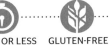

10 PIECES   **30 MIN OR LESS**   **GLUTEN-FREE**   **MEATLESS**

PER SERVING 77 CALORIES | 4 G TOTAL FAT (2 G SATURATED FAT) | 11 MG CHOLESTEROL | 121 MG SODIUM | 5 G CARBOHYDRATE | 0 G FIBER | 7 G PROTEIN

Crispy Calamari Rings
Calamari "fritti"

IT WASN'T JUST THE SCENT OF FISH THAT was *the* giveaway Mom was preparing a batch of fried seafood. Once you walked into the kitchen, the haze of flour dust over a peaked pile of just-dredged fish usually gave it away even before the smell drifted throughout the entire house. Pasty remnants sometimes made it to Mom's face like the war paint soldiers donned before battle, and we awaited the ensuing bonanza from the deep fryer. While this recipe can't guarantee the absence of floured faces or soiled aprons, what it will promise is that loved ones will be anxiously awaiting batch after batch.

¼ cup	egg whites
½ cup	whole wheat dry breadcrumbs
¼ cup	cornmeal
¼ tsp	baking soda
½ tsp	sea salt
Pinch	freshly ground black pepper
19 oz	(550 g) frozen large calamari (squid) rings, thawed

Lemon wedges for garnish

➤ Preheat oven to 450°F. Line a large baking sheet with foil and coat with cooking spray.

➤ Place egg white in a shallow bowl or pie plate. In another shallow bowl, combine breadcrumbs, cornmeal, baking soda, salt and pepper.

➤ Pat calamari dry. In batches, dip entire calamari rings into egg whites, then coat well with breadcrumb-cornmeal mixture. Shake off any excess crumbs and place dredged rings side by side on baking sheet. Coat calamari with cooking spray for 3 seconds. Cook in preheated oven for 15 minutes, turning halfway through cooking.

➤ Serve hot with lemon wedges or a Quick Marinara Sauce (*see recipe, page 13*).

⇆ VARIATION Squid tentacles or a combination of squid mixed species can be substituted for squid rings.

⌂ HIGH IN...PROTEIN

Like most seafood, squid contains a significant amount of protein, almost one-third of the recommended amount a day in one serving of these baked calamari. Squid is also loaded with B vitamins, including niacin (B3), cyanocobalamin (B12) and riboflavin (B2), which help the body metabolize fats. The high-protein content comes with minimal amounts of fat, only 1 gram in 3 ounces of squid.

6-8 SERVINGS   30 MIN OR LESS   MEATLESS

PER SERVING(8) 118 CALORIES | 1 G TOTAL FAT (0 G SATURATED FAT) | 160 MG CHOLESTEROL | 236 MG SODIUM | 13 G CARBOHYDRATE | 1 G FIBER | 13 G PROTEIN

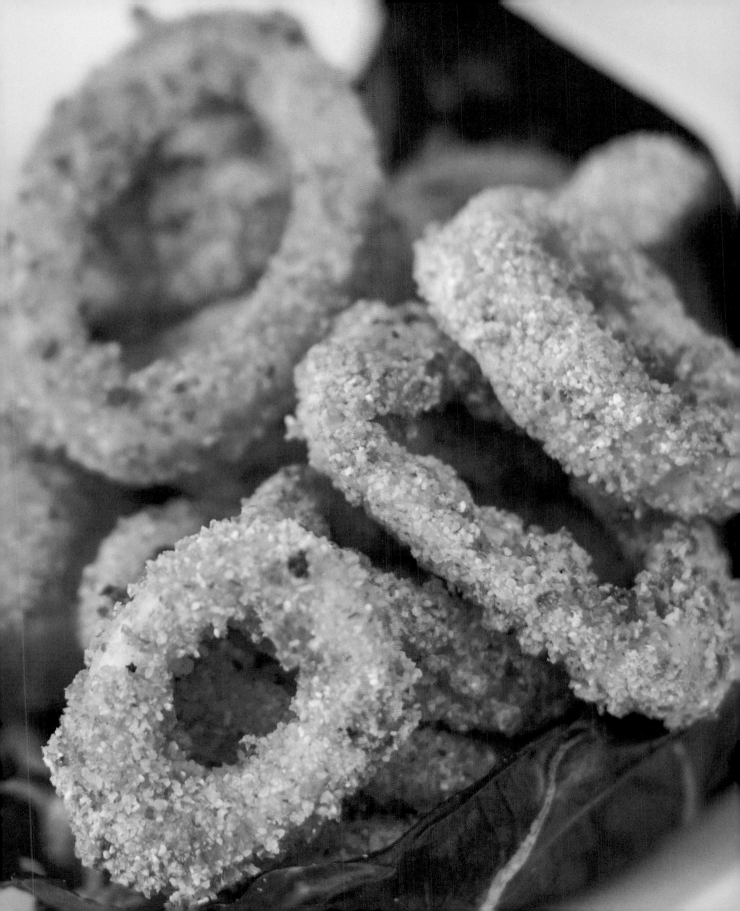

Grilled Artichokes
Carciofi alla griglia

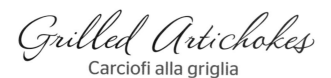

LIKE BUILDING THE PERFECT CAMPFIRE, setting up *la griglia a carbone* (or the charcoal grill) is an exercise in patience and if there was anyone I know who best exemplifies that quality, it's my dad. It's no surprise then that Dad was always the flame-keeper — at home, the cottage or a Sunday picnic — carefully stacking charcoal and wood chips, then nurturing the flame first with gentle puffs of breath and then later with huge waves of air from an honorary piece of cardboard. An hour into it and the fiery heat from the grill was ready to do its job, whether it was to perfectly sear a juicy steak, tender shrimp or fresh vegetables.

2 tsp	sea salt
1 tbsp	extra-virgin olive oil
4	cloves garlic (whole)
Juice of 1 lemon	
6	medium artichokes

Marinade

3 tbsp	extra-virgin olive oil
3 tbsp	each: red wine vinegar and white balsamic vinegar
Juice and zest of ½ lemon	
4	cloves garlic, minced or pressed
¼ tsp	sea salt
Freshly ground black pepper to taste	
2 tbsp	minced fresh parsley for garnish

➤ In a medium pot of cold water (about 2 cups), add salt, olive oil, garlic and lemon juice.

➤ Trim the stems of each artichoke and about one-quarter of each top with a serrated knife. Remove tough, brown outer leaves and discard. Cut artichoke in half, lengthwise. Quickly add artichokes into the pot of seasoned water, making sure artichokes are fully submerged. Bring to a boil, then reduce heat to medium and simmer until leaves are tender and easy to pull, about 25 minutes. Use tongs to remove artichokes.

➤ In a deep pie plate, combine olive oil, vinegars, lemon juice and zest, garlic, salt and pepper. Add cooked artichokes, mix gently to fully coat and let sit for 30 minutes.

➤ Preheat grill to medium setting. Grill artichokes for 4 to 5 minutes on each side, basting with marinade in between cooking time, until artichokes begin to brown. Remove from grill and drizzle with any leftover marinade and sprinkle parsley before serving.

MAKE AHEAD Boil artichokes and marinate for several hours or up to overnight before grilling.

⌂ HIGH IN...FIBER

Artichokes are an excellent source of fiber, boasting more than a quarter of the recommended daily intake in one of these servings. That's more fiber than a bowl of oatmeal or 1 cup of broccoli. Artichokes also contain a bit of plant-based protein with no fat and few calories.

6 SERVINGS   GLUTEN-FREE   MEATLESS   MAKE AHEAD

PER SERVING 143 CALORIES | 9 G TOTAL FAT (1 G SATURATED FAT) | 0 MG CHOLESTEROL | 318 MG SODIUM | 14 G CARBOHYDRATE | 7 G FIBER | 4 G PROTEIN

Shrimp Skewers with Gremolata
Spiedini di gamberi con gremolata

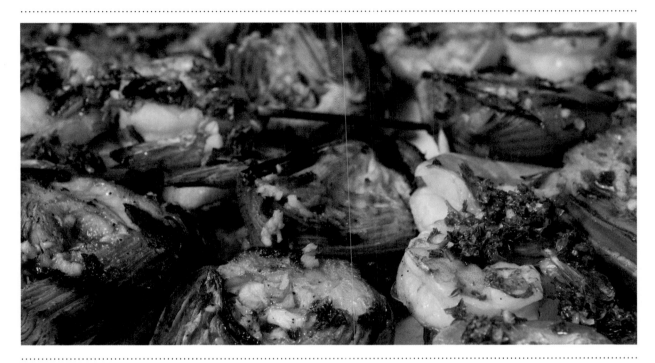

Gremolata

1 cup	packed chopped fresh Italian (flat-leaf) parsley
2	cloves garlic, chopped
Zest of 1 lemon	
1 tsp	freshly squeezed lemon juice
¼ tsp	sea salt
Pinch	freshly ground black pepper
1 tbsp	extra-virgin olive oil

Shrimp Skewers

10	8-inch bamboo skewers
1 lb	(454 g) frozen raw large shrimp, peeled, deveined and thawed
1 tbsp	extra-virgin olive oil
Lemon slices for garnish	

➤ To make the gremolata, combine all gremolata ingredients, except olive oil, in the bowl of a food processor and pulse until all ingredients are well chopped. Add to a bowl and stir in olive oil.

➤ Soak wooden sticks in warm water for at least 10 minutes. Remove from water and pat dry. Preheat grill to medium-high setting.

➤ Finish thawing out shrimp by running them under cold water. Pat dry and skewer 4 shrimp per stick. Spray skewers lightly with cooking spray. Place shrimp on preheated grill rack that has been brushed lightly with oil and grill until opaque and pink, about 4 to 5 minutes on each side.

➤ Place skewers on a serving platter and spoon gremolata evenly over them while hot. Serve with lemon slices.

⇆VARIATION Substitute chicken breast pieces for shimp on these skewers. Make gremolata less tangy by adding 1 tbsp minced green olives.

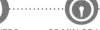
 10 SKEWERS   30 MIN OR LESS   GLUTEN-FREE   MEATLESS

PER SKEWER 74 CALORIES I 4 G TOTAL FAT (1 G SATURATED FAT) I 69 MG CHOLESTEROL I 129 MG SODIUM I 1 G CARBOHYDRATE I 0 G FIBER I 9 G PROTEIN

Eggplant Caponata Dip
Caponata

WHEN DAD PROUDLY BROUGHT in a freshly picked eggplant from his garden, there would always be a mini-conference with Mom about what recipe she'd make with it. Eggplant was a staple when they were growing up so inspiration was never an issue. Dad always let Mom decide, but when ripe tomatoes, a handful of celery stalks, spring onions and fresh herbs accompanied the eggplant in the basket, it was clear he was casting his vote for this Sicilian specialty that combines salty and sweet ingredients to make a deliciously creamy mixture served over crunchy bread or on its own.

2 lbs	(1 kg) eggplant (about 2 large eggplants)
Sea salt	
2 tbsp	extra-virgin olive oil
1	large onion, chopped (about 1½ cups)
3	cloves garlic, minced
1 cup	thinly sliced celery, filaments removed
1 cup	canned no-salt-added whole peeled tomatoes, drained and chopped, or 2 ripe tomatoes, peeled and chopped
2 tbsp	no-salt-added tomato paste
1 tsp	granulated sugar
¾ cup	no-salt-added vegetable or chicken broth
⅓ cup	small green olives packed in brine, pitted and halved
3 tbsp	red wine vinegar
2 tbsp	chopped fresh parsley
1½ tbsp	capers in brine, rinsed and patted dry
½ tsp	sea salt
Freshly ground black pepper to taste	
¼ cup	chopped fresh basil for garnish
¼ cup	toasted pine nuts for garnish

TIP Can also be served warm as a side dish.

▶ Trim ends of eggplant (do not remove skin) and chop into medium-sized cubes. (Cooking eggplant with the skin on gives this dish its great texture.) Sprinkle eggplant lightly with salt. Let stand in a colander for 15 minutes to "sweat" out bitterness. Rinse and pat dry.

▶ In a very large non-stick skillet, heat olive oil over high heat. Add eggplant and toss well with oil to coat, stirring often until pieces soften and brown on all sides, about 8 to 10 minutes. Remove eggplant and set aside.

▶ Coat the same saucepan with cooking spray and add onion, garlic and celery and cook over medium-high heat until softened, about 2 to 3 minutes. Add tomatoes, tomato paste and sugar until well combined. Add broth, reserved eggplants, olives, wine vinegar, parsley, capers, salt and pepper. Let simmer on low heat, covered, for about 20 to 25 minutes, stirring occasionally. Add a little water if the eggplants are drying up. Eggplants should be falling apart and mixture should have a creamy texture.

▶ Let cool and refrigerate for at least 4 hours or overnight to soak in flavors. Serve chilled with chopped basil and pine nuts, along with thick slices of toasted whole-grain bread or crostini.

MAKE AHEAD Best served the next day. Keeps refrigerated for three to four days.

⋂ HIGH IN...ANTIOXIDANTS

Aside from a multitude of vitamins and fiber, eggplant has a unique antioxidant found on the skin called nasunin, which protects brain cells from damaging free radicals. Other powerful antioxidants — the most notable is chlorogenic acid — protect against viruses, cardiovascular disease, rheumatoid arthritis and certain cancers.

6 CUPS GLUTEN-FREE MEATLESS MAKE AHEAD

PER ½ CUP 84 CALORIES | 5 G TOTAL FAT (1 G SATURATED FAT) | 2 MG CHOLESTEROL | 223 MG SODIUM | 9 G CARBOHYDRATE | 4 G FIBER | 2 G PROTEIN

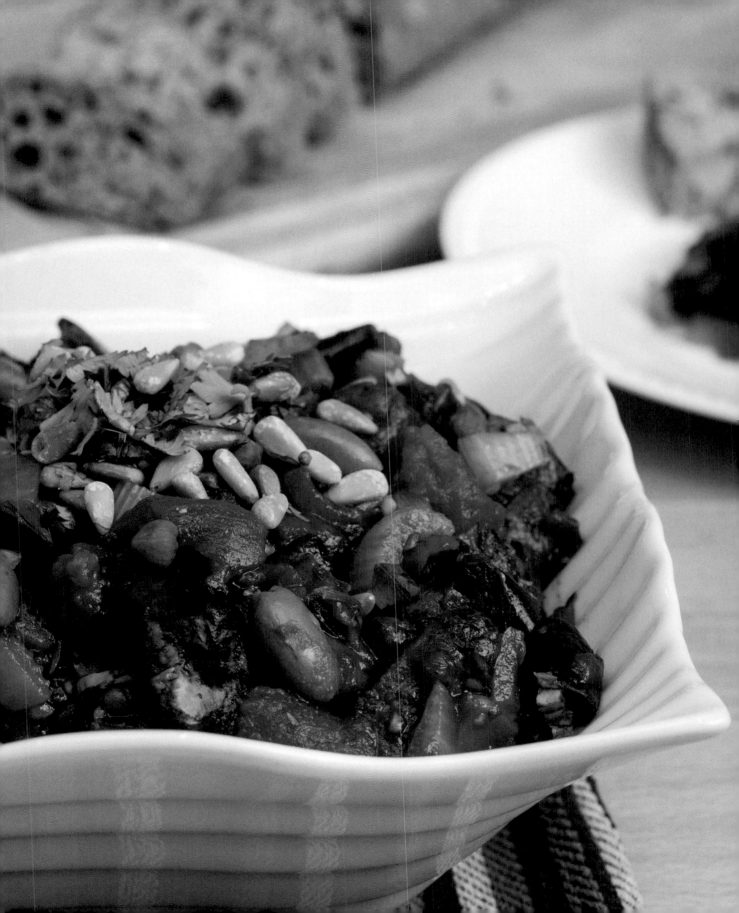

Belgian Endive & Treviso Radicchio with Gorgonzola & Candied Walnuts

Fior di insalata con gorgonzola e noci candite

DAD'S ASSORTMENT OF HOMEGROWN LETTUCE has always been food for admiration. Tucked in between his staked tomato and pepper plants, neat rows of verdant and red-tinged lettuce leaves gently wave in the wind as if to assert their presence. In fact, at their growing peak, I forgo the grocery store and take a stroll in Dad's lettuce aisles with shopping bags in tow to take advantage of the fresh bounty. In any year, there's an impressive crop of romaine, green radicchio, escarole, curly endive, arugula and additional crunchy long leaves that we enjoy either tossed in a light vinaigrette or as edible spoons that scoop up other delights.

2 tsp	extra-virgin olive oil
2 tsp	brown sugar
1 tsp	ground cinnamon
Pinch	sea salt
Pinch	freshly ground black pepper
½ cup	walnut pieces
1	head Belgian endive (about 12 pieces)
1	small head Treviso radicchio (about 12 pieces), (see tip)
4 tbsp	Gorgonzola cheese (about 3.5 oz/100 g)

➤ Preheat oven to 350°F. In a small bowl, combine olive oil, brown sugar, cinnamon, salt and pepper. Toss walnut pieces into mixture and stir until well coated. Place on a baking sheet on the *middle* oven rack and bake for about 7 to 8 minutes, stirring once halfway through cooking time.

➤ Separate leaves of endive and radicchio and add about ½ tsp of Gorgonzola on the ends of each leaf. Press a good pinch of coated walnuts on top of Gorgonzola and alternate leaves on a platter to create a pretty flower-petal pattern. The cupped leaves of endive and radicchio make perfect edible finger foods.

TIP Treviso radicchio, unlike the more common Chioggio radicchio (ball-shaped maroon type), has long, slender leaves that resemble the shape of Belgian endive and aren't as bitter tasting as other radicchios. Treviso radicchio is also great grilled on its own, as a pizza topping or in a stir-fry.

⇆ VARIATION The rich, creamy and pungent taste of Gorgonzola is a perfect accompaniment to these tender leaves but if you prefer a more subtle flavor, substitute goat's cheese (there are even lower-fat varieties available).

 24 PIECES   30 MIN OR LESS   GLUTEN-FREE MEATLESS

PER PIECE 40 CALORIES | 3 G TOTAL FAT (1 G SATURATED FAT) | 3 MG CHOLESTEROL | 63 MG SODIUM | 2 G CARBOHYDRATE | 1 G FIBER | 2 G PROTEIN

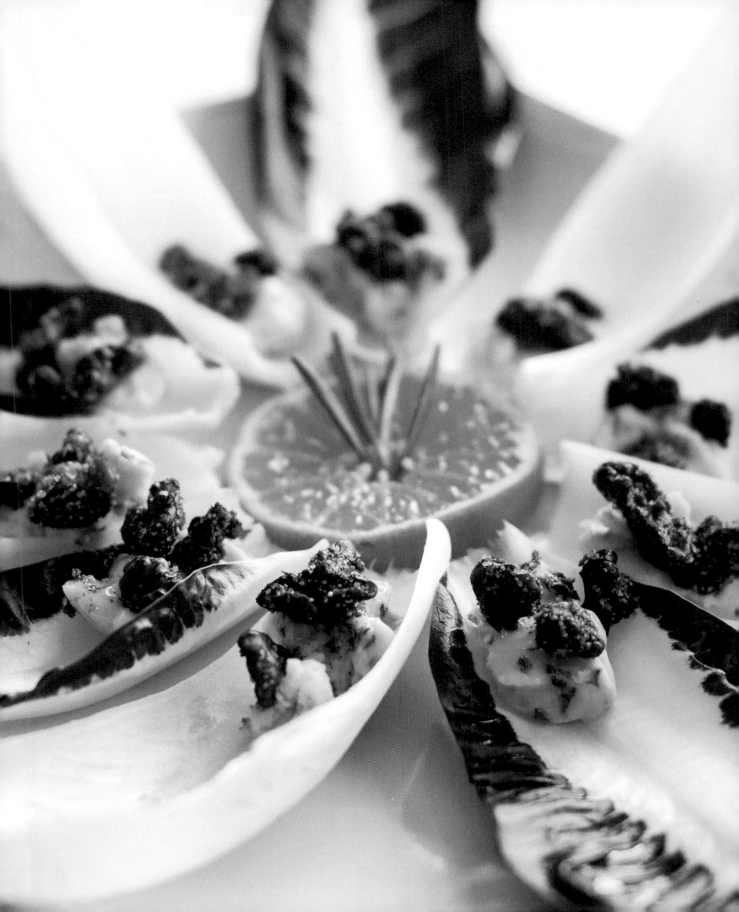

Glazed Fig Bruschetta
Bruschetta di ficchi

IT'S NOT HARD FOR ME TO OVERINDULGE IN FIGS, especially when they're fresh. But it wasn't until my husband first visited my late grandfather's land in Italy that he truly understood my passion for the fruit. Situated on arid sloping terrain punctuated by olive trees, a lemon orchard and prickly pear-bearing cacti, the fig trees stood out like Christmas trees embellished with aubergine and pale green ornaments. His wide-eyed expression said it all as he bit into the plump fruit and slurped up the juice. I'm taken back to this moment when I make this recipe. Roasted figs, piled high on creamy goat's cheese, brings out that lusciously decadent sweetness I so love.

12	slices whole-grain baguette or Vienna loaf*
3 tsp	extra-virgin olive oil, divided
¼ tsp	Italian herb seasoning
3	large black figs
1 tbsp	balsamic vinegar
2 tsp	honey
Pinch	sea salt
Freshly ground black pepper to taste	
1	small log (5 oz/130 g) light goat's cheese (see tip)

➤ Preheat oven to 350°F.

➤ Cut baguette into thin slices, about ½ inch (1 cm) thick. Combine 2 tsp olive oil with Italian seasoning in a small bowl and brush both sides of bread slices. Place on a baking sheet and bake in oven for 8 minutes, turning halfway during cooking.

➤ Trim tops of figs and cut each one into quarters. In a small bowl, combine remaining 1 tsp olive oil, vinegar, honey, salt and pepper; toss figs gently to coat. On each slice of toasted baguette, place a thin slice of goat's cheese and top with a wedge of glazed fig. Drizzle remaining glaze over figs.

➤ Place bruschetta slices on a baking sheet and cook in *middle* rack of preheated oven for 12 minutes. Let cool for 5 minutes before serving.

TIP To thinly slice goat's cheese to a thickness of ¼ inch (0.5 cm), use unflavored dental floss to prevent it from crumbling.

⇆VARIATION Use dried figs if you're having a hard time finding fresh figs. Thinly slice a dried fig, season it as directed and let it sit for about 10 minutes before topping the goat's cheese.

MAKE AHEAD Prepare bread toasts the day before.

6 SERVINGS   30 MIN OR LESS   GLUTEN-FREE* REPLACE WITH GF BREAD   MEATLESS   MAKE AHEAD

PER SERVING 164 CALORIES | 6 G TOTAL FAT (2 G SATURATED FAT) | 8 MG CHOLESTEROL | 265 MG SODIUM | 23 G CARBOHYDRATE | 2 G FIBER | 6 G PROTEIN

Bocconcini, Prosciutto, Tomato & Melon Skewers

Spiedini di bocconcini, prosciutto, pomodorini e melone

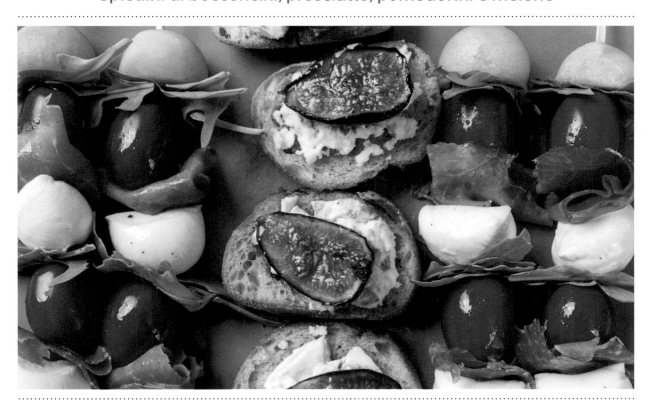

24	mini (cherry) light bocconcini
24	ripe cherry or grape tomatoes
2 tsp	extra-virgin olive oil
Pinch	each: sea salt and freshly ground black pepper
½	cantaloupe melon
6	very thin slices prosciutto (1.75 oz/50 g)
12	bamboo skewers
1 cup	baby arugula leaves

➤ In a medium bowl, combine bocconcini and cherry tomatoes and toss with olive oil, salt and pepper. Use a melon baller to shape 24 cantaloupe balls. Tear each prosciutto slice into 4 equal pieces to make 24 pieces.

➤ To thread each skewer, assemble with: 1 piece cantaloupe, 2 to 3 pieces arugula, 1 tomato, 1 prosciutto piece, 1 bocconcini, and again with the same amounts of arugula, tomato, prosciutto, bocconcini, arugula and cantaloupe. Repeat with remaining skewers.

➤ Refrigerate until ready to serve.

⇆ VARIATION Any sweet melon works, so substitute other sweet orange melons or honeydew. Or replace melon with fresh figs, cut in half.

12 SKEWERS   30 MIN OR LESS   GLUTEN-FREE

PER SKEWER 57 CALORIES | 3 G TOTAL FAT (1 G SATURATED FAT) | 7 MG CHOLESTEROL | 145 MG SODIUM | 4 G CARBOHYDRATE | 1 G FIBER | 4 G PROTEIN

Venetian Cod Mantecato Dip
Baccalà mantecato alla Veneziana

IT WAS NEVER A HOST'S PRACTICE TO SERVE colorful bowls of dips as appetizers when we were growing up. But in modern-day Italy, they've become the norm. I first got a taste for freshly whipped dips while there several years ago. My aunt treated me to a *rinfresco* (the equivalent of happy hour) at a local bar. I was quite content to skip dinner that night and indulge in a smorgasbord of tapenades and dips, much like these regional favorites, along with fresh cheeses, soppressata, olives, breadsticks and a little Chianti. Dip in!

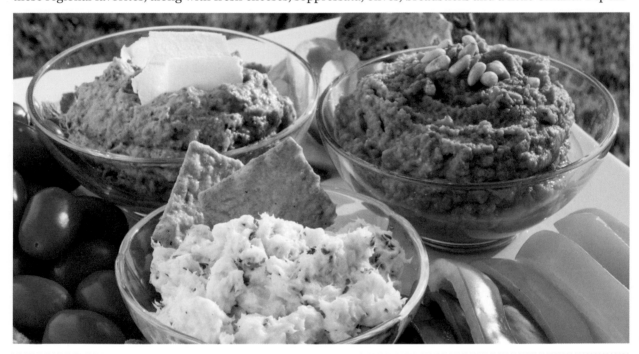

14 oz	(400 g) fresh or frozen (thawed) skinless, boneless cod fillets
2	bay leaves
2	cloves garlic, chopped
¼ cup	low-fat plain Greek yogurt
¼ cup	light cream cheese
1 tbsp	freshly squeezed lemon juice
2 tbsp	chopped fresh parsley
¼ tsp	sea salt
Freshly ground black pepper to taste	

➤ Cut cod into large pieces and add to a medium pot of water along with bay leaves. Bring to a boil, reduce heat to medium-high and cook for about 10 minutes, just until cod pieces are starting to flake. Drain, reserving some liquid. Remove and discard bay leaves.

➤ Place cod and remaining ingredients into the bowl of a food processer and pulse until it forms a chunky paste. If mixture seems dry, add 2 to 3 tbsp of reserved liquid. Place dip into a bowl and serve with whole-grain crackers.

MAKE AHEAD You can boil the cod the day before and refrigerate it. Pulse with remaining ingredients before serving.

 2 CUPS
 30 MIN OR LESS
 GLUTEN-FREE
 MEATLESS
 MAKE AHEAD

PER ¼ CUP 54 CALORIES | 1 G TOTAL FAT (1 G SATURATED FAT) | 28 MG CHOLESTEROL | 267 MG SODIUM | 1 G CARBOHYDRATE | 0 G FIBER | 9 G PROTEIN

Fava Bean Dip
Puré di fave

2 cups	fresh or frozen fava (broad) beans (see tip)
1 tbsp	extra-virgin olive oil
1 tbsp	low-fat plain Greek yogurt
½	avocado
2	cloves garlic, minced
¼ cup	chopped fresh basil
¼ cup	chopped fresh mint
¼ tsp	sea salt
Freshly ground black pepper to taste	
Ricotta insalata cheese shavings (about 0.7 oz/20 g) for garnish (see tip)	

➤ Bring a medium pot of water to boil. Add the fava beans and cook for about 10 minutes or until beans are tender-crisp. Drain (reserving some liquid), rinse with cold water and quickly remove shells.

➤ Place fava beans and remaining ingredients, except ricotta insalata, into the bowl of a food processor and pulse for about 1 to 2 minutes, until mixture is creamy but slightly chunky. If mixture seems dry, add 3 to 4 tbsp of reserved liquid. Top dip with ricotta insalata and serve with fresh vegetables or crostini.

TIPS You'll find fresh fava beans in their pods during spring and summer months in grocery stores. Remove bean seeds from pods. If you can't find them fresh, use frozen or canned beans, although they may not taste as fresh. Be sure to shell the beans once they've been boiled.
➤ Ricotta insalata (meaning "salted ricotta") is a cheese made with sheep's milk. The ricotta is pressed, salted and aged.

⌂ HIGH IN...FIBER

Compared to other varieties of beans and lentils, fava beans are lower in calories yet are a rich source of dietary fiber. A half cup cooked offers just over 3 grams of fiber (almost four times that amount when eaten raw). They're particularly known for their soluble fiber, the type of fiber that turns gel-like when water is added to help you feel full longer and lower bad cholesterol.

| 1½ CUPS | 30 MIN OR LESS | GLUTEN-FREE | MEATLESS |

PER ¼ CUP 82 CALORIES | 5 G TOTAL FAT (1 G SATURATED FAT) | 1 MG CHOLESTEROL | 123 MG SODIUM | 5 G CARBOHYDRATE | 3 G FIBER | 3 G PROTEIN

Tuscan Hummus Dip
Puré di ceci Toscana

1 can	(19 oz/540 mL) no-salt-added chickpeas, gently rinsed and drained
½ cup	canned no-salt-added whole peeled tomatoes, drained and chopped
⅓ cup	water
1 tbsp	freshly grated Parmigiano-Reggiano or Pecorino Romano cheese
Juice of 1 small lime	
1 to 2	cloves garlic, chopped
1 tbsp	each: chopped fresh basil and fresh parsley
1 tsp	dried oregano
½ tsp	Italian herb seasoning
2 tbsp	extra-virgin olive oil
¼ tsp	sea salt
Freshly ground black pepper to taste	
Pinch	crushed red pepper flakes (optional)
Toasted pine nuts for garnish	
Paprika for garnish	

➤ Place all ingredients except pine nuts and paprika into the bowl of a food processor and whirl for about 10 minutes or until smooth. Chill for 1 to 2 hours before serving. Top dip with pine nuts and a dash of paprika and serve with fresh vegetables, whole-grain crostini, crackers or pita wedges.

⇄ VARIATIONS For a tangier dip, substitute ¼ cup sun-dried tomatoes for peeled tomatoes.
➤ For a more intense garlic flavor, cook garlic with olive oil until slightly golden before adding to the mix.

| 4 CUPS | 30 MIN OR LESS | GLUTEN-FREE | MEATLESS |

PER ¼ CUP 45 CALORIES | 2 G TOTAL FAT (0 G SATURATED FAT) | 0 MG CHOLESTEROL | 152 MG SODIUM | 5 G CARBOHYDRATE | 1 G FIBER | 2 G PROTEIN

Grilled Portobello Mushrooms & Polenta
Polenta e funghi portobello alla griglia

WITH SO MANY OF US CLAIMING THE CHEF'S HAT in my family, our *cucina* has always been a "test kitchen" of sorts. Many passed-along recipes instantly earned a permanent page in our scrapbook of favorites — there's the crab salad from our friend Rosanna, rabbit stew from my dad's work colleague and from our late neighbor the famous sponge cake that appears at every birthday. And so one day when a batch of polenta produced more than we could consume, we took inspiration to grill polenta from a Northern Italian friend who makes the regional specialty regularly. A crunchy exterior with creamy center is now the base for so many appetizers that welcome guests to our home, but the most preferred is this one.

1	recipe Sweet Potato Polenta (*see recipe, page 22*) or 1 cylinder store-bought polenta
6	large portobello mushrooms, stems detached
1½ tbsp	extra-virgin olive oil
	Sea salt and freshly ground black pepper to taste
1	small log (5 oz/130 g) light goat's cheese
6	fresh basil leaves, thinly sliced

➤ Cook polenta as per recipe. Spread out hot polenta to about ¾ inches (2 cm) thickness on a platter. Let cool and cut out 6 pieces with a 3.5-inch (9-cm) cookie cutter, or use a glass with a similar diameter as a guide and a sharp knife to cut into 6 disks. (If you're using a store-bought cylinder of already-made polenta, cut 6 disks, ¾ inch (2 cm) thick.)

➤ Preheat grill to medium-high setting.

➤ Brush mushroom caps and polenta disks with olive oil on both sides. Season portobello with salt and pepper.

➤ Place polenta disks on one side of preheated grill rack that has been brushed lightly with oil and grill for 7 to 8 minutes per side. You'll want to see some grill marks. On the other side of the grill rack, place mushrooms and cook for 4 to 5 minutes per side, until juices are running and mushrooms are tender. Place polenta on a serving platter and top each with a grilled mushroom.

➤ Cut goat's cheese log into 6 medallions, about ½ inch (1 cm) thick. Place in the center of grilled portobello while hot. Top with basil slices and serve.

⇆ **VARIATION** Substitute basil pesto or sun-dried tomato pesto for fresh slices of basil.

MAKE AHEAD Prepare the polenta the day before and refrigerate until ready to use.

6 SERVINGS

GLUTEN-FREE

MEATLESS

MAKE AHEAD

PER SERVING 274 CALORIES | 9 G TOTAL FAT (2 G SATURATED FAT) | 9 MG CHOLESTEROL | 345 MG SODIUM | 40 G CARBOHYDRATE | 9 G FIBER | 9 G PROTEIN

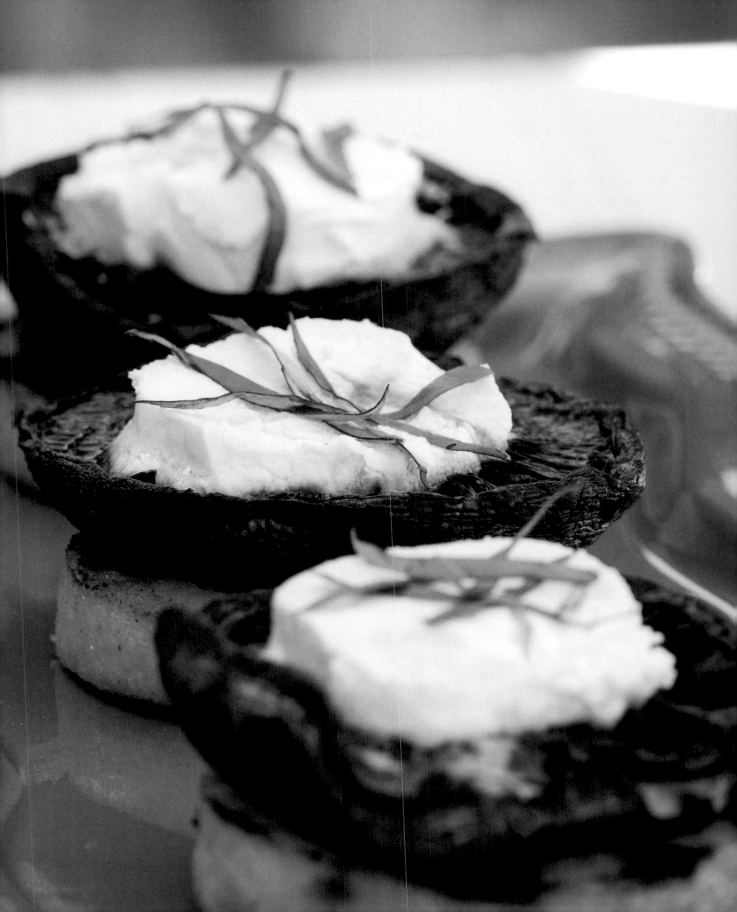

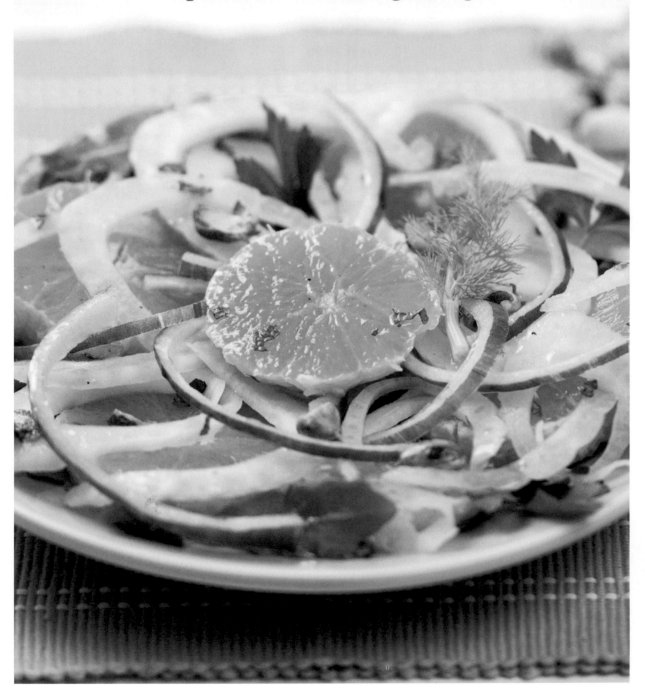

Some might consider fennel an exotic ingredient, but it has been part of my cooking repertoire since the beginning

Salads

Insalate

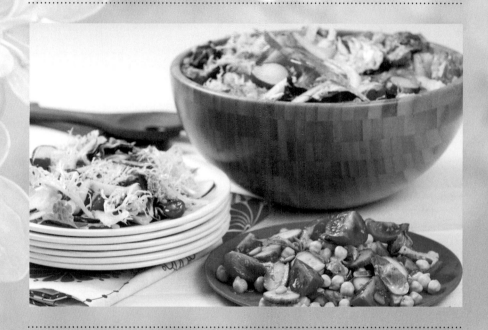

He has been making it since, well, I remember eating salad. You might call him a salad sommelier, if there was such a thing

Tuna, Green Bean & Tomato Salad

Insalata di tonno, fagioli e pomodori

MY MOM HAS ALWAYS BEEN A BIG FAN of canned tuna for its ease of use, but she only discovered it after emigrating to Canada, despite the abundance of bluefin tuna surrounding the coastal waters of her native Sicily. Back in her day, if you lived high up in the mountains (her village is 900 meters above sea level) in the center of a large island, access to fresh fish was almost impossible. For those of us who can't boast living by the coast or don't have time to get to the fish market, this salad is a protein-packed meal all on its own.

Salad

2 cups	greens beans, sliced in half
2	small cans (3 oz/80 g each) chunk tuna in olive oil, drained (see tip)
1½ cups	quartered campari tomatoes (or halved cherry tomatoes)
½ cup	sliced celery
¼ cup	thinly sliced red onions
2	hard-boiled eggs, quartered or sliced
2 tbsp	chopped fresh Italian (flat-leaf) parsley or mint for garnish

Dressing

Juice of 1 lemon	
1 tbsp	white balsamic vinegar
1 tbsp	extra-virgin olive oil
1 tsp	light mayonnaise
¼ tsp	dried oregano
Sea salt and freshly ground black pepper to taste	

➤ In a pot of boiling water, cook beans until tender-crisp. Drain, run under cold water to stop them from cooking and let cool.

➤ In a large bowl, combine beans, tuna, tomatoes, celery and red onions.

➤ Whisk together all dressing ingredients in a small bowl or measuring cup. Pour over vegetables and tuna, toss gently and top with eggs and parsley before serving.

TIP I've chosen an oil-packed tuna instead of water-packed tuna for flavor. But make sure you're using a brand that uses a good-quality oil like olive and low-mercury tuna, such as skipjack or yellowfin tuna. To keep things healthier, the amount of oil added to the dressing has been cut back.

⌂ HIGH IN... PROTEIN

Tuna can bolster your intake of protein without a high amount of calories. A serving of this salad has almost one-quarter of your daily recommended intake.

4 SERVINGS   **30 MIN OR LESS**   **GLUTEN-FREE**   **MEATLESS**

PER SERVING 185 CALORIES | 10 G TOTAL FAT (2 G SATURATED FAT) | 107 MG CHOLESTEROL | 216 MG SODIUM | 11 G CARBOHYDRATE | 3 G FIBER | 11 G PROTEIN

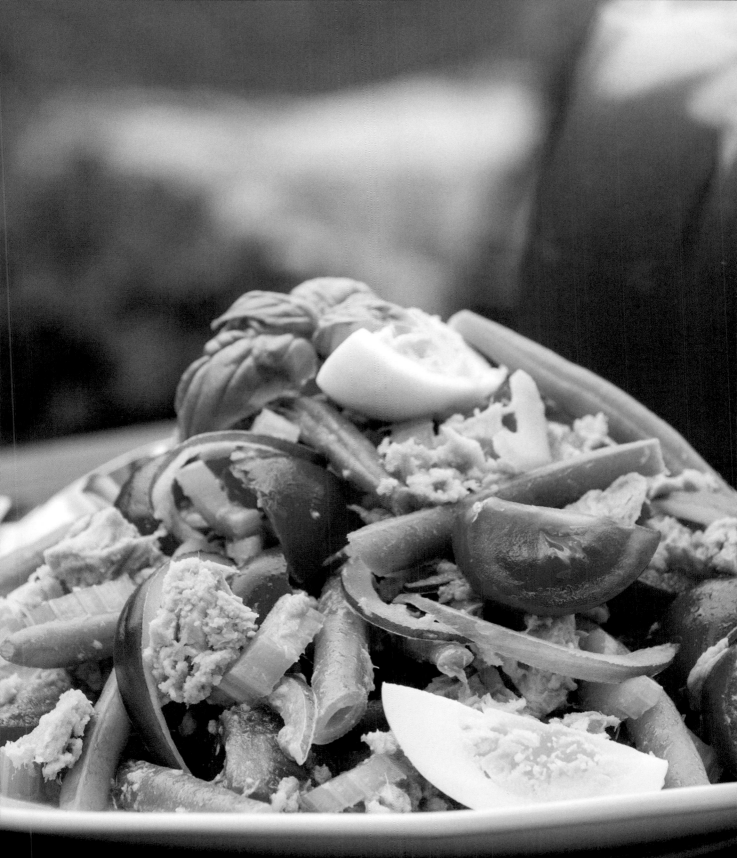

Mixed Greens & Radicchio Salad with Pomegranate

Insalata di verdure miste e melagrana

CHRISTMAS WAS NEVER A BIG GIFT-EXCHANGE holiday when I was young. Besides, my parents grew up with the tradition of receiving presents — usually limited to only one or two — on the Feast of the Epiphany on January 6, or on the 12th day of Christmas. In Italy, even today, it's La Befana, an old kind witch, and not jolly Saint Nick who fills kids' stocking with toys and sweets. Christmas at our house is more about food. This is my sister's "gift" to us — an ode to the North American tradition of red, green and white during this time. It complements all the trimmings on my table along with my menu of lamb, lasagna and cardoons.

Dressing

2 tbsp	pomegranate juice
1½ tbsp	extra-virgin olive oil
1 tbsp	white balsamic vinegar
¼ tsp	sea salt
Freshly ground black pepper to taste	

Salad

2 cups	packed torn romaine lettuce
2 cups	packed torn escarole lettuce
1 cup	baby spinach leaves
½ cup	torn radicchio leaves
3 tbsp	pomegranate seeds
2 tbsp	crumbled light goat's cheese (1 oz/28 g)

➤ Whisk together all dressing ingredients in a small bowl or measuring cup.

➤ In a large salad bowl, combine romaine, escarole, spinach and radicchio leaves. Add dressing and toss well. Sprinkle salad with pomegranate seeds and toss lightly. Top with goat's cheese and serve.

⇆ VARIATION Throw in a couple spoonfuls of red walnuts for even more cheer. Red walnuts are slightly sweeter than regular walnuts and are an excellent source of heart-healthy omega-3 fatty acids, which are found only in a limited number of foods.

⌒ HIGH IN...ANTIOXIDANTS

Spinach, radicchio and pomegranates are a potent trio high in antioxidants, such as vitamins A, C and E, as well as plant nutrients like carotenoids and flavonoids, all of which protect the body from cell-damaging oxidation caused by free radicals. A diet high in antioxidants can boost your immunity, prevent aging and lower your risk of life-threatening diseases like heart disease, diabetes and certain cancers.

 4 SERVINGS

 30 MIN OR LESS

 GLUTEN-FREE

 MEATLESS

PER SERVING 84 CALORIES | 6 G TOTAL FAT (1 G SATURATED FAT) | 3 MG CHOLESTEROL | 198 MG SODIUM | 5 G CARBOHYDRATE | 2 G FIBER | 2 G PROTEIN

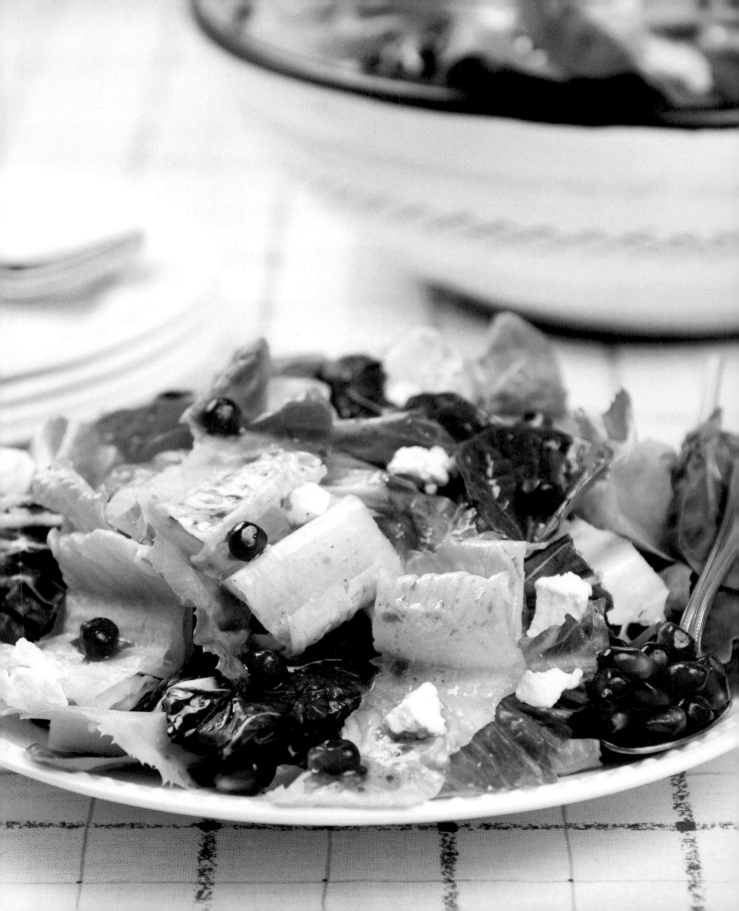

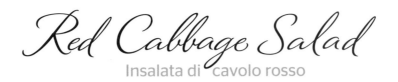

Red Cabbage Salad

Insalata di cavolo rosso

THIS SALAD HAS BECOME my most popular barbecue salad. Every time I serve it, there's always someone in the crowd that exclaims, "I never thought cabbage could taste so good!" While the Dutch first made the use of shredded cabbage in salads commonplace, the Italians use a wide variety of this popular vegetable — from the loose- and smoother-leafed cabbage to head varieties — in salads, soups and stews or stuffed. My family is no exception, gobbling it up throughout all the seasons.

Dressing

3 tbsp	red wine vinegar
3 tbsp	white balsamic vinegar or apple cider vinegar
2 tbsp	extra-virgin olive oil
1 tbsp	sesame seed oil
¼ tsp	sea salt
¼ tsp	freshly ground black pepper

Salad

4 cups	packed thinly sliced red cabbage (about ½ to ¾ large head)
¾ cup	chopped fresh parsley
2 tbsp	minced fresh mint
2	green onions, chopped (white and green parts)
1 tbsp	capers in brine, rinsed and patted dry
3 tbsp	raw sunflower seeds

➤ Whisk together all dressing ingredients in a small bowl or measuring cup.

➤ Combine all salad ingredients, except sunflower seeds, in a large bowl. Pour dressing over cabbage, toss well and let stand for 30 minutes to let flavors soak in. Give it a good toss before, sprinkle with sunflower seeds and serve.

⇆VARIATION Add a can of tuna to this salad, serve with a slice of whole-grain bread and you've got a fantastic lunch plate. Or give it a more exotic taste and substitute more of the sesame oil for the olive oil, replace the capers with a couple handfuls of dried cranberries or currants and add 1 tsp of ground cinnamon.

MAKE AHEAD Tastes even better when made a few hours or the day before. Toss, taste and adjust seasoning just before serving.

↻LOW IN...CALORIES

This colorful salad gives any meal a lift, both because of its vibrant color and antioxidant powers. But what's most impressive about its main ingredient — red cabbage — is the amount of fiber it contains with very few calories (1 packed cup of red cabbage alone equals about 2 grams of fiber and has only 30 calories). One serving of this salad also offers about 100 percent of your daily recommended amount of vitamins C and K.

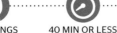

6 SERVINGS	40 MIN OR LESS	GLUTEN-FREE	MEATLESS	MAKE AHEAD

PER SERVING 139 CALORIES | 9 G TOTAL FAT (1 G SATURATED FAT) | 0 MG CHOLESTEROL | 172 MG SODIUM | 8 G CARBOHYDRATE | 2 G FIBER | 2 G PROTEIN

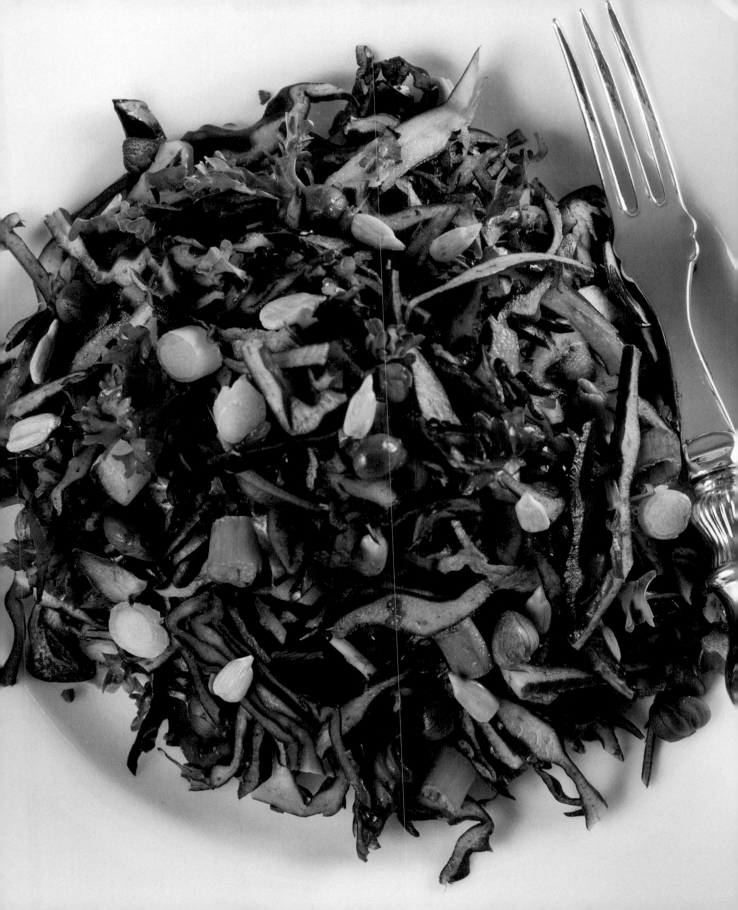

Frisée & Romaine Salad

Insalata riccia e lattuga Romana

THIS CRUNCHY MIX IS MY DAD'S CREATION. He's been making it since, well, I remember eating salad. You might call him a salad sommelier, if there is such a thing. Even when another family member puts some lettuce leaves together, at the very least, Dad is designated salad dresser and tosser. He has a perfect palate for the right blend of seasoning. So much so that he has inspired other men who have joined the family (read: my hubby) to pick up the salad servers.

Dressing

1½ tbsp	extra-virgin olive oil
2 tbsp	red wine vinegar
1 tbsp	balsamic vinegar
Pinch	Italian herb seasoning
¼ tsp	sea salt
Freshly ground black pepper to taste	

Salad

3 cups	torn romaine lettuce hearts
2 cups	torn frisée lettuce (see tip)
1 cup	torn radicchio
1 cup	thinly sliced fennel bulb
4	radishes, thinly sliced
½ cup	halved ripe cherry tomatoes

➤ Whisk together all dressing ingredients in a small bowl or measuring cup. Set aside.

➤ In a large salad bowl, combine torn lettuces, fennel, radishes and cherry tomatoes. Add dressing and toss well. Let salad stand for at least 5 minutes before serving to better absorb all the flavors.

TIP Frisée is a lettuce with pale green frayed or shredded edges and a thick white center. It belongs to the chicory family and has a mildly bitter taste.

 4-5 SERVINGS 30 MIN OR LESS GLUTEN-FREE MEATLESS

PER SERVING(5) 57 CALORIES | 4 G TOTAL FAT (1 G SATURATED FAT) | 0 MG CHOLESTEROL | 139 MG SODIUM | 4 G CARBOHYDRATE | 2 G FIBER | 1 G PROTEIN

Tomato-Cucumber Salad with Chickpeas

Insalata di pomodori e cetrioli con ceci

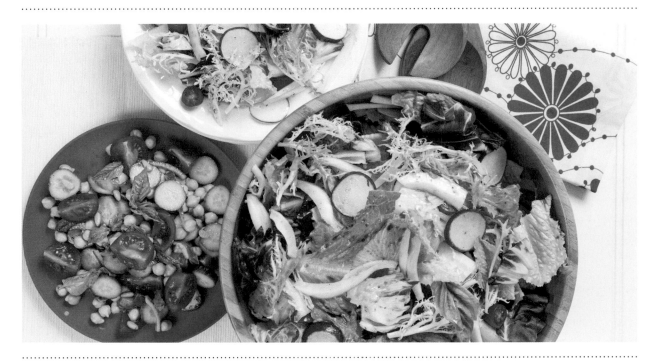

Dressing

2 tbsp	extra-virgin olive oil
1 tbsp	white balsamic vinegar
½ tsp	dried oregano
	Sea salt and freshly ground black pepper to taste

Salad

1 cup	canned no-salt-added chickpeas, rinsed and drained
2 cups	chopped fresh tomatoes
2 cups	diced mini cucumbers
2 tbsp	thinly sliced red onion
2 tbsp	chopped fresh basil
1 tbsp	toasted pine nuts for serving (see tip)

➤ Whisk together all dressing ingredients in a small bowl or measuring cup.

➤ In a large bowl, combine all salad ingredients except pine nuts. Add dressing and toss well. Let salad stand for at least 10 minutes to better absorb all the flavors. Stir again and serve topped with nuts.

TIP Keep a close eye on pine nuts when toasting them. Toss them in a non-stick skillet on medium heat for 30 seconds.

∩ HIGH IN...FIBER

The addition of chickpeas to this simple classic adds some notable fiber clout. Just one serving enables you to meet 15 percent of the daily value of fiber, and it comes in both soluble and insoluble fiber. Soluble fiber ferries dietary cholesterol out of the body before it can be absorbed into the bloodstream, while insoluble fiber adds bulk to your diet and prevents constipation by helping foods pass through the digestive tract more quickly. Chickpeas are also a good source of inexpensive, meatless protein.

 4-5 SERVINGS   30 MIN OR LESS   GLUTEN-FREE   MEATLESS

PER SERVING(5) 131 CALORIES | 8 G TOTAL FAT (1 G SATURATED FAT) | 0 MG CHOLESTEROL | 139 MG SODIUM | 12 G CARBOHYDRATE | 3 G FIBER | 4 G PROTEIN

Warm Beet & Spinach Salad

Insalata di barbabietole e spinaci

ANY WAY THEY'RE SERVED, I devour beets and tuck them into a meal whenever I can. So do the home cooks of Italy's Dolomites area, who are best known for their beet-stuffed ravioli (*casunziei*). My affection for these brilliant root veggies extends beyond taste and texture — they remind me of those late summer Sundays when we visited my husband's nonno, who always had a few in his garden for the kids to dig up.

Dressing

2 tbsp	extra-virgin olive oil
2 tbsp	balsamic vinegar
½ tsp	honey
½ tsp	Italian herb seasoning
¼ tsp	freshly ground black pepper
Pinch	sea salt

Salad

6	medium beets (about 1 lb/ 454 g)
4 cups	packed baby spinach leaves (about 5 oz/142 g)
¼ cup	thinly sliced red onions
1 tbsp	minced fresh mint

➤ Preheat oven to broil setting.

➤ Whisk together all dressing ingredients in a small bowl or measuring cup. Set aside.

➤ Peel beets and cut them into ¾-inch (2-cm) slices. Toss in a large bowl with half of the dressing until well coated. Reserve the other half of the dressing for later. Place dressed beets with dressing on a foil-lined baking sheet and place on the middle oven rack. Cook for 30 to 35 minutes or until tender, turning once halfway through cooking. Be careful that beets don't char or they'll taste bitter.

➤ Let beets cool down for about 5 to 10 minutes and cut them in half. Add them to a large bowl along with spinach, red onions and mint. Pour in remaining dressing and toss well to fully coat.

➤ Serve warm.

⇆VARIATION Sprinkle salad with some chia seeds or hemp seeds. Both of these nutritious powerhouses are a perfect way to increase your intake of omega-3 and omega-6 fatty acids. Both seeds also contain a complete protein (all nine essential amino acids), which will leave you feeling full longer.

⌂ HIGH IN...FOLATE

The deep red-purple pigment of beets comes from a set of unique phytonutrients, which deliver a host of benefits to combat degenerative diseases in the body. But what makes beets a standout is folate, a B vitamin that is crucial for making red blood cells, building muscle and, most importantly for pregnant women, reducing the risk of neural defects in fetuses. Together the beets and spinach in just one serving of this salad deliver about a third of the daily recommended intake of folate. If your beets are attached to green tops, save them for another dish. Beet greens are rich in vitamin A and are great in soups, braised with some olive oil or topped on pizza.

 4 SERVINGS

 GLUTEN-FREE
 MEATLESS

PER SERVING 86 CALORIES | 5 G TOTAL FAT (1 G SATURATED FAT) | 0 MG CHOLESTEROL | 175 MG SODIUM | 10 G CARBOHYDRATE | 3 G FIBER | 2 G PROTEIN

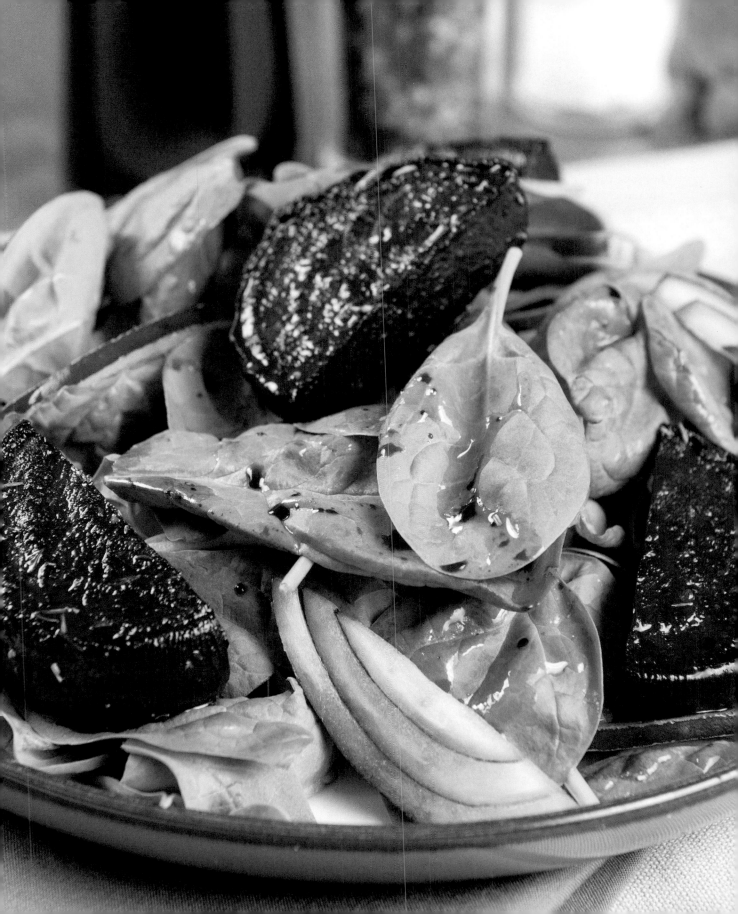

Flat Green Bean & Sweet Potato Salad

Insalata di fagiolini e patate dolci

IF I WERE TO GIVE MY DAD A BLUE RIBBON for one of the vegetables he grows in his garden it would be his flat green beans. He not only artfully coaxes the bean vines to climb his handmade stakes-and-twine trellis, but also gives them daily tender care. In short, his beanstalks rival the best farmers'. By harvest time, a bounty of prized beans fill baskets and we, the beneficiaries, find lots of ways to fill our plates — either enjoying them on their own, in soups or tossed among sweet potatoes.

Dressing

1 tbsp	red wine vinegar
1 tsp	extra-virgin olive oil
1 tbsp	chopped fresh basil
½ tsp	dried oregano
¼ tsp	sea salt

Freshly ground black pepper to taste

Salad

1 lb	(454 g) flat green beans
3 cups	cubed sweet potato (about 1 to 1½ large sweet potatoes)
1 tbsp	extra-virgin olive oil
3	green onions, chopped
3 tbsp	reduced-sodium vegetable broth

➤ Whisk together all dressing ingredients in a large bowl. Set aside.

➤ Cut beans into bite-sized pieces — you'll have about 4 cups. Bring a large pot of water to a boil. Add sweet potato and cook for 10 minutes. Add beans to pot during the last 5 minutes of cooking time to blanch them. Drain vegetables, run under cold water, drain again.

➤ In a large non-stick skillet, heat oil over medium-high heat and cook green onions for 1 minute. Add cooked potato, beans and chicken broth. Cook for 7 to 8 minutes, stirring several times until potatoes and beans have softened. Let cool for 10 minutes.

➤ Transfer potatoes and beans to bowl with dressing and toss until well coated. Serve at room temperature or chilled.

⇆ VARIATION Add some crunch with diced celery, bell pepper or sliced red onion and serve chilled. Or make this versatile recipe a side dish and substitute 1 or 2 tbsp basil pesto for the dressing (*see recipe, page 18*).

MAKE AHEAD Steam vegetables the day before and refrigerate. Cook them with green onions and toss in dressing on the day you're serving this salad.

⋒ HIGH IN...VITAMINS A AND C

A take on the classic green beans and potato salad, this version replaces regular white potatoes with vitamin C-rich sweet potatoes. From the deep orange hue of the sweet potatoes, you've probably already guessed that they're high in vitamins A and C but green beans also get big points for their abundance of the same vitamins, making the two veggies a great match in this recipe.

6 SERVINGS	40 MIN OR LESS	GLUTEN-FREE	MEATLESS	MAKE AHEAD

PER SERVING 180 CALORIES | 3 G TOTAL FAT (1 G SATURATED FAT) | 0 MG CHOLESTEROL | 150 MG SODIUM | 35 G CARBOHYDRATE | 6 G FIBER | 4 G PROTEIN

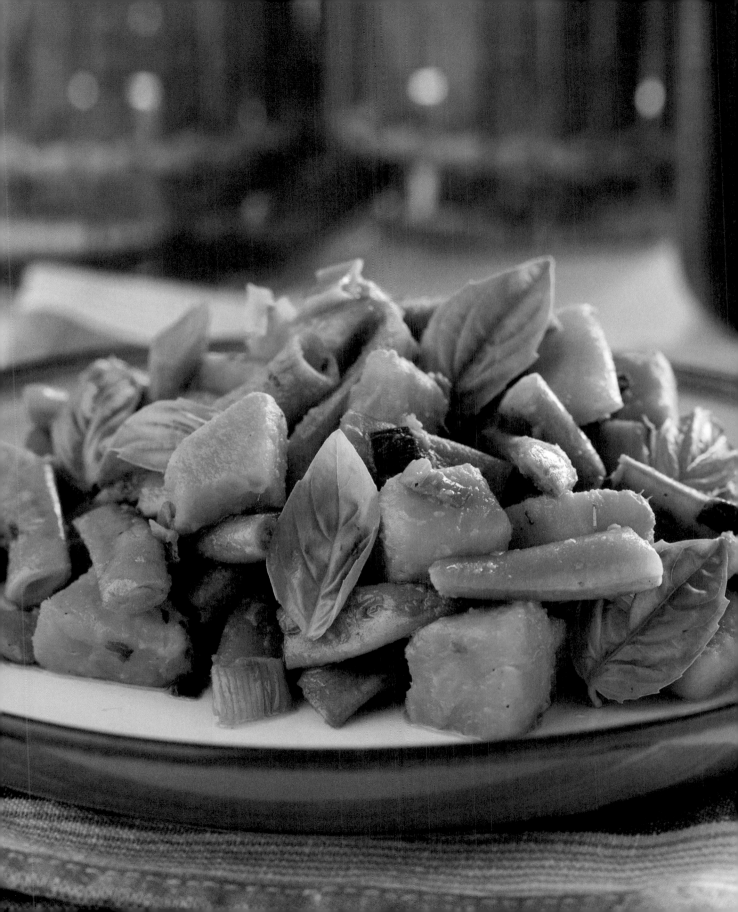

Arugula-Radicchio Salad with Figs, Prosciutto & Cantaloupe

Insalata di arugula e radicchio con fichi prosciutto e melone

YOU MIGHT THINK THE PAIRING OF MELON AND PROSCIUTTO is a mismatch but it is as customary to me as fries and hamburgers. History tells us that the two foods were first put together centuries ago to help aid in the digestion of "chilled" melon. It's more than custom that compels me to include it here — together with fresh figs and arugula in my own updated version of the classic companions, the sweet and salty collision is an explosion of flavor unlike any other.

Salad

3	large black figs
5 cups	packed baby arugula leaves (about 4 oz/125 g)
2 cups	chopped Treviso radicchio (see tip)
1 cup	cubed cantaloupe
2 tbsp	shredded red onions
3	very thin slices prosciutto, torn (0.9 oz/25 g)

Dressing

2 tbsp	extra-virgin olive oil
1½ tbsp	good-quality balsamic vinegar
½ tsp	honey
Sea salt and freshly ground black pepper to taste	

➤ Cut each fig in half, then each half in thirds so you have 6 wedges (18 in total), a good bite-sized piece.

➤ Trim tops of figs. In a large bowl, combine figs with arugula, radicchio, cantaloupe and red onions. Toss gently.

➤ Whisk together all dressing ingredients in a small bowl or measuring cup. Pour dressing over salad and toss gently. Top with prosciutto and serve immediately.

TIP If you can't find Treviso radicchio, the variety with long, slender leaves (*for more information, see page 42* see page 42), I don't recommend substituting regular, ball-shaped radicchio since it may be too bitter and tough for this salad. Instead, replace with Belgian endive, a variety of lettuce with tender leaves that tastes less bitter than radicchio.

⌒ HIGH IN...VITAMINS K AND C

Like many leafy greens, both arugula and radicchio are excellent sources of vitamin K, which is important for bone growth and regular blood clotting. Toss in cantaloupe to the mix and this salad boasts a healthy dose of vitamin C — almost one-quarter of the recommended daily intake.

6 SERVINGS · 30 MIN OR LESS · GLUTEN-FREE

PER SERVING 92 CALORIES | 5 G TOTAL FAT (1 G SATURATED FAT) | 2 MG CHOLESTEROL | 172 MG SODIUM | 9 G CARBOHYDRATE | 1 G FIBER | 2 G PROTEIN

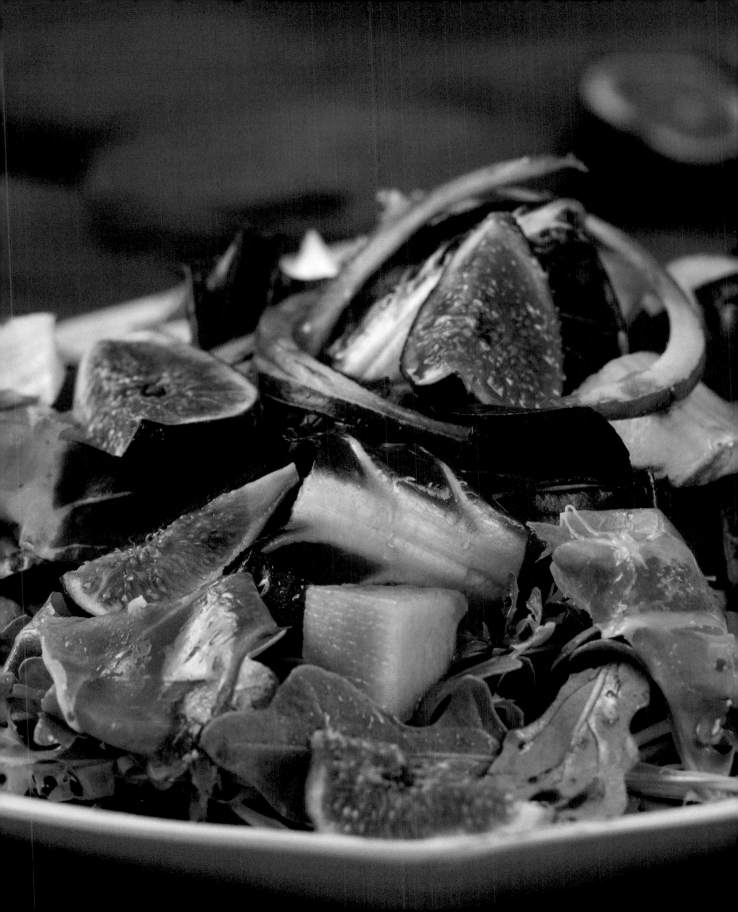

Potato Herb Salad

Insalata di patate ed erbe

ONE OF THE FONDEST MEMORIES of my childhood summers was the Sunday family picnic, organized at a nearby conservation area. By 7:30 a.m., the phone would already be ringing off the hook and the women would be confirming the "menu." Someone was always assigned to bring a big bowl of boiled potatoes, dressed later with fresh herbs and a simple vinaigrette to accompany the steaks grilled on the charcoal barbecue. This recipe takes me back to those precious days.

Salad

1½ lbs	(525 g) mini red, white or yellow potatoes, skin on
2	sprigs fresh rosemary
1 cup	thinly sliced fennel bulb
3 tbsp	chopped red onions
2 tbsp	each: chopped fresh parsley, basil and mint
2 tbsp	green olive slices

Dressing

2 tbsp	extra-virgin olive oil
3 tbsp	reduced-sodium vegetable or chicken broth
1 tbsp	freshly squeezed lemon juice
1	clove garlic, minced or pressed
¼ tsp	dried oregano
¼ tsp	sea salt

Freshly ground black pepper to taste

➤ Place potatoes and rosemary sprigs in a pot of water and bring to a boil. Cook until tender, about 18 to 20 minutes. Run them under cold water for about 30 seconds, let drain and cool for about 10 minutes. Discard rosemary stems and cut potatoes in half.

➤ In the meantime, add fennel, red onions, fresh herbs and olives in a large bowl. Toss with the potatoes.

➤ Whisk together all dressing ingredients in a small bowl or measuring cup. Pour dressing over potato-herb mixture and toss gently to evenly coat. Let stand for at least 20 to 30 minutes to absorb flavors before serving. Toss again before serving.

MAKE AHEAD Boil potatoes the day before and refrigerate until they're ready to be dressed.

⌒ HIGH IN...FIBER AND POTASSIUM

Potatoes often get a bad rap for being too starchy, too fattening. But it's how you cook them (read: fried!) or what you put on top of them (like sour cream and bacon) that gives you the unwanted calories. Small potatoes with their skin offer considerable fiber, like in this recipe, and are low in calories and fat with more potassium per serving than a banana.

6 SERVINGS · 40 MIN OR LESS · GLUTEN-FREE · MEATLESS · MAKE AHEAD

PER SERVING 119 CALORIES | 5 G TOTAL FAT (1 G SATURATED FAT) | 0 MG CHOLESTEROL | 186 MG SODIUM | 17 G CARBOHYDRATE | 3 G FIBER | 2 G PROTEIN

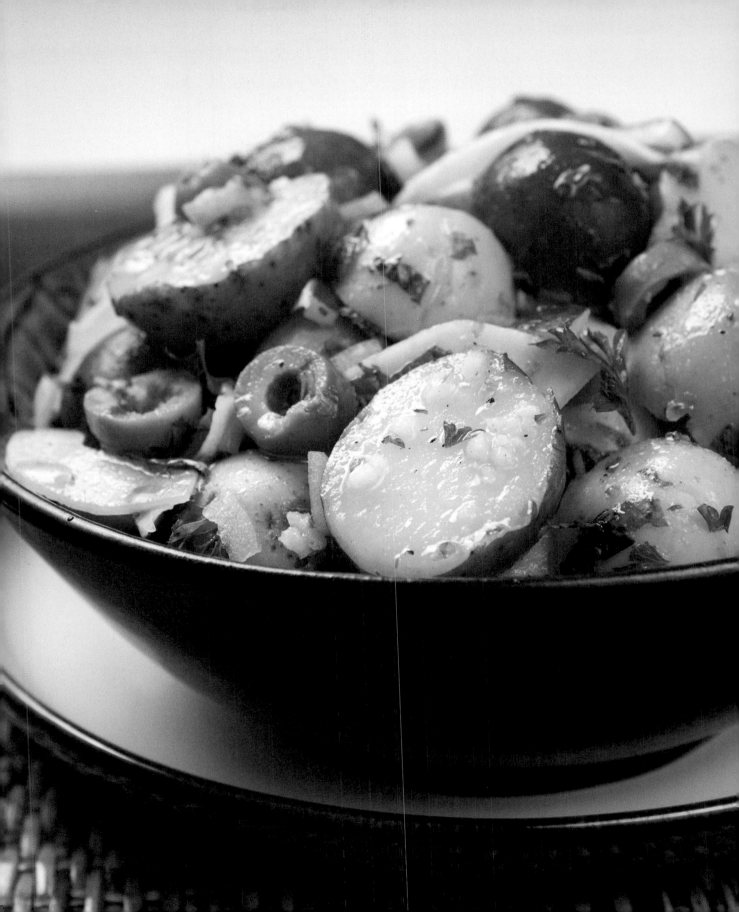

"Reinforced" Cauliflower Salad
Insalata di rinforzo

LIKE THE NEAPOLITAN INSALATA DI RINFORZO, my mother's "appetizer salad" includes an assortment of vegetables in brine — olives, pickles, cauliflower, carrots and eggplant. The salad is "reinforced" (English of *rinforzo*) with pantry ingredients that are always at the ready when company drops in, which happens regularly in Italian homes. Taking the reinforced theme a little further, I've bolstered it with more crunchy goodness — the kind that comes from the produce aisle.

Dressing

4 tbsp	red wine vinegar
2 tbsp	extra-virgin olive oil
1	clove garlic, pressed or minced
¼ tsp	sea salt
Freshly ground black pepper to taste	

Salad

1	small head cauliflower
⅓ cup	white vinegar
2 cups	shredded romaine lettuce
1 cup	cubed red bell peppers
½ cup	sliced mini cucumbers
½ cup	coarsely grated carrots
¼ cup	sliced celery
8 to 9	pickled onions, rinsed and halved
1 tsp	capers in brine, rinsed and halved
12	small black olives in brine, rinsed and drained
2 tbsp	chopped fresh parsley

➤ Whisk together all dressing ingredients in a small bowl or measuring cup. Set aside.

➤ Remove and discard leaves and large stalk from cauliflower. Pull apart florets to make several small to medium-sized pieces. Combine about 5 cups of water with vinegar in a large pot and bring to a boil. Add cauliflower florets and let cook till tender-crisp, about 6 to 7 minutes. Drain and let cool in a large bowl. Pour half of the dressing over the cauliflower and toss gently to fully coat.

➤ On a large serving platter, spread romaine lettuce over entire platter. Arrange dressed cauliflower over lettuce. Scatter red peppers, cucumbers, carrots, celery, pickled onions, capers and olives on top of cauliflower. Drizzle remaining dressing over vegetables.

➤ Sprinkle with parsley and serve.

⇆ VARIATION Substitute 2 anchovy fillets, rinsed, patted dry and chopped, for black olives.

MAKE AHEAD Can be refrigerated for two to three hours before serving. Hold back half the dressing and pour on salad just before serving.

⌒ HIGH IN...VITAMIN C

Admit it, what's the first food you think of when I tell you it's loaded with vitamin C? Did you know that 1 cup of steamed cauliflower has roughly the same amount of vitamin C as an orange and that just ¾ cup of chopped red peppers has double the amount? Orange you glad I asked? In fact, just one serving of this salad contains almost your entire daily recommended amount of vitamin C, which is between 75 and 90 milligrams a day.

 6 SERVINGS

 30 MIN OR LESS

 GLUTEN-FREE

 MEATLESS

 MAKE AHEAD

PER SERVING 78 CALORIES | 5 G TOTAL FAT (1 G SATURATED FAT) | 0 MG CHOLESTEROL | 226 MG SODIUM | 6 G CARBOHYDRATE | 2 G FIBER | 2 G PROTEIN

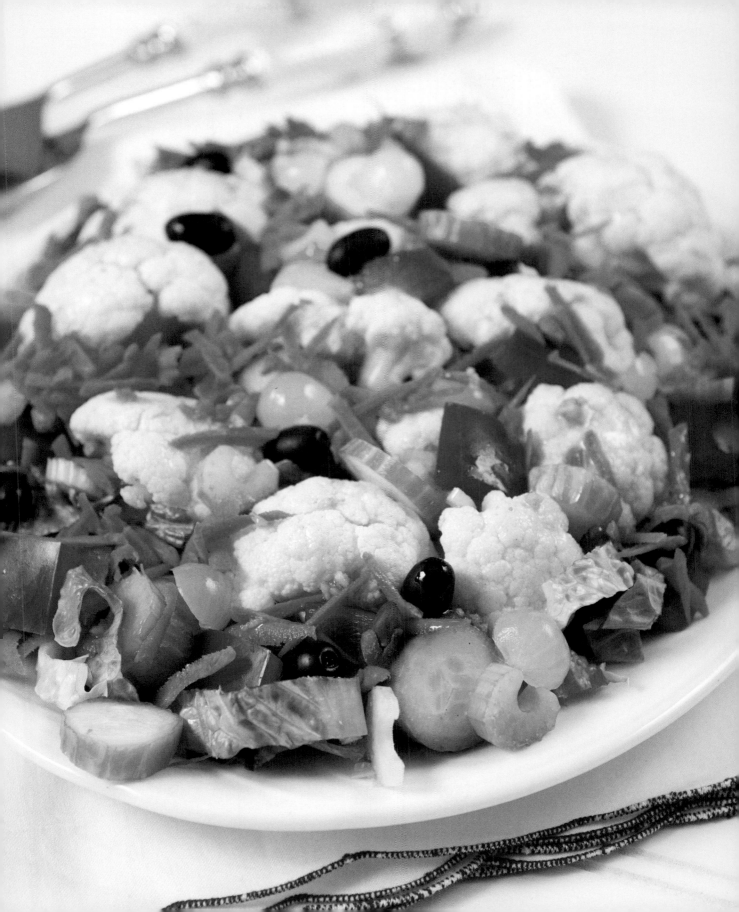

Couscous Salad with Tomatoes, Dried Currants & Pine Nuts

Insalata di couscous con pomodorini, ribes e pinoli

PASTA SALADS WEREN'T TYPICAL when we were growing up. The only time we ever really ate cold pasta was when we grabbed the leftovers from the fridge. But by the time I was ready to pick up my own cutting board and ladle, I developed quite a liking for pasta salads of all types, and there was an abundance in modern Italian cuisine to inspire, such as the revamped ones on these pages. Alternative grains take the place of pasta here — whether it's to add more fiber or protein — but that won't stop you from opening the fridge and indulging in them — that is, if there are any leftovers.

Salad

1 cup	uncooked whole wheat couscous (see tip)
2 cups	packed baby arugula leaves
1½ cups	halved ripe cherry tomatoes
3 tbsp	dried currants
2	green onions, chopped
3.5 oz	(100 g) light Friulano cheese, cut into small cubes (see tip)
2 tbsp	toasted pine nuts

Dressing

1½ tbsp	extra-virgin olive oil
1 tbsp	white balsamic vinegar
Zest of ½ lemon	
¼ tsp	sea salt
Freshly ground black pepper to taste	

➤ In a saucepan, add 1¼ cups of water and bring to a boil. Stir in couscous, cover and remove from heat. Let stand for 5 minutes while covered. Fluff with fork and let cool.

➤ In a large bowl, combine arugula, tomatoes, currants, green onions and cooked couscous.

➤ Whisk together all dressing ingredients in a small bowl or measuring cup. Pour over couscous mixture and toss well until fully coated. Once couscous is at room temperature, toss in cheese cubes and top with pine nuts.

TIPS Couscous is made of miniature pasta-like granules that are produced using durum wheat.
➤ Friulano is a firm cheese with a subtle nutty flavor. Cheesemakers in Italy's Frioul region have been making the well-known cheese for centuries. If you can't find it, replace it with white Cheddar.

 5-6 SERVINGS   30 MIN OR LESS   MEATLESS

PER SERVING(6) 262 CALORIES | 10 G TOTAL FAT (3 G SATURATED FAT) | 8 MG CHOLESTEROL | 236 MG SODIUM | 36 G CARBOHYDRATE | 6 G FIBER | 11 G PROTEIN

Chicken Pesto & Artichoke Barley Salad

Insalata d'orzo con pollo pesto e carciofi

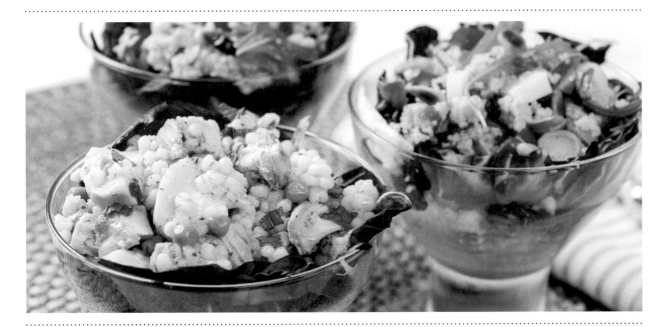

Salad

¾ cup	pot barley, rinsed
½ cup	frozen green peas, thawed
1 can	(14 oz/398 mL) artichoke hearts (packed in water), drained and chopped
1 cup	cubed cooked chicken breast
2 tbsp	each: minced fresh mint and chopped fresh parsley

Dressing

¼ cup	reduced-sodium chicken broth
1 tbsp	extra-virgin olive oil
3 tbsp	basil pesto (*see recipe, page 18*) or store-bought basil pesto
Pinch	sea salt
¼ tsp	dried oregano
Freshly ground black pepper to taste	

> In a medium pot, bring 3 cups of water to boil. Stir in barley and simmer on medium-low heat until slightly chewy, about 20 to 25 minutes. Add thawed peas to pot during last 5 minutes of cooking time. Drain and let cool.

> In a large bowl, combine artichoke hearts and chicken; add barley, peas, mint and parsley and toss well to combine.

> Whisk together all dressing ingredients in a small bowl or measuring cup. Pour over barley mixture, toss and serve.

⌒ HIGH IN...FIBER

The combination of barley, green peas and artichokes contributes up to 8 grams of fiber per serving.

  5-6 SERVINGS 40 MIN OR LESS

PER SERVING(6) 189 CALORIES | 5 G TOTAL FAT (1 G SATURATED FAT) | 22 MG CHOLESTEROL | 199 MG SODIUM | 24 G CARBOHYDRATE | 6 G FIBER | 13 G PROTEIN

Kale Salad with Grilled Pear, Goat's Cheese & Pecans

Insalata di cavolo nero con pera grigliata, formaggio di capra e pecan

LONG BEFORE THE FUSION OF SWEET AND SAVORY was adopted by foodies, my mom had embraced it. Her Mediterranean roots exposed her to pairings of fruit with other atypical ingredients. In fact, ever since I was a kid, I remember her gazing out the window while snacking on pears or grapes, a couple leaves of lettuce, a slice of bread and a few chunks of cheese for good measure. She was usually taking a quiet break from the roaring sewing machine that as a seamstress demanded her attention for hours at a time. I'm equally drawn to dishes like this that offer a mix of surprises for the palate — and judging from the reaction this salad gets, I'm not the only one.

Dressing

1½ tbsp	extra-virgin olive oil
1½ tbsp	each: freshly squeezed lemon juice and red wine vinegar
1 tsp	pure maple syrup
¼ tsp	sea salt

Freshly ground black pepper to taste

Salad

6 cups	packed shredded kale (see tip)
1	ripe Bartlett pear
4 to 5 tbsp	crumbled light goat's cheese (2 oz/56 g)
2 tbsp	chopped pecans

⇆ **VARIATION** Combine pear with shaved piave cheese instead of goat's cheese. Piave, a hard cow's milk cheese whose slightly sweet taste intensifies with age, is similar to a young Parmigiano-Reggiano and comes in vecchio or stravecchio, meaning "old" or "extra old." It's named after the Piave River near Veneto, an area rich with vineyards.

➤ Whisk together all dressing ingredients in a small bowl or measuring cup.

➤ In a large salad bowl, toss kale with dressing. Don't be afraid to get your hands in there — once oil coats kale, it's especially soothing to toss it with your hands, so enjoy the free therapy! Refrigerate for 20 minutes (or up to 3 hours) to let kale absorb flavors.

➤ Preheat grill to medium setting. Cut pear into ½-inch (1-cm) slices; lightly coat them with cooking spray. Grill pears for 2 minutes on each side or until grill marks appear. Slice pear into thin strips.

➤ Just before serving, remove kale from fridge and toss well. Serve topped with pear slices, goat's cheese and pecans.

TIPS Remove tough rib in the center of the leaf by folding it and slicing off greens from stalk. Discard ribs and slice kale thinly into long strips.
➤ Baby kale, which is tender, bite-sized leaves, is starting to make an appearance in grocery stores. Great news if you want to cut down on preparing this salad and eliminate the work of cutting out the tough rib in each leaf. Look for it in the salad section where you'll find boxed salads.

🎧 HIGH IN...VITAMIN A

Kale is a powerhouse of vitamins, antioxidants, fiber and calcium. It's especially high in vitamin A, with a whopping 200 percent of the amount needed a day in just one serving of this salad. That's great news for individuals who want to maintain healthy eyes and teeth, keep skin looking young and prevent oral and lung cancers. An excellent source of the antioxidant lutein, kale also protects the eyes from damaging UV rays. Its respectable dose of fiber — a little more than lettuce — promotes regularity.

 4-5 SERVINGS
 40 MIN OR LESS
 GLUTEN-FREE
 MEATLESS
 MAKE AHEAD

PER SERVING(5) 139 CALORIES | 8 G TOTAL FAT (2 G SATURATED FAT) | 4 MG CHOLESTEROL | 208 MG SODIUM | 15 G CARBOHYDRATE | 3 G FIBER | 5 G PROTEIN

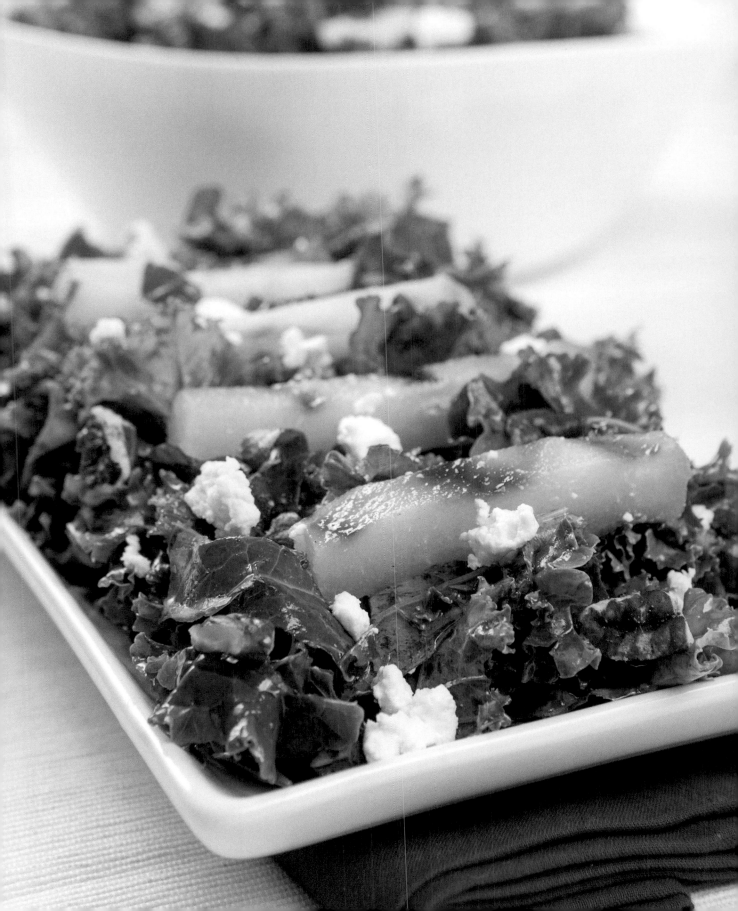

Fennel & Orange Salad

Insalata di finocchio e arance

WHILE SOME MIGHT CONSIDER FENNEL an exotic ingredient, it's been part of my cooking repertoire since the beginning. My Sicilian roots have naturally made me open to plenty of Mediterranean foods, including the flavors of this licorice-tasting vegetable. My entire family often gnaws on it either with mandarins or on its own as a sort of digestive after big holiday dinners. It's also taught me that by balancing its taste — here, with the tangy sweetness of oranges — it can form a unique union that completely changes the flavor of a dish.

Salad

1½ cups	packed baby arugula leaves
2	large oranges, peeled and seeded
1	medium fennel bulb
2 tbsp	thinly sliced red onions
2 tbsp	minced fresh mint
1 tbsp	torn fresh Italian (flat-leaf) parsley
3 tbsp	unsalted dry-roasted pistachios, shelled

Dressing

2 tbsp	almond, walnut or olive oil
2 tbsp	apple cider vinegar
Juice of ½ orange or mandarin	
¼ tsp	sea salt
Freshly ground black pepper to taste	

➤ Arrange arugula on a serving platter. Cut whole oranges crosswise into thin slices, ¼-inch (0.5-cm) thick. Lay flat in a single layer over arugula.

➤ Remove top core of fennel bulb. Slice thinly, reserving the fronds. Layer fennel on top of orange slices; layer red onions on top of fennel. Sprinkle evenly with mint and parsley.

➤ Whisk together all dressing ingredients in a small bowl or measuring cup and drizzle evenly over salad. Top with pistachios. Garnish with reserved fronds and serve chilled.

⌂ HIGH IN...VITAMIN C

You'd expect a dish with oranges to be high in vitamin C but fennel is no slouch when it comes to contributing. In this salad, it offers more than 10 percent of the total amount in the recipe.

4 SERVINGS · **30 MIN OR LESS** · **GLUTEN-FREE** · **MEATLESS**

PER SERVING 130 CALORIES | 8 G TOTAL FAT (1 G SATURATED FAT) | 0 MG CHOLESTEROL | 180 MG SODIUM | 14 G CARBOHYDRATE | 4 G FIBER | 3 G PROTEIN

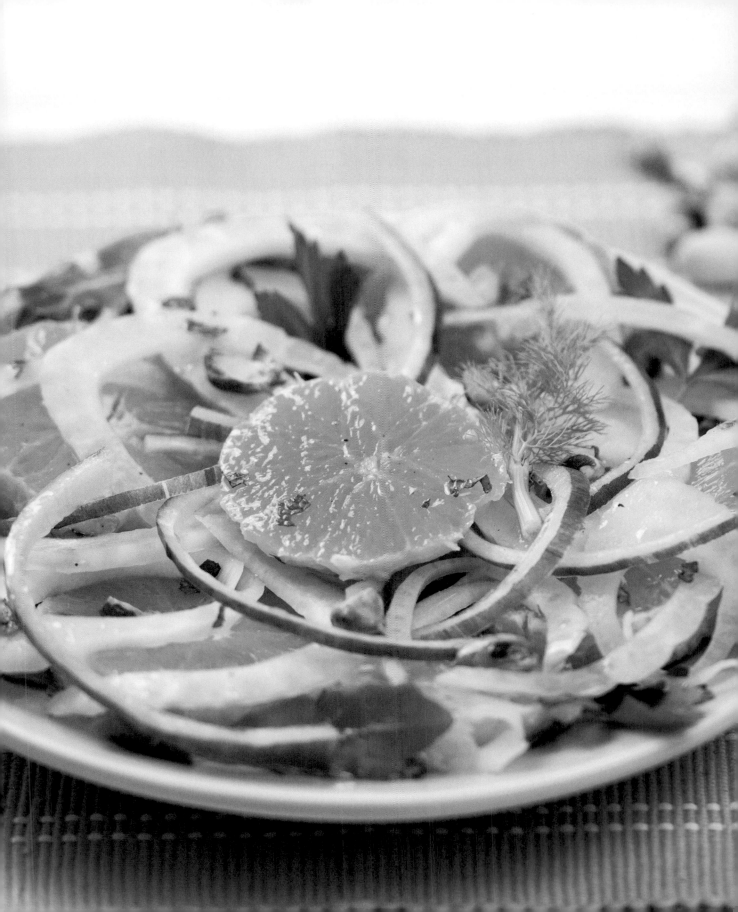

Marinated Octopus Salad

Insalata di polpo marinato

IT'S CUSTOMARY FOR ALMOST ALL REGIONS OF ITALY to celebrate Christmas Eve with an extravagant fish dinner. The Scroppos have marked it in their own special way — our gang typically approaches the table with excitement, anticipating the ensuing feast of fish, from the crispy battered cod that is prepared over two days, to the bread-and-caper-stuffed squid to the tomato-sauce-drenched mussels to the simple fast-fry smelts. But the much-anticipated salad, the pièce de résistance, *l'insalata favoloso* is this fish classic, which gets better as it soaks up the vinegary dressing. Can you tell I *really* like this salad? It is unequivocally the favorite among young and old.

Salad

4 cups	water
2 cups	white vinegar
1½ lbs	(680 g) fresh whole octopus (1 to 2 small to medium size)
1 cup	chopped fennel bulb
¾ cup	each: chopped red bell peppers and yellow bell peppers
½ cup	sliced celery

Dressing

2½ tbsp	extra-virgin olive oil
2	cloves garlic, minced
¼ cup	white vinegar
½ cup	minced fresh parsley
¼ tsp	sea salt
¼ tsp	freshly ground black pepper
Juice of 1 lemon	

⇆ VARIATION For those watching their sodium intake, substitute fresh squid rings (calamari) for half the octopus.

➤ In a large pot, combine water and vinegar and bring to a boil.

➤ Add octopus and let cook for 8 to 10 minutes until tender and bright pink. Don't overcook it or it'll be rubbery. Drain, rinse for a few seconds under cold water and let cool for a few minutes before handling. Cut octopus into ½-inch (1-cm) pieces, discarding the eye and inside of the head, and combine the pieces with vegetables in a large bowl.

➤ Whisk together all dressing ingredients in a small bowl or measuring cup. Pour evenly over octopus and vegetables and toss well. Refrigerate and let sit for 2 to 4 hours, tossing occasionally, or overnight to let octopus absorb flavors.

MAKE AHEAD Keeps for up to one week in the refrigerator. You may need to top up with oil and vinegar.

⌂ HIGH IN...B VITAMINS

Octopus delivers heaping doses of most B vitamins, in particular B12, which is offered five-fold the daily amount recommended in one serving of this salad. Octopus delivers other B vitamins as well. B vitamins play a key role in the body's metabolism of energy sources and the brain's neurotransmitters, such as serotonin, norepinephrine and dopamine, which affect mood and depression and feelings of anxiety.

6 SERVINGS

GLUTEN-FREE

MEATLESS

MAKE AHEAD

PER SERVING 112 CALORIES | 1 G TOTAL FAT (0 G SATURATED FAT) | 54 MG CHOLESTEROL | 383 MG SODIUM | 5 G CARBOHYDRATE | 1 G FIBER | 17 G PROTEIN

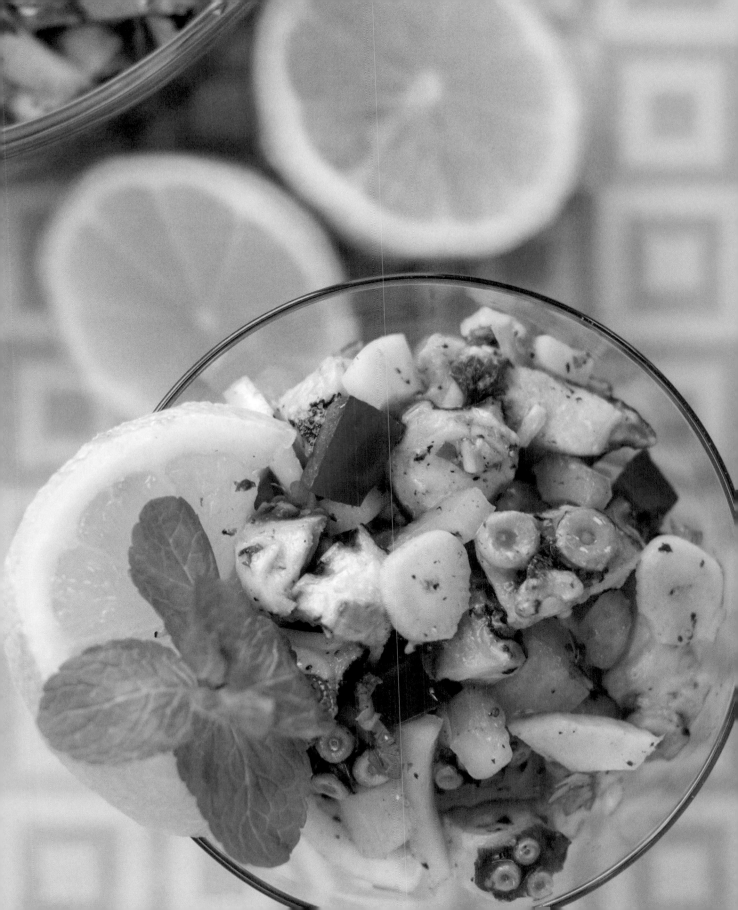

Quinoa Mediterranean Salad

Insalata Mediterranea con quinoa

IF THERE WAS AN IDEAL CLASSIC SALAD FOR KIDS AND ADULTS ALIKE, I'd have to say it's the bocconcini-tomato salad (opposite). Not only because I've eaten it since the beginning of my time, but also because each morsel is the perfect bite size. Fresh soft cheese, tangy tomatoes and fragrant basil blending in a balsamic vinaigrette — it's a match unparalleled by other salads. It was always served in our home with chunks of crusty bread with a spongy center, which mopped up the delicious juices left behind. But a refresh with protein-packed quinoa does a wonderful job of mingling with the dressing before coating every morsel. I make quinoa the star ingredient in many of the salads I've been eating for years, including the one on this page — where pasta, bread or grains once filled the bowl — and it always delivers a fine performance.

1 cup	uncooked quinoa, rinsed
2 cups	reduced-sodium vegetable broth
1	bay leaf
2 cups	packed coarsely chopped baby spinach leaves
¾ cup	canned brown lentils, rinsed
5	pieces sun-dried tomatoes, reconstituted and cut into strips (*see tip, page 234*)
¼ cup	black olive slices, rinsed and drained
¼ cup	chopped fresh basil
2 tbsp	chopped fresh parsley
Zest of ½ lemon	
2 tbsp	freshly squeezed lemon juice
1½ tbsp	extra-virgin olive oil
Sea salt and freshly ground black pepper to taste	
2 tbsp	crumbled light goat's cheese (1 oz/28 g)

➤ In a large pot, combine quinoa, vegetable broth and bay leaf and bring to a boil. Reduce heat to medium-low and simmer for 12 to 15 minutes, or until all liquid is absorbed. Remove and discard bay leaf and place quinoa in large bowl while hot. Mix in spinach leaves until they wilt from the heat. Let cool.

➤ Add lentils, sun-dried tomatoes, olives, basil, parsley, lemon zest and juice, olive oil, salt and pepper and toss until well combined. Sprinkle in goat's cheese, toss and serve.

MAKE AHEAD Cook quinoa, toss with spinach and refrigerate the day before. Bring to room temperature and toss with remaining ingredients just before serving.

⌂ HIGH IN...PROTEIN

So what gives quinoa its mother-of-all-grains status? Lots. By the way, it's technically a seed but often referred to as an ancient grain. One thing that makes it superior is its quality and quantity of protein. It's a protein with all nine essential amino acids ("essential" meaning something the body can't produce on its own), making it an important protein source for vegetarians. All nine essential amino acides is pretty rare to find in a plant source. Quinoa contains more than double the amount of protein of other healthy grains.

    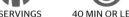

6 SERVINGS   **40 MIN OR LESS**   **GLUTEN-FREE**   **MEATLESS**   **MAKE AHEAD**

PER SERVING 173 CALORIES | 7 G TOTAL FAT (1 G SATURATED FAT) | 2 MG CHOLESTEROL | 136 MG SODIUM | 22 G CARBOHYDRATE | 4 G FIBER | 7 G PROTEIN

Bocconcini–Tomato Salad with Quinoa
Caprese con quinoa

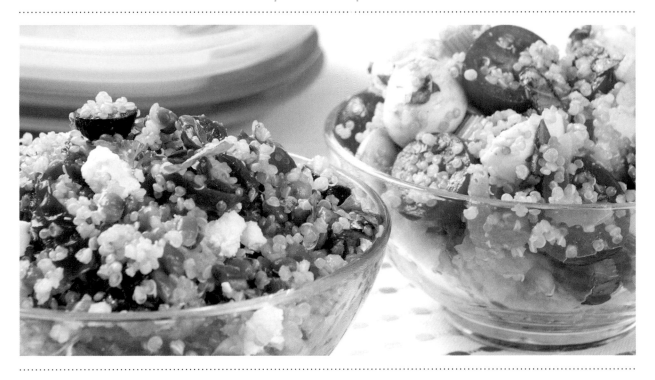

Salad

¾ cup	uncooked quinoa
1½ cups	reduced-sodium vegetable broth
2 cups	halved ripe cherry tomatoes
1½ cups	halved mini (cherry) light bocconcini (about 200 g)
1 cup	sliced celery
¼ cup	chopped fresh basil

Dressing

2 tbsp	extra-virgin olive oil
1 tbsp	good-quality balsamic vinegar (see tip)
Pinch	sea salt

Freshly ground black pepper to taste

➤ In a medium pot, combine quinoa and broth and bring to a boil. Reduce heat to medium-low and simmer for 12 to 15 minutes or until all liquid is absorbed. Fluff with a fork. Set aside.

➤ Combine tomatoes, bocconcini, celery and basil in a large bowl. Add the quinoa and toss until well coated.

➤ Whisk together all dressing ingredients in a small bowl or measuring cup. Pour over salad and toss well to coat. Refrigerate until ready to serve.

TIP Choose an aged balsamic vinegar for a more exquisite flavor. The finest balsamic comes from Modena, Italy, considered the birthplace of this distinctive vinegar.

  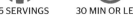

4-5 SERVINGS   30 MIN OR LESS   GLUTEN-FREE   MEATLESS

PER SERVING(5) 187 CALORIES | 9 G TOTAL FAT (4 G SATURATED FAT) | 20 MG CHOLESTEROL | 105 MG SODIUM | 11 G CARBOHYDRATE | 2 G FIBER | 13 G PROTEIN

Grilled Zucchini Scapece Salad

Zucchine alla scapece

MAKING HOMEMADE PICKLED VEGETABLES is no easy feat. When Mom and Dad made our annual batch of marinated eggplants, for example, it would take days and a sizable amount of low-tech equipment — pails to house the vegetables, tea towels to add in between the tower of layers, and bricks to squeeze out the water from the vegetables before they sat in a salty brine. This salad, which has its roots in the city of Napoli, is prepared Scapece-style with a marinade of oil, vinegar, garlic and fresh mint. It requires very little equipment and effort, yet it's still big on taste.

Marinade

¼ cup	chopped fresh mint
2½ tbsp	red wine vinegar
1½ tbsp	extra-virgin olive oil
1 tbsp	chopped fresh basil
2 tsp	freshly squeezed lemon juice
3	cloves garlic, crushed or minced
¼ tsp	sea salt

Freshly ground black pepper to taste

Salad

3	medium green zucchini
2	medium yellow zucchini

⇆ VARIATION Add some protein and more texture to this salad with 1 or 2 cups of cooked quinoa. Cut up zucchini slices, drizzle with dressing and toss with quinoa.

➤ Preheat grill to medium-high setting.

➤ Combine all marinade ingredients in a small bowl. Toss well and set aside to let herbs and spices infuse the liquid.

➤ Slice zucchini lengthwise into thin strips, about ¼ inch (0.5 cm), with a mandoline or a sharp knife. Coat zucchini lightly with cooking spray before placing on preheated grill. Grill for about 4 to 5 minutes on each side — you want them to have light grill marks but not cooked so much that they fall apart.

➤ Place grilled zucchini in a medium bowl and let cool for 5 minutes.

➤ Toss marinade ingredients once more and pour over zucchini. Gently stir zucchini until well coated and let sit for 10 minutes before serving.

MAKE AHEAD This salad tastes even better the next day when the flavors really soak in. Make it the night before, refrigerate it and bring it to room temperature before serving.

⌂ HIGH IN...MANGANESE

Zucchini is a terrific source of the mineral manganese. So how is something you've hardly ever heard about good for you? Manganese can offer significant benefits for women: it can slow down bone loss, decrease premenstrual symptoms and help produce sex hormones. You'll get about a quarter of the daily recommended intake in one serving. Zucchini is a good source of potassium, which is important for healthy blood pressure regulation. Here, zucchini retains its low-cal status by avoiding the traditional scapece method of deep-frying veggies before dipping into a marinade.

 4 SERVINGS 40 MIN OR LESS GLUTEN-FREE MEATLESS MAKE AHEAD

PER SERVING 91 CALORIES | 6 G TOTAL FAT (1 G SATURATED FAT) | 0 MG CHOLESTEROL | 154 MG SODIUM | 8 G CARBOHYDRATE | 2 G FIBER | 3 G PROTEIN

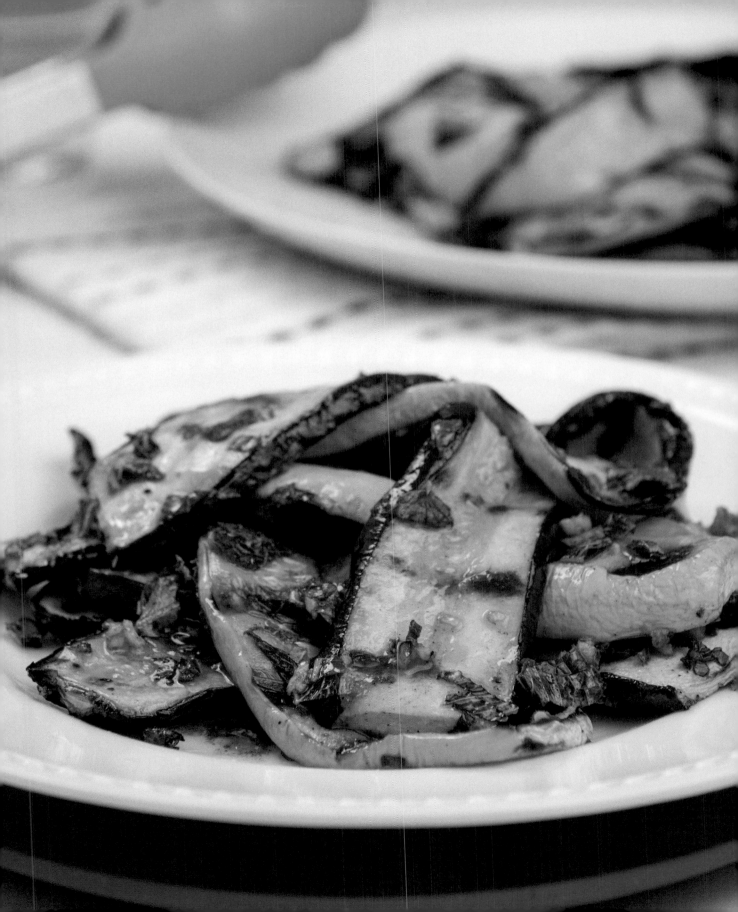

Gluten-Free Pasta Salad

Insalata di pasta senza glutine

MY SISTER'S YUMMY PASTA SALAD tells the story of how far we've come from the time she was first diagnosed with Celiac disease decades ago. Besides the difficulty in finding gluten-free pasta, sourcing commercial salad dressings and sauces void of gluten was nearly impossible — full of fillers and thickeners abound in them — so she couldn't trust eating food prepared outside the home. If friends invited her to a barbecue, she'd volunteer to bring her own food, along with this hearty salad — combining all the ingredients she loves from the sunny Mediterranean. Now friends request it, and it's always such a big hit, she has to make sure there are enough helpings for everyone!

16 oz	(454 g) gluten-free brown rice fusilli or rotini pasta
1 cup	thinly sliced sun-dried tomatoes (3 oz/85 g) (*see tip, page 228*)
2 tbsp	chopped fresh basil
1	clove garlic, chopped
1 tbsp	extra-virgin olive oil
1¼ cups	diced red bell peppers
¾ cup	black olive slices, rinsed and drained
1 tbsp	capers in brine, rinsed and chopped (see tip)
4 tbsp	basil pesto (*see recipe, page 18*) or store-bought gluten-free basil pesto
2 tbsp	chopped fresh parsley

➤ In a large pot, bring a pot of water to a boil and cook pasta according to package directions. Drain pasta but set aside a ladle of pasta water.

➤ In the meantime, pulse sun-dried tomatoes with basil and garlic in the bowl of a food processor until well minced. Scrape down sides. Stream in olive oil.

➤ Place sun-dried tomato mixture into a large bowl, along with red peppers, black olives and capers.

➤ Add cooked pasta to bowl; toss well with basil pesto and other ingredients until fully combined. Add reserved pasta water to moisten pasta and coat well. Top with parsley.

➤ Serve immediately or at room temperature.

TIPS One tiny caper packs a whole lot of flavor so you don't need many to add zing to this salad. You'll find them in the pickle section of your grocery store.
➤ If you're bringing this salad to a barbecue (it's great accompanied with ribs), reserve half the sun-dried tomato mixture and basil pesto, along with some pasta water, and toss into pasta just before serving.

 8 SERVINGS   40 MIN OR LESS   GLUTEN-FREE   MEATLESS

PER SERVING 264 CALORIES | 5 G TOTAL FAT (1 G SATURATED FAT) | 0 MG CHOLESTEROL | 104 MG SODIUM | 50 G CARBOHYDRATE | 4 G FIBER | 5 G PROTEIN

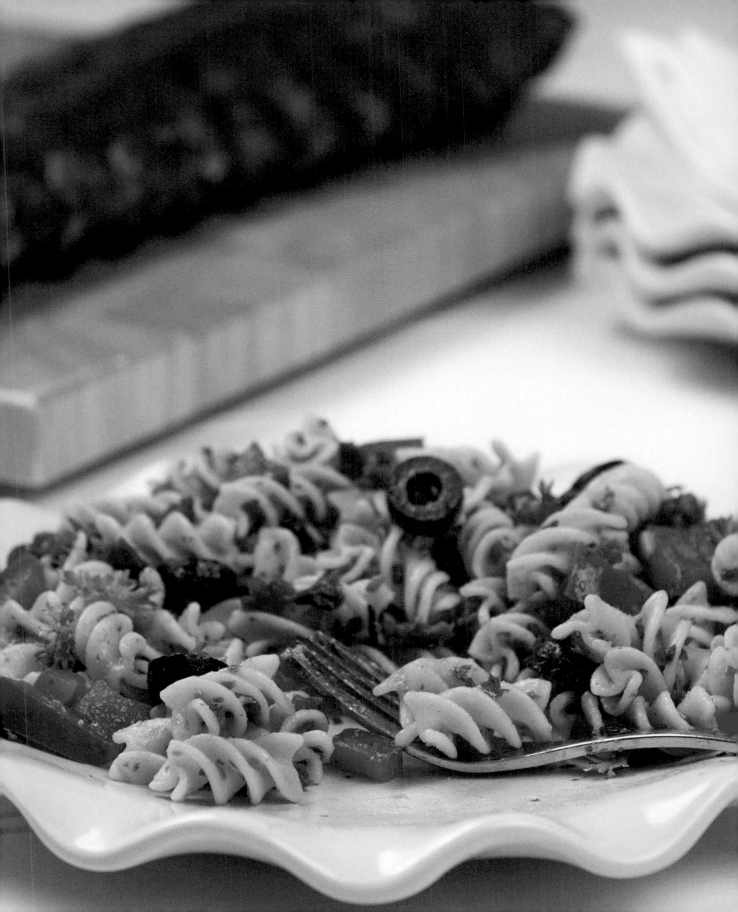

Traditional "Summer" Rice Salad

Insalata di riso d'estate

I HAVE NO IDEA WHY AN ICONIC "summer" salad in Italy rarely contains fresh vegetables, especially when every region grows an abundance of them. I think its popularity has more to do with the fact that it's bursting with so many textures and flavors, making it the perfect accompaniment to grilled meats or enjoyed on its own al fresco when temperatures soar. Whatever the reason, I serve it all year-round and throw in some "unbottled" ingredients.

Salad

1 cup	uncooked long-grain brown rice
1 can	(6 oz/170 g) flaked light tuna (skipjack or yellowfin preferably) in water, drained
2	slices reduced-sodium extra-lean deli-style prosciutto cotto or ham, chopped (about 1.2 oz/35 g)
12	sweet pickled onions, halved
¾ cup	marinated artichoke hearts, drained and chopped
½ cup	chopped red or yellow peppers or combined
⅓ cup	black olive slices, rinsed and drained
3 tbsp	chopped fresh Italian (flat-leaf) parsley

Dressing

2 tbsp	extra-virgin olive oil
1 tbsp	Worcestershire sauce
	Juice of ½ lemon
	Freshly ground black pepper to taste

➤ Cook rice in a medium pot according to package directions. Drain and let cool.

➤ In a large bowl, combine rice, tuna, prosciutto cotto, onions, artichoke hearts, red peppers, olives and parsley. Toss until well combined.

➤ Whisk together all dressing ingredients in a small bowl or measuring cup. Pour dressing over rice and mix well. Serve at room temperature or chill for 2 to 4 hours before serving.

⇄ VARIATION Substitute about ½ cup of summer fresh peas for the prosciutto cotto and make this salad meatless. For a gluten-free and vegetarian alternative, replace the Worcestershire sauce (not available as a gluten-free product in Canada and it's made with anchovies) with Bragg Liquid Soy Seasoning, which is also a lower-sodium alternative to soy sauce.

MAKE AHEAD Can be made one to two days before serving. Hold back the tuna until just before serving.

⋃ LOW IN...SODIUM

If I was following a traditional recipe, I might be adding more cured meats like hotdogs, pickles and fontina cheese, but these ingredients are laden with sodium. In fact, you'd be taking in 500 to 600 milligrams more sodium per serving — that's about one-third of the daily recommended intake.

6 SERVINGS   **30 MIN OR LESS**   **MAKE AHEAD**

PER SERVING 245 CALORIES | 10 G TOTAL FAT (1 G SATURATED FAT) | 11 MG CHOLESTEROL | 251 MG SODIUM | 32 G CARBOHYDRATE | 4 G FIBER | 11 G PROTEIN

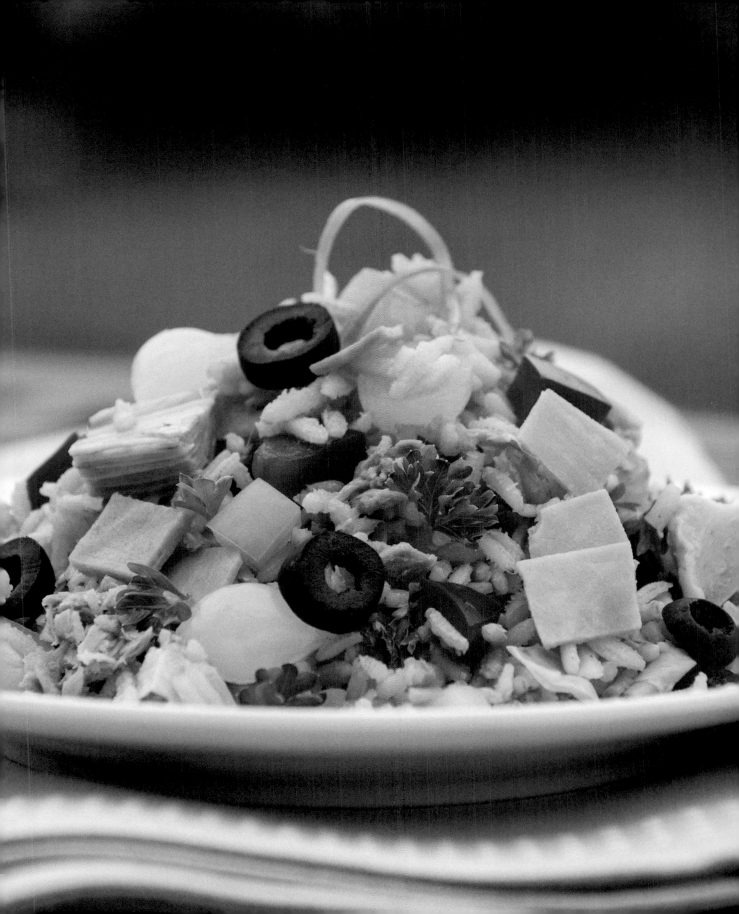

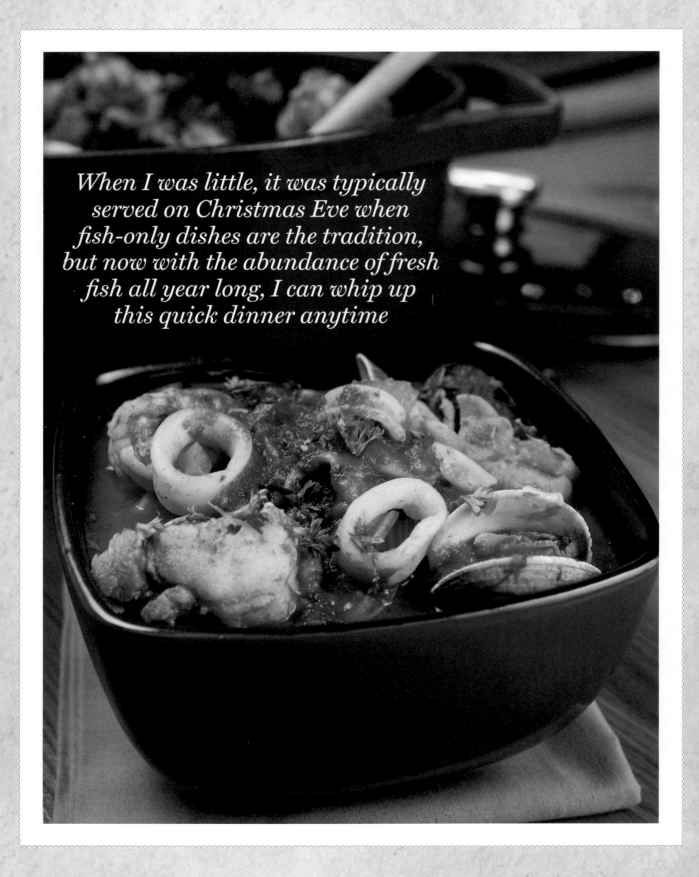

When I was little, it was typically served on Christmas Eve when fish-only dishes are the tradition, but now with the abundance of fresh fish all year long, I can whip up this quick dinner anytime

Soups & Stews

Minestroni e zuppe

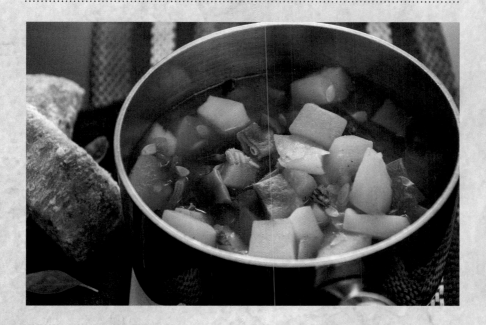

At local competitions, my dad's Italian squash never earned a top prize, but they were delicious and the basis for so many great dishes

Tomato, White Bean & Cauliflower Soup with Spaghettini

Minestra di pomodoro, fagioli bianchi e cavolfiore con spaghettini spezzati

WHEN WE WERE GROWING UP, making a quick and healthy meal meant adding to what already worked well. In most cases, it was building a dish on the prevalent go-to ingredients of pasta and tomato sauce. The cold cellar shelves were already neatly stocked with Mason jars of homemade tomato sauce and cupboard space was plentiful of dry pasta, so together they formed the basis for so many other tantalizing dishes. This one was one of them, which first comes together with an intoxicating sizzle of garlic followed by fresh ingredients that simmer gently until the heavyweights — beans and pasta — enter the pot for bulk. It's a simple combination yet it's filling enough to get the family through soccer practice, dance class or a bike ride.

1 ½ tbsp	extra-virgin olive oil
4	cloves garlic, sliced
½ cup	chopped celery
2 cups	chopped cauliflower florets
1 can	(28 oz/796 mL) no-salt-added whole peeled tomatoes with purée or juice
3 cups	reduced-sodium vegetable broth
½ cup	red wine
1 tbsp	no-salt-added tomato paste
1 can	(540 mL/19 oz) no-salt-added cannellini beans (or white kidney or navy beans), rinsed and drained, divided
2 tbsp	minced fresh sage leaves
3 tbsp	chopped fresh basil
1	bay leaf
½ tsp	sea salt
Freshly ground black pepper to taste	
6 oz	(175 g) whole-grain spaghettini*
Freshly grated Pecorino Romano cheese for serving (optional)	

➤ In a large pot, heat olive oil over medium heat. Add garlic and cook until lightly browned, about 2 minutes. Add celery and cauliflower and stir continuously until they start to soften, about 3 to 4 minutes.

➤ In the meantime, pulse the canned tomatoes, along with purée, in the bowl of a food processor or blender until smooth and add to pot. Stir in broth, wine, tomato paste, half the beans, sage, basil, bay leaf, salt and pepper. Mash by hand the remaining beans and add to pot — this will add a bit of creaminess to broth. Bring to a boil.

➤ Reduce heat to medium-low, cover and simmer for 20 minutes, stirring occasionally.

➤ Over a small bowl, use your hands to break spaghettini into 1-inch (2.5-cm) pieces. Add to pot and cook for another 8 minutes, or until pasta is al dente, stirring occasionally. Remove and discard bay leaf. Ladle soup into bowls and serve hot with freshly grated cheese, if using.

⌒ HIGH IN...FIBER

There is a trio of fiber-rich foods packed into this soup — cannellini beans, cauliflower and whole-grain pasta. They alone provide 30 percent of the daily recommended intake of fiber. This soup is also low in fat and delivers a hefty amount of vitamin B1, vitamin C and protein.

6 SERVINGS

40 MIN OR LESS

GLUTEN-FREE*
REPLACE WITH GF SPAGHETTINI

MEATLESS

PER SERVING 316 CALORIES | 6 G TOTAL FAT (1 G SATURATED FAT) | 0 MG CHOLESTEROL | 276 MG SODIUM | 51 G CARBOHYDRATE | 13 G FIBER | 14 G PROTEIN

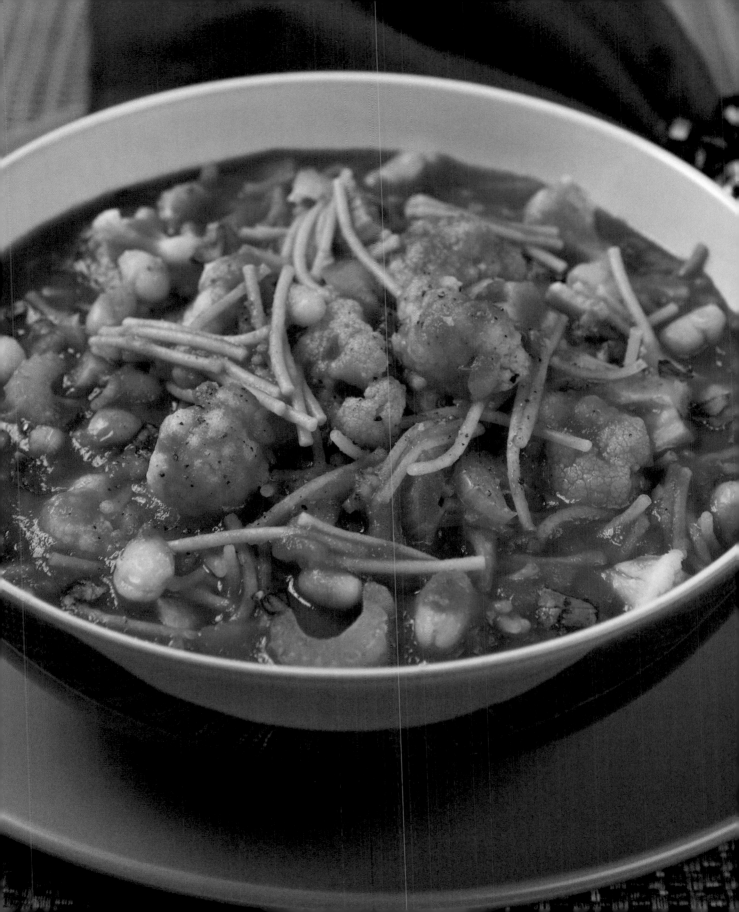

Kale, Sausage & White Bean Soup

Zuppa di cavolo nero con salsiccia e fagioli bianchi

SAUSAGE IS ONE OF THE PREPARED MEATS of choice in Italian cooking so it often makes its way into main courses, pizzas, frittatas and, as here, in soups. A blend of aromatic spices — like the ones my parents always added to their homemade sausages, including garlic, paprika, peppercorns, sea salt and red chili peppers — uplift any cream-based soup, including this variation that has its foundations in Northern Italy.

1	small bunch kale
1 tbsp	extra-virgin olive oil
2	turkey sausages*, casings removed (about 7 oz/200 g)
½ cup	chopped onions
4	cloves garlic, minced
¼ cup	white wine
2	bay leaves
1	medium zucchini, cubed
7 cups	no-salt-added chicken broth
½ tsp	sea salt
¼ tsp	crushed red pepper flakes
1 cup	canned no-salt-added white kidney beans or cannellini, rinsed and drained
¼ cup	2% evaporated milk
	Freshly grated Parmigiano-Reggiano cheese (optional)

➤ Remove the kale's tough rib at the center of the leaves. Shred leaves to yield about 6 cups kale.

➤ In a large pot, heat olive oil over medium-high heat. Add sausage meat, breaking up pieces as you stir to cook it. Continue to cook until almost no longer pink, about 3 to 4 minutes. Add onions and garlic and cook until onions are softened. Reduce heat to medium and add white wine and bay leaves, stirring until almost all the liquid has evaporated.

➤ Add the remaining ingredients, except the beans, evaporated milk and cheese. Cover, reduce heat to medium and continue to cook for 25 minutes, stirring occasionally. Remove and discard bay leaves. Add in beans during the last 5 minutes of cooking. Stir in evaporated milk. Ladle hot soup into bowls and sprinkle with grated cheese, if using.

ʊLOW IN...FAT

Turkey sausages replace the pork variety while milk replaces cream to make this recipe 30 percent lower in fat. The abundance of nutrients in kale, such as vitamins C and A, minerals and fiber, add a heaping dose of antioxidants and flavor.

6 SERVINGS

40 MIN OR LESS

GLUTEN-FREE*
CHECK LABELS

PER SERVING 200 CALORIES | 6 G TOTAL FAT (2 G SATURATED FAT) | 27 MG CHOLESTEROL | 479 MG SODIUM | 21 G CARBOHYDRATE | 4 G FIBER | 16 G PROTEIN

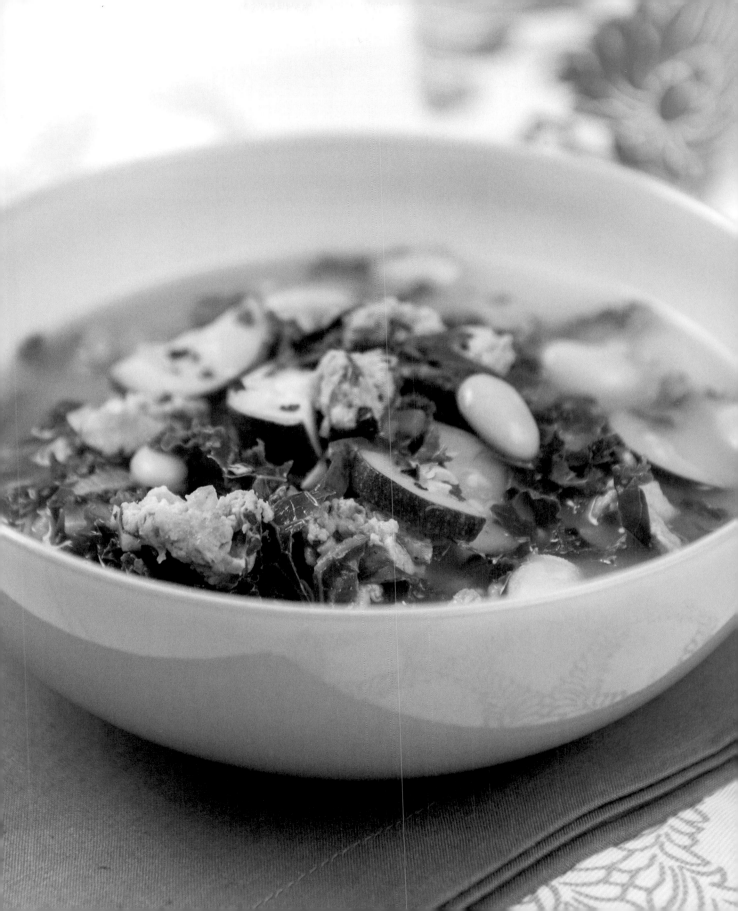

Tortellini & Escarole Soup

Tortellini al brodo con scarola

IN OUR HOUSE WHEN I WAS GROWING UP, there was no such thing as greens for soups and greens for salads. Each was used interchangeably for both types of dishes. My mother taught me that a leafy green like escarole gives broths like this hearty classic more complexity and depth. For me, it also means more flexibility in my kitchen, using up ingredients for more than just one purpose.

1 tbsp	extra-virgin olive oil
2 cups	finely chopped leeks
2	cloves garlic, minced
6 cups	chopped escarole
1 cup	thinly sliced celery
6 cups	reduced-sodium chicken broth
¼ cup	minced fresh parsley
Sea salt and freshly ground black pepper to taste	
1 pkg	(1 lb/454 g) fresh or frozen whole-grain or whole wheat cheese tortellini
4 tsp	freshly grated Parmigiano-Reggiano cheese

➤ In a large pot, heat olive oil over medium-high heat. Add leeks and garlic and cook until leeks are softened, about 2 minutes. Add escarole and celery and stir continuously until softened. Add broth, parsley, salt and pepper to taste. Cover, reduce heat to medium-low and simmer for 20 minutes.

➤ In the meantime, cook tortellini according to package directions in a separate pot. When cooked to al dente, drain and add to broth pot. Ladle soup into bowls and serve hot, topped equally with cheese.

⇆ VARIATION You can substitute spinach or collard greens for escarole if you prefer a milder flavor.

⌂ HIGH IN...FIBER

Escarole, a broad-leafed endive with curly green leaves, is an excellent source of roughage. Just 2 cups of escarole offers 3 grams of fiber and only 17 calories. While this leafy green helps to flush the body of toxins, it also offers an excellent source of vitamins A, C and K, as well as folate.

5-6 SERVINGS   30 MIN OR LESS

PER SERVING(6) 312 CALORIES | 9 G TOTAL FAT (1 G SATURATED FAT) | 28 MG CHOLESTEROL | 390 MG SODIUM | 44 G CARBOHYDRATE | 5 G FIBER | 15 G PROTEIN

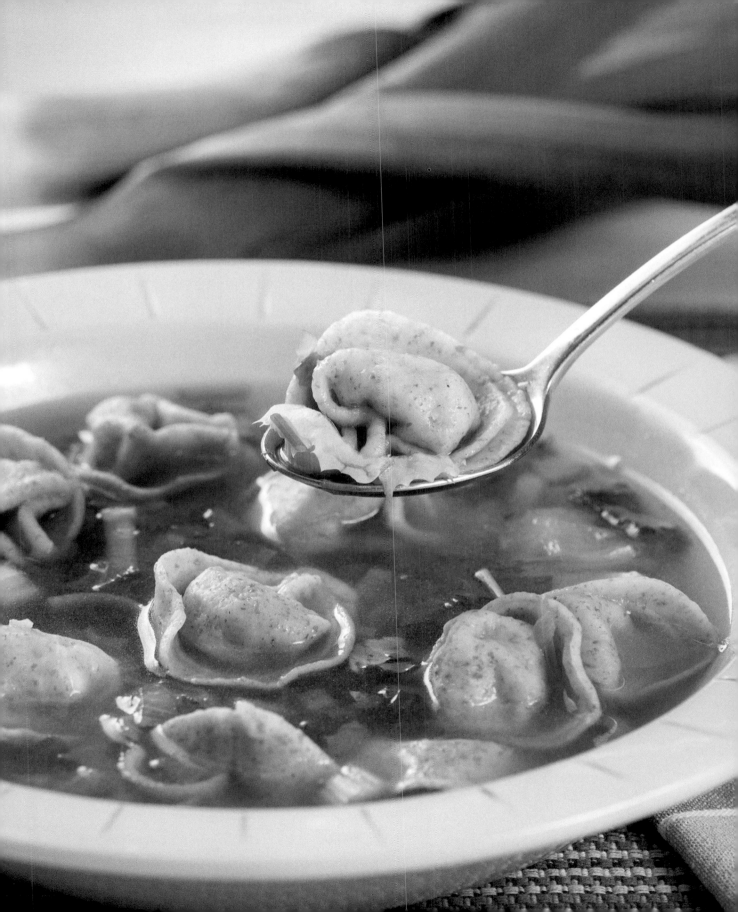

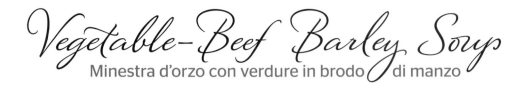

Vegetable-Beef Barley Soup

Minestra d'orzo con verdure in brodo di manzo

EVERY TIME I COOK A SOUP WITH BARLEY, it reminds me of "la cuccia," a dish using wheat berries that we ate, along with townspeople from southern Italy, to commemorate the feast day of Santa Lucia. Almost identical in taste and texture, barley is a more suitable substitute for a hearty soup like this since it takes a lot less time to cook and can offer similar nutritional benefits — plus, you don't have to wait until the feast on December 13th to serve it.

1 tbsp	extra-virgin olive oil
3	slices turkey bacon-style, chopped (2.8 oz/80 g)
1	onion, chopped
1 cup	each: diced celery and squash
½ cup	diced carrots
¾ cup	pot barley (see tip)
7 cups	no-salt-added beef broth
3	sprigs fresh thyme
2 tbsp	chopped fresh parsley
1	bay leaf
½ tsp	sea salt
Freshly ground black pepper to taste	
2 tsp	light butter
Freshly grated Parmigiano-Reggiano cheese (optional)	

➤ In a large pot, heat olive oil over medium-high heat. Add bacon and onion. Stir continuously until onion has softened and bacon pieces are lightly browned, about 3 to 4 minutes.

➤ Add celery, squash, carrots and barley and stir for 1 minute until barley is well coated. Slowly add broth, a little at a time for the first 5 minutes of cooking until vegetables begin to soften. Add remaining broth, along with thyme, parsley, bay leaf, salt and pepper.

➤ Bring to a boil, cover, reduce heat to medium-low and simmer for 35 to 40 minutes, stirring occasionally. When soup is finished cooking, remove and discard bay leaf and thyme stems, and stir in butter until melted. Ladle hot soup into bowls and serve with freshly grated cheese, if desired.

TIP If you can't find pot barley, pearl barley is a suitable replacement, although it doesn't offer the same bounty of fiber. Substitute 1 cup of pearl barley and reduce cooking time by 10 minutes.

↻ LOW ON...THE GLYCEMIC INDEX

Barley, one of the oldest cultivated grains, has been labelled by some dietitians as a super food for its nutritional properties; among them is its ranking on the Glycemic Index (GI). It's a grain with one of the lowest GIs on the scale, posting between 25 and 35, depending on the type of barley. Foods with a low GI (55 or less) release carbohydrates into the blood stream at a slower rate, which means blood sugar levels are more stable over a longer period of time and your body will experience fewer cravings.

6 SERVINGS   GLUTEN-FREE

PER SERVING 187 CALORIES | 4 G TOTAL FAT (1 G SATURATED FAT) | 9 MG CHOLESTEROL | 389 MG SODIUM | 31 G CARBOHYDRATE | 6 G FIBER | 7 G PROTEIN

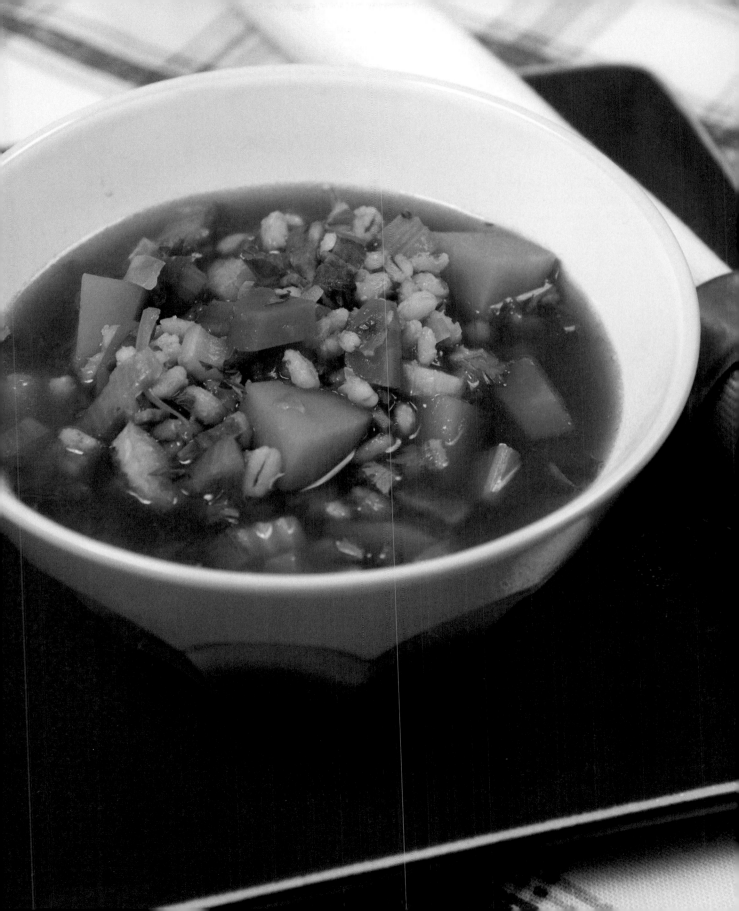

Romano & Cannellini Bean Soup with Swiss Chard

Minestra di farro e fagioli

DECADES AGO, THE GARAGE WAS WHERE A LOT OF ITALIANS did their prep work before crafting ingredients into divine dishes. Family and friends usually offered a helping hand since it seemed like there was always a rotation of picking, cleaning or canning fresh produce among the community. In my friend Anna's garage, it was bushels brimming with hand-picked Romano beans that awaited our help to manually peel away their pods and scoop out the speckled red-and-white bean seed. It was labor-intensive but we didn't mind it — the silly jokes and laughter helped keep our minds off the monotonous work. Besides, the reward of a creamy *pasta e fagioli* soup was worth it! The same ingredients mingle in this soup but it gets a refresh with farro instead of pasta.

2 tsp	extra-virgin olive oil
1	onion, chopped
1 cup	sliced celery
2	cloves garlic, minced
3	slices turkey bacon-style, chopped (2.8 oz/80 g)
3 cups	chopped Swiss chard
8 cups	reduced-sodium vegetable broth
1 cup	pre-soaked dried or canned Romano beans, rinsed (see tip)
1 cup	pre-soaked dried or canned cannellini beans (or other white beans such as navy or white kidney), rinsed
2 tbsp	each: minced fresh parsley and fresh basil
1 tsp	dried thyme
	Salt and freshly ground black pepper to taste
1 cup	semi-pearled farro (see tip)

▸ In a large pot, heat olive oil over medium-high heat. Add onion, celery and garlic and cook until softened, about 2 to 3 minutes. Add bacon and stir continuously until bacon starts to shrink up, about 2 minutes. Toss in Swiss chard. Add remaining ingredients, except farro, and bring to a boil.

▸ Reduce heat to medium, cover and simmer for 40 to 45 minutes, stirring occasionally. Add farro to pot during the last 25 minutes of cooking time. Ladle soup into bowls and serve hot.

TIPS Dried beans that have been soaked the night before in cold water typically have more flavor than canned beans. Always use a fresh package to guarantee beans will soften. One cup of dried beans usually yields up to three times the quantity after soaking. Use any extra to make a tasty salad later in the week. If you're using canned beans, buy a brand that offers reduced-sodium beans, rinse well and add them into this recipe when there's only 15 minutes left of cooking time, or they may fall apart.
▸ Farro takes the place of the traditional orecchiette (small oval pasta) here. Farro, an ancient grain used in southern Europe for centuries, is known to have less gluten and twice the fiber of wheat.

MAKE AHEAD If you're using dried beans, soak them the night before.

6 SERVINGS   MAKE AHEAD

PER SERVING 255 CALORIES | 5 G TOTAL FAT (1 G SATURATED FAT) | 8 MG CHOLESTEROL | 224 MG SODIUM | 38 G CARBOHYDRATE | 6 G FIBER | 16 G PROTEIN

Farro Soup

Zuppa di farro

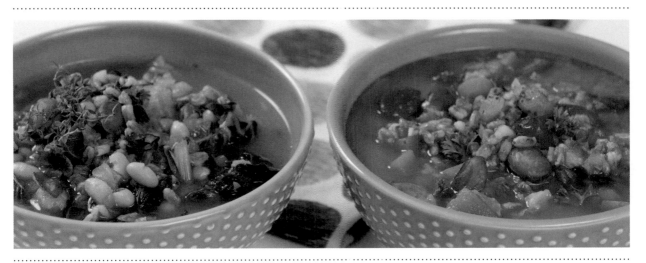

1 tbsp+2 tsp extra-virgin olive oil, divided

1½ cups chopped onions, divided

2 cloves garlic, minced

1 cup cubed butternut squash

½ cup each: chopped celery, chopped carrots and chopped ripe tomatoes

4 cups water

2 tbsp chopped fresh parsley

½ tsp sea salt

Freshly ground black pepper to taste

1 can (19 oz/540 mL) reduced-sodium Romano beans, well rinsed and drained (see tip)

1 cup semi-pearled farro

1 tbsp chopped fresh sage

3 cups reduced-sodium vegetable broth

Pinch crushed red pepper flakes (optional)

Olive oil for drizzle (optional)

➤ In a large pot, heat 1 tbsp olive oil over medium-high heat. Add 1 cup onions and garlic; cook until onions are softened, about 1 to 2 minutes. Add squash, celery, carrots and tomatoes and stir continuously until they start to soften, about 4 to 5 minutes. Add water and season with parsley, salt and pepper. Bring to a boil, reduce heat to medium-low and simmer for 25 minutes. Stir in beans during last 15 minutes of cooking time.

➤ While vegetables are cooking, heat remaining 2 tsp olive oil in a medium pot over medium-high heat. Add remaining ½ cup onions and cook until softened. Add farro and sage. Stir continuously for 1 minute. Add broth, bring to a boil and reduce heat to medium. Stir occasionally and cook for about 20 minutes or until farro is al dente. You'll have two pots of ingredients cooking simultaneously.

➤ Carefully transfer half of the cooked vegetables and beans to the bowl of a food processor or use a stick hand blender to purée them until smooth. Add vegetable-bean purée back to pot. Pour farro and any remaining broth from one pot into the vegetable-bean pot and cook for 2 to 3 more minutes to blend all flavours. Ladle into bowls and serve hot with crushed red pepper flakes and olive oil, if using.

TIP Romano beans are ideal for soups because of their thin skin and creamy texture. They're typically known as borlotti beans in Italy.

 6 SERVINGS 40 MIN OR LESS   MEATLESS

PER SERVING 302 CALORIES | 6 G TOTAL FAT (1 G SATURATED FAT) | 0 MG CHOLESTEROL | 251 MG SODIUM | 50 G CARBOHYDRATE | 10 G FIBER | 13 G PROTEIN

Chickpea Paprika Soup
Minestra di ceci e paprika

ONCE I GOT TO HIGH SCHOOL, we had a rule in our house: whoever got home first — mom, sister, brother, father — had command of our kitchen. If it was my brother, who is also a passionate home cook, I could predict that he'd be browning up some garlic slices in a sea of olive oil with a dollop of paprika to pour over a bed of capellini (angel hair pasta). This is an ode to his dish, made here as a soup, and its wafting aroma that reminds me of that famed after-school special.

1½ tbsp	extra-virgin olive oil
5	cloves garlic, thinly sliced
1 tbsp	ground paprika (see tip)
¼ tsp	crushed red pepper flakes
2 cups	chopped broccoli florets
1 can	(19 oz/540 mL) no-salt-added chickpeas, rinsed and drained
6 cups	no-salt-added vegetable broth (*for an easy way to make your own, see page 6*)
¼ cup	no-salt-added tomato paste
¾ tsp	sea salt
Freshly ground black pepper to taste	
1	bay leaf
2 tbsp	chopped fresh parsley
Freshly grated Pecorino Romano cheese (optional)	

▶ In a large pot, heat olive oil over medium-high heat. Add garlic and stir. Reduce heat to medium-low after 1 minute and continue to slowly cook garlic until light brown, about 2 to 3 minutes. Stir in paprika until dissolved. Toss in crushed red pepper flakes, broccoli and chickpeas and cook until well coated and fragrant, about 1 to 2 more minutes.

▶ Pour in vegetable broth. Dissolve tomato paste in broth while stirring. Season with salt, pepper and bay leaf; bring to a boil. Reduce heat to medium and simmer for 20 minutes. Remove and discard bay leaf.

▶ Serve hot in each bowl with a sprinkle of chopped parsley and cheese, if using.

⇄ VARIATION Substitute 2 cups sliced zucchini for chopped broccoli florets. Add more fiber to this soup by tossing in a fistful of cut-up whole-grain capellini or spaghettini pasta with 10 minutes left in cooking time. You can also add more texture by puréeing half the soup in the bowl of a food processor and returning it to the pot.

TIP For more zing, use smoked paprika instead of the sweet variety.

⌒ HIGH IN...VITAMINS C AND A

Paprika isn't just a pretty garnish that gives color and depth to dishes. This spice, which is ground from peppers of the *Capsicum annuum* family, is very high in vitamin C. By weight, it has significantly more vitamin C than citrus fruits or tomatoes. And just 1 tablespoon of paprika has about 70 percent of the daily recommended intake of vitamin A. Like peppers, it's also abundant in capsaicin, a compound that helps fight infection and calm inflammation.

4 SERVINGS

30 MIN OR LESS

GLUTEN-FREE

MEATLESS

PER SERVING 313 CALORIES | 9 G TOTAL FAT (1 G SATURATED FAT) | 0 MG CHOLESTEROL | 476 MG SODIUM | 49 G CARBOHYDRATE | 11 G FIBER | 14 G PROTEIN

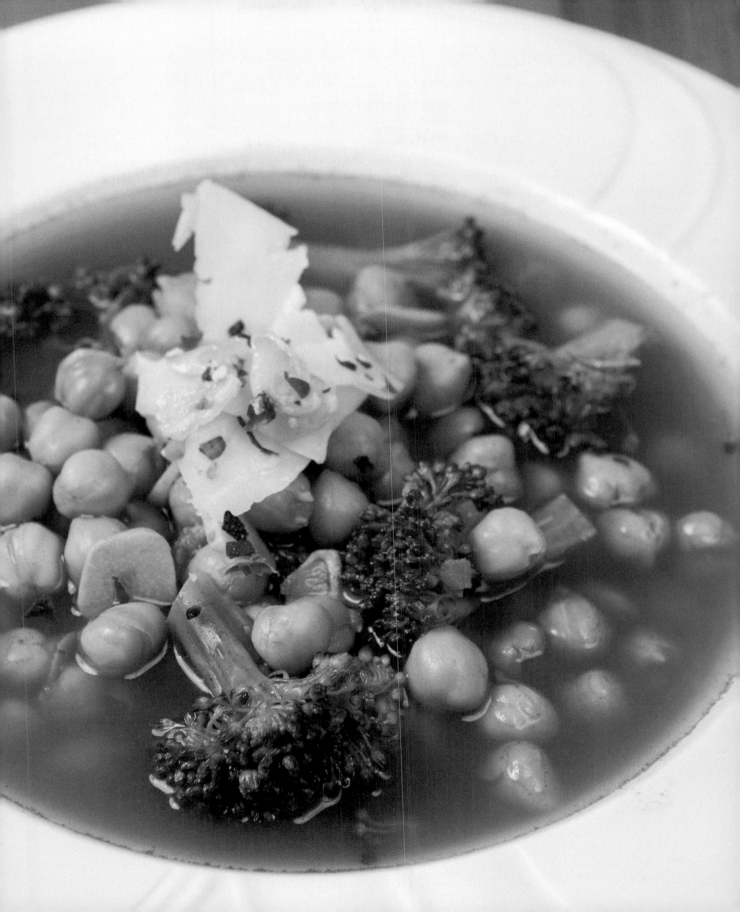

Canederli (Ball) Soup
Zuppa di canederli

I WAS FIRST INTRODUCED TO THIS BREAD-BALL SOUP more than 20 years ago and it was love at first taste. My husband's family, who brought the recipe over with them when they emigrated from Italy to Canada in the 1930s, has been making this recipe for festive occasions for 80 years. It's now a tradition in our home and it receives the same attention when the balls are being scooped into bowls.

1	loaf (24 oz/675 g) day-old whole-grain bread, crusts removed, cubed (about 7 to 8 cups)
¾ cup	1% milk
2 tsp	extra-virgin olive oil
1 tsp	light butter
1	onion, minced
1	egg, beaten
¼ cup	freshly grated Parmigiano-Reggiano cheese
½ cup	minced deli-sliced extra-lean cooked capocollo (about 2 oz/56 g), (see tip)
½ cup	minced fresh parsley
¼ tsp	freshly ground black pepper
8 cups	no-salt-added chicken broth (see tip)
Sea salt to taste	
Freshly grated Parmigiano-Reggiano cheese (optional)	

MAKE AHEAD Prepare the bread balls 2 to 3 weeks before they're needed. Place them on a parchment-lined baking sheet and freeze for 1 hour. Transfer balls to a freezer storage bag, seal and keep frozen until ready to use. Increase the soup's cooking time by 8 to 10 minutes.

➤ Place cubed bread in a very large bowl. Pour milk in slowly, tossing bread well to absorb. Set aside.

➤ Heat oil and butter on medium-low heat in a large non-stick skillet. Add onion and cook, stirring frequently, until lightly golden, about 5 minutes. Let cool and add to bread mixture.

➤ Add egg, cheese, capocollo, parsley and black pepper to bread mixture and work in well (use your hands!). Dampen hands and portion out 1 cup of mixture, squeezing mixture together as tightly as possible, to form each ball, for a total of 6 balls. Place balls on a glass or ceramic plate and refrigerate for 1 hour.

➤ In a large pot, bring chicken broth to a boil and slowly drop in balls, one at a time. Don't stir. Reduce heat to medium, cover and simmer until all the balls float to the top, about 10 minutes. Once balls rise, cook for 2 to 3 more minutes. Taste soup and add salt if needed. Ladle soup with one ball into each bowl and serve hot with freshly grated cheese, if desired.

TIPS Capocollo, also known as capicolo, is a deli meat similar to dry-cured prosciutto or ham. It's seasoned with a blend of garlic and spice but is more tender than salami or prosciutto. The lean type retains most of the flavor with considerably less fat and often less sodium.
➤ This soup demands a good-quality chicken broth. There are some delicious broths on store shelves today but if you prefer the taste of a homemade broth, prepare it the day before using chicken pieces, onion, carrots, celery, parsley and bay leaves. Be sure to strain broth well before bringing it to a boil and adding in the bread balls.

↻ LOW IN...FAT

Swapping out Italian pork salami for a leaner deli meat like this capocollo cuts the fat down by more than 90 percent (55 grams of salami has 20 grams of fat compared to only 1.5 grams of fat in the same amount of lean capocollo) yet it has a similar great taste. Using whole-grain instead of the traditional white bread also triples the amount of fiber in this recipe.

6 SERVINGS

MAKE AHEAD

PER SERVING 293 CALORIES | 9 G TOTAL FAT (3 G SATURATED FAT) | 42 MG CHOLESTEROL | 479 MG SODIUM | 35 G CARBOHYDRATE | 5 G FIBER | 20 G PROTEIN

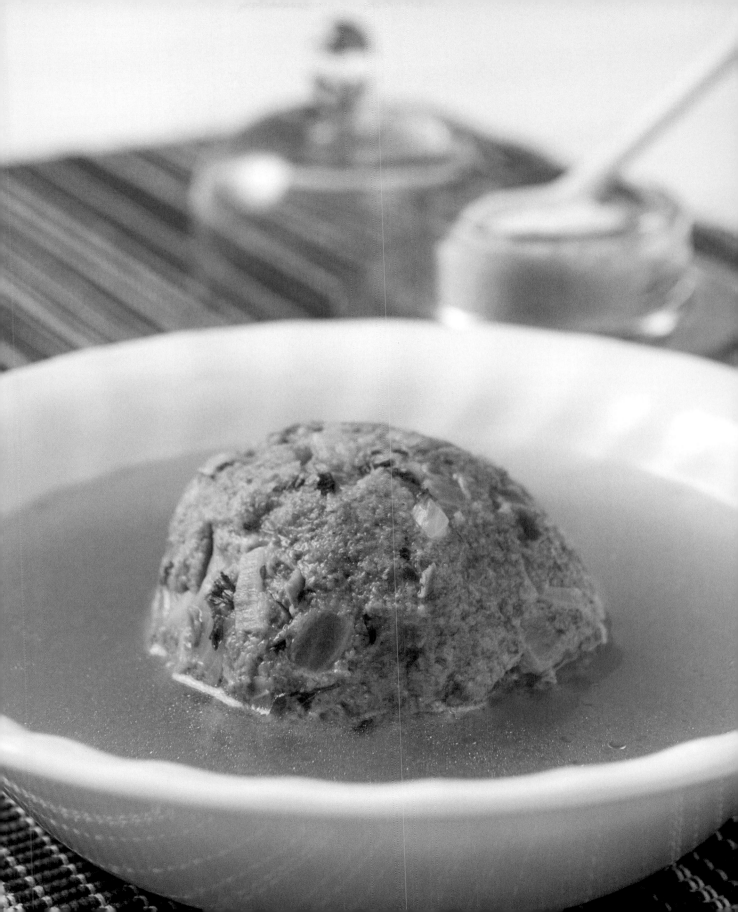

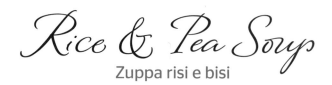

Rice & Pea Soup
Zuppa risi e bisi

RICE AND PEAS ARE A FAMILIAR CULINARY MATCH in many kitchens worldwide. This particular recipe has its roots from a centuries-old Venetian risotto dish that is a standout for its meaty broth and fresh peas. The Venetians are very proud of it and so they should be — while in Venice, a waiter once insisted I add it to my order of a slow-braised veal shank. That was advice I was glad I followed! The dish gets a revamp here from a delectable risotto to a savory soup: I took notes from my mom who often uses rice in place of pasta in soups for its creamier texture. A handful is often enough to give sustenance when it's slurped up with a broth of fresh vegetables and herbs.

2 tsp	extra-virgin olive oil
1 tsp	light butter
1	large onion, chopped
2	slices turkey bacon-style, chopped (1.8 oz/52 g)
1 cup	brown short-grain rice
6 cups	no-salt-added chicken broth
1½ cups	fresh green peas (see tip)
2 tbsp	minced fresh mint
1 tbsp	chopped fresh basil
½ tsp	sea salt

Freshly ground black pepper to taste

Freshly grated Parmigiano-Reggiano or Pecorino Romano cheese (optional)

➤ In a large pot, heat oil and butter over medium-high heat. Add onion and bacon and cook until onion is softened, about 2 minutes.

➤ Add rice and stir continuously to coat well, about 1 minute. Add 2 cups of broth slowly, one ladle at a time to allow liquid to be partially absorbed before stirring and adding more for the first 5 minutes. Add remaining broth, peas, mint, basil, salt and pepper and bring to a boil. Cover, reduce heat to medium-low and cook for 25 minutes until rice is al dente but tender.

➤ Stir in cheese, if using, before serving.

TIP Use fresh green peas if possible. They're sweeter and creamier than the frozen variety although large frozen peas will still work well for this recipe. Avoid canned peas, which will turn into a green mush in this dish.

6 SERVINGS   40 MIN OR LESS   GLUTEN-FREE

PER SERVING 105 CALORIES | 3 G TOTAL FAT (1 G SATURATED FAT) | 6 MG CHOLESTEROL | 341 MG SODIUM | 16 G CARBOHYDRATE | 3 G FIBER | 5 G PROTEIN

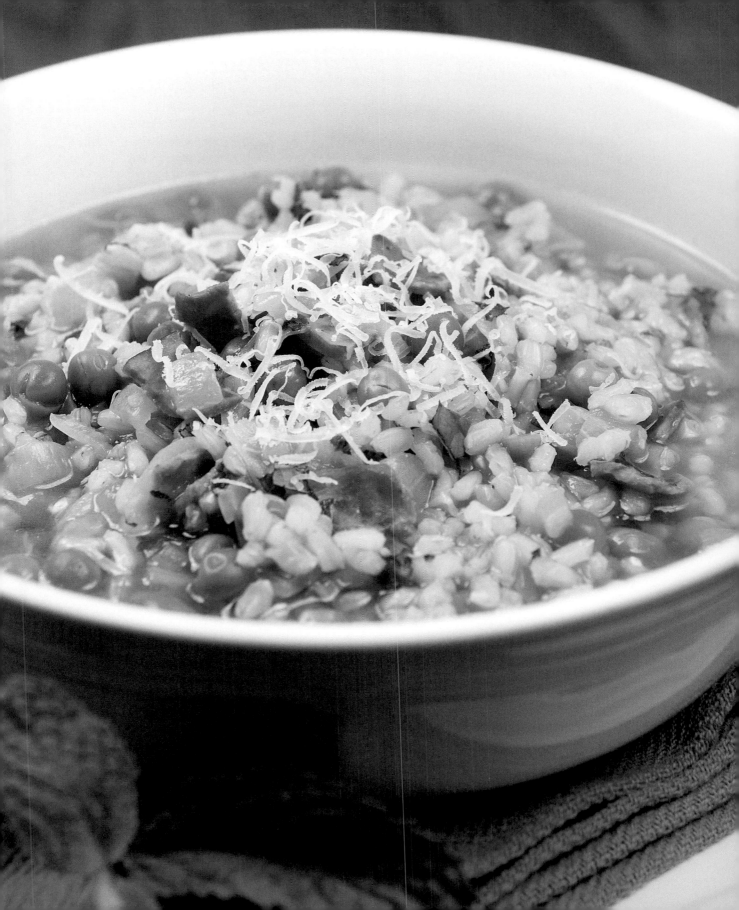

Brown & Red Lentil Soup

Zuppa di lenticchie marrone e rosse

WHEN I MENTION LENTILS, most people assume I'm only referring to the flat brown-shelled lentils that are packed in cans. But there are so many more varieties of dried lentils and legumes worth exploring, including the teeny red ones in this soup. For the longest time, I never knew my mom was adding them to soups because they melted away, leaving behind incredible flavor and lots of fiber. The fact that they cook so quickly makes them even more prized in this dish.

1 tbsp	extra-virgin olive oil
1	large onion, chopped
2	cloves garlic, minced
1½ cup	chopped celery with leaves
¾ cup	diced carrots
1¼ cups	canned no-salt-added diced tomatoes, drained
7 cups	reduced-sodium vegetable broth
2 cups	coarsely chopped baby spinach leaves
⅔ cup	dried brown lentils, rinsed
⅔ cup	dried red lentils, rinsed
2 to 3	bay leaves (see tip)
2 tbsp	minced fresh parsley
Pinch	crushed red pepper flakes
Freshly grated Parmigiano-Reggiano cheese (optional)	

➤ In a large pot, heat oil over medium-high heat. Add onion and garlic and cook until onions are softened, about 2 minutes. Add celery and carrots and stir continuously until they start to soften, about 2 to 3 minutes. Add diced tomatoes, simmer for 4 to 5 minutes and stir in remaining ingredients, except cheese.

➤ Reduce heat to medium, cover and simmer for 25 to 30 minutes, stirring occasionally. Remove and discard bay leaves. Ladle soup into bowls and serve hot with freshly grated cheese, if desired.

TIP Don't skip the bay leaves. They impart a wonderfully unique taste that helps give this soup its full character. Look for them where either fresh herbs or dried spices are sold at your local grocery store.

∩ HIGH IN...PROTEIN

Protein doesn't just come from meat. While lentils are one of the smallest members of the legume family, they're a mighty provider of both protein — here they offer 8 grams per 1 cup — and iron, with virtually no fat. Their rich fiber content also helps stabilize blood sugar so you feel full for longer.

 6 SERVINGS   **40 MIN OR LESS**   **GLUTEN-FREE**   **MEATLESS**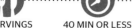

PER SERVING 197 CALORIES | 2 G TOTAL FAT (0 G SATURATED FAT) | 0 MG CHOLESTEROL | 149 MG SODIUM | 34 G CARBOHYDRATE | 8 G FIBER | 11 G PROTEIN

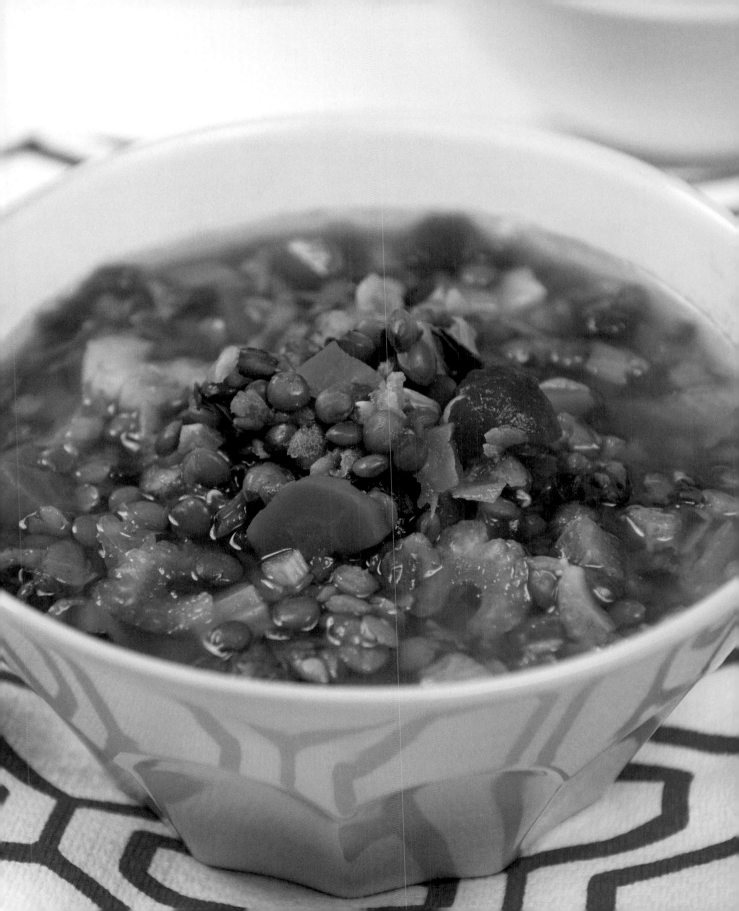

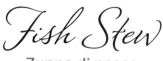

Fish Stew
Zuppa di pesce

MY SONS AND NEPHEWS, who are all admitted fish-avours, devour this meal when I occasionally make it on Friday fish nights. When I was little, it was typically served on Christmas Eve when fish-only dishes are the tradition, but now with the abundance of fresh fish all year long at grocers' fish counters, I can whip up this easy and quick dinner anytime. Fish Fridays are now Fast Fridays.

1 lb	(454 g) mussels, cleaned
1 lb	(454 g) clams, cleaned
1 lb	(454 g) monkfish fillet
1 tbsp	extra-virgin olive oil
4	cloves garlic, chopped
2 cups	chopped ripe tomatoes
1 cup	chopped celery
½ cup	white wine (see tip)
2 cups	no-salt-added tomato purée (passata)
2 cups	water
3 tbsp	no-salt-added tomato paste
¼ cup	chopped fresh parsley + 2 tbsp for garnish
3 tbsp	chopped fresh basil
½ tsp	sea salt
½ tsp	crushed red pepper flakes
Freshly ground black pepper to taste	
14 oz	(400 g) frozen mixed seafood (includes squid rings, mini octopus, shrimp, mussel or clam meat)

➤ Make sure the mussels and clams are on ice and refrigerated until you're ready to use them. Run mussels and clams under cold water to remove any grit and debeard them (you'll want to remove the little threads that are attached to them if they aren't already removed). Discard any open mussels. Set aside. Cut monkfish fillet into large pieces and set aside.

➤ In a large pot, heat olive oil over medium-high heat. Add garlic and cook until lightly browned, about 1 to 2 minutes. Add tomatoes and celery and cook until softened, about 2 minutes. Stir in wine and cook for 1 minute. Stir in tomato purée, water and tomato paste until paste is completely dissolved. Add monkfish pieces, ¼ cup parsley, basil, salt, crushed red pepper flakes and black pepper. Reduce heat to medium-low and simmer for 5 minutes.

➤ Add mussels, clams and mixed seafood. Cover, reduce heat to medium-low and cook for another 15 to 20 minutes, or until mussels and clams have opened. Ladle soup, along with mussel and clam shells, into bowls. Sprinkle with additional chopped parsley.

TIP If you don't have any white wine on hand, substitute beer, which works equally well.

⌒ HIGH IN...VITAMIN B12 AND IRON

This combination of seafood is a powerhouse of vitamins and minerals. Among the most potent is the content of vitamin B12; surpassing the daily recommended intake in just one serving of this stew. B12 is vital in keeping the body's nerve and blood cells healthy. Mussels and clams are also an excellent source of iron, essential in the formation of red blood cells. And while you might be consuming only vegetables and fruit for their antioxidant benefits, consider that selenium — which comes in a big dose here — is a mineral with antioxidant properties that protects the body's cells from damage and plays a key role in metabolism.

 6 SERVINGS   **40 MIN OR LESS**   **GLUTEN-FREE**   **MEATLESS**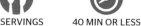

PER SERVING 237 CALORIES | 6 G TOTAL FAT (1 G SATURATED FAT) | 188 MG CHOLESTEROL | 412 MG SODIUM | 15 G CARBOHYDRATE | 3 G FIBER | 29 G PROTEIN

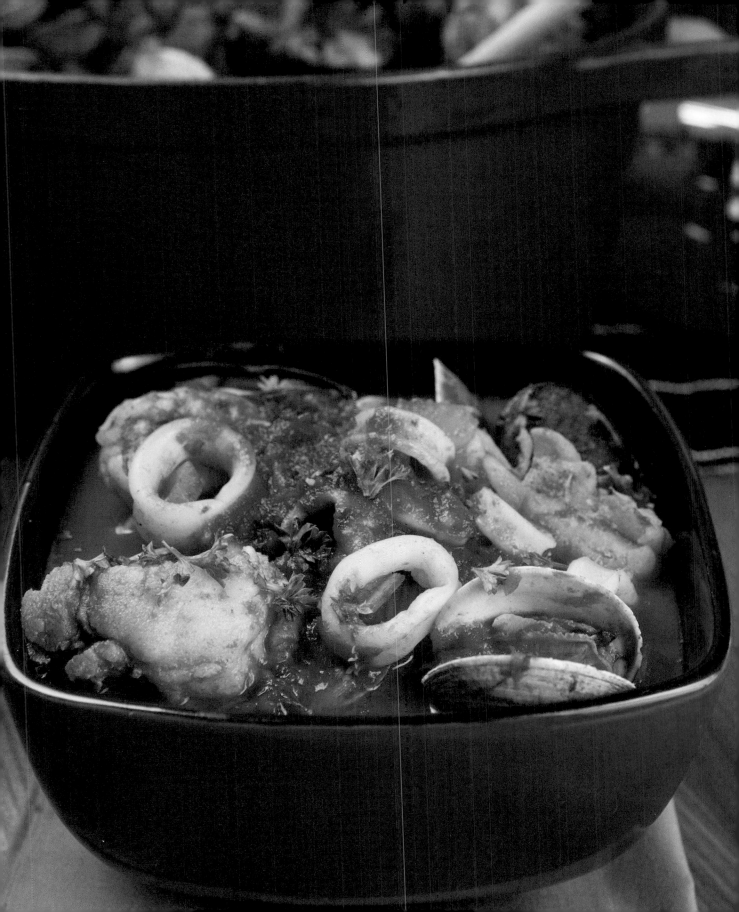

Garden Vegetable Stew
Zuppa del giardino

THE PRIDE OF ANY GARDENER'S PLOT is the abundance of his harvest, but if you're Italian, chances are it's the length of your *cucuzzas* (Italian squash also known as vegetable marrow). So much so that through the years, I've been witness to many organized local competitions that gave Italian hobby farmers a chance to show off their best, usually carried to the competition tied onto wooden planks or loaded onto pick-up trucks. While my dad's cucuzzas never earned a top prize, they were delicious, and the basis for so many great dishes, including this one.

2 tbsp	extra-virgin olive oil
4	green onions, chopped (reserve some greens for garnish)
2	white or yellow potatoes, peeled and chopped into ¾-inch/2-cm cubes
6 cups	peeled and chopped vegetable marrow (cut into 1-inch/2.5-cm chunks)
2 cups	chopped ripe tomatoes, preferably Roma or San Marzano variety
1 cup	chopped flat green beans
2 cups	reduced-sodium vegetable broth
	Sea salt and freshly ground black pepper to taste
¼ cup	coarsely chopped fresh basil

➤ In a large pot, heat olive oil over medium-high heat. Add onions and cook until softened, about 1 to 2 minutes. Add potatoes and stir continuously for 3 to 4 minutes to prevent them from sticking while they soften slightly; add remaining vegetables and mix well. Stir in vegetable broth and season with salt and pepper to taste.

➤ Cover, reduce to medium and simmer for 25 minutes, stirring regularly. Ladle soup into bowls, sprinkle with basil and reserved onion greens and serve hot with crusty whole-grain Calabrese Italian bread on the side.

☋ LOW IN...CALORIES

An elogated squash with a patchy green skin and milky cream flesh, vegetable marrow adds lots of bulk to stews like this one without adding the calories or carbohydrates of more starchy vegetables like potatoes, corn or peas.

 6 SERVINGS 40 MIN OR LESS GLUTEN-FREE MEATLESS

PER SERVING 142 CALORIES | 5 G TOTAL FAT (1 G SATURATED FAT) | 0 MG CHOLESTEROL | 76 MG SODIUM | 21 G CARBOHYDRATE | 5 G FIBER | 5 G PROTEIN

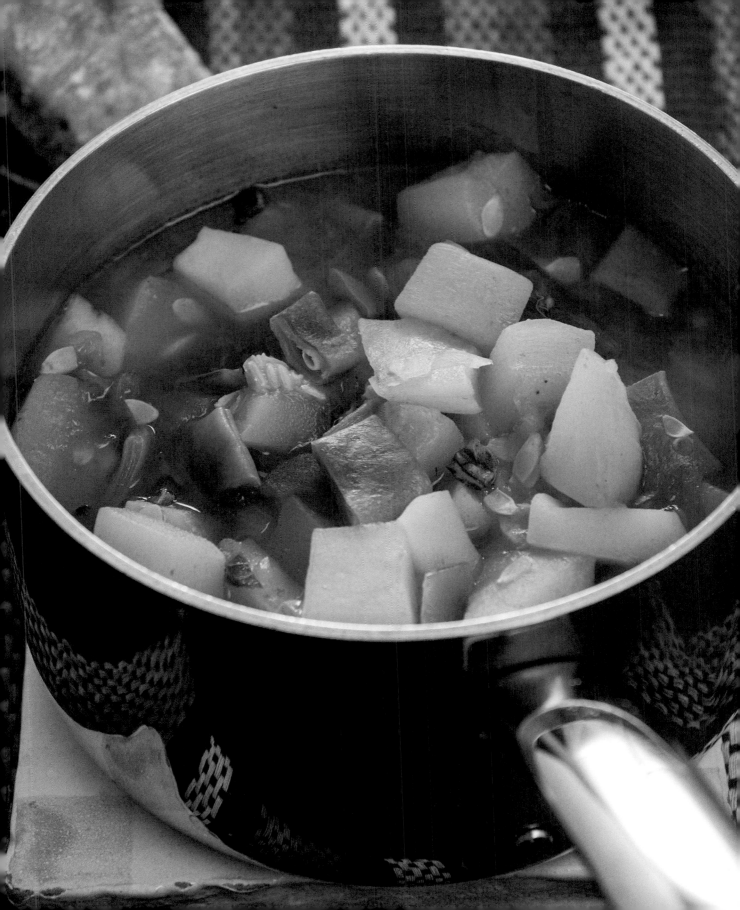

Egg-Drop Spinach Soup

Stracciatella con spinaci

FUNNY THING IS THAT I DON'T EVER REMEMBER having a meatball soup at any Italian wedding I've attended; rather it's been the brothy Stracciatella soup (below) that typically fills bowls when soup is on the menu. But what this "wedding" soup has been for me is my go-to recipe when family and friends have needed some comfort — either because they're grieving a loved one, they're recovering from an illness or they've just brought a newborn home from the hospital.

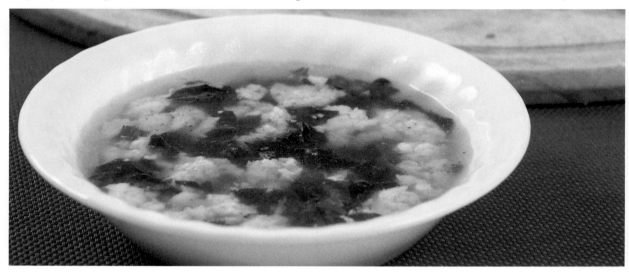

2	eggs
2	egg whites
3 tbsp	freshly grated Parmigiano-Reggiano or Pecorino Romano cheese
Freshly ground black pepper to taste	
1 tsp	extra-virgin olive oil
¼ cup	chopped onions
6 cups	no-salt-added chicken broth
½ tsp	sea salt
¼ cup	whole wheat couscous
1 cup	coarsely chopped baby spinach leaves
2 tbsp	chopped fresh parsley

➤ Beat eggs, egg whites, cheese and black pepper in a large bowl until well combined. Set aside.

➤ In a large pot, heat olive oil over medium-high heat. Add onions and cook until softened, about 1 to 2 minutes. Add chicken broth and salt and bring to a boil. Stream in egg mixture as you gently stir. Break up large pieces of egg with a fork as they form. Add couscous and spinach; stir and cook for 2 more minutes. Ladle in bowls and serve with parsley.

⇄ **VARIATION** Make this a gluten-free option or change the flavor by using brown rice couscous by Lundberg or a rice or corn pastina. Substitute vegetable broth for chicken broth to make this a meatless dish.

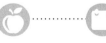

4 SERVINGS   **30 MIN OR LESS**   **GLUTEN-FREE*** SEE VARIATION

PER SERVING 177 CALORIES | 7 G TOTAL FAT (2 G SATURATED FAT) | 95 MG CHOLESTEROL | 201 MG SODIUM | 15 G CARBOHYDRATE | 1 G FIBER | 15 G PROTEIN

Italian Wedding Soup
Minestra maritata

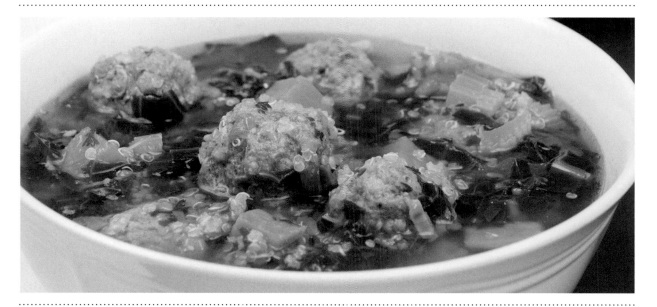

2 tsp	extra-virgin olive oil
3	green onions, chopped
1 cup	diced sweet potatoes
1 cup	chopped celery
7 cups	no-salt-added chicken broth
4 cups	thinly sliced collard greens, center stalks removed
1 tbsp	chopped fresh parsley
¾ tsp	sea salt
30	mini meatballs (*see recipe, page 12*)
½ cup	uncooked quinoa
	Freshly grated Parmigiano-Reggiano cheese

MAKE AHEAD Prepare meatballs a few days ahead and freeze until ready to use in this soup.

➤ In a large pot, heat olive oil over high heat. Add green onions, sweet potatoes and celery. Stir for 2 minutes until vegetables have slightly softened.

➤ Pour in broth; add collard greens and parsley. Stir, cover and bring soup to a boil. Once boiling, drop in mini meatballs, one at a time. Cover and let meatballs rise to the top; reduce heat to medium and simmer for 20 minutes. Add quinoa to the soup and cook for another 12 to 15 minutes.

➤ Ladle soup into bowls and serve hot with grated cheese.

⌂ HIGH IN...VITAMINS A AND K

Collard greens replace spinach here for a huge nutritional boost. Collards are a cruciferous vegetable, along with broccoli, cabbage and Brussels sprouts, and are an off-the-nutritional-chart source of vitamin K, as well as an excellent source of vitamin A and other disease-fighting antioxidants. Here's one more reason to include this green in your soup: it offers a helpful dose of calcium, about 15 percent of the daily recommended intake in one serving.

6 SERVINGS   GLUTEN-FREE   MAKE AHEAD

PER SERVING 153 CALORIES | 5 G TOTAL FAT (1 G SATURATED FAT) | 5 MG CHOLESTEROL | 419 MG SODIUM | 19 G CARBOHYDRATE | 3 G FIBER | 10 G PROTEIN

Tuscan Spring Vegetable Stew

Zuppa garmugia Lucchese

THIS SOUP HAILS FROM THE TUSCAN CITY OF LUCCA, and was served as far back as the 6th century. It uses springtime verdant vegetables commonly grown throughout the region's rolling hills for a chunky stew that is distinctly from these parts. Every time I indulge in this dish, I'm reminded of the magnificent Tuscan countryside. Sturdy sunflowers covered the landscape in a swath of bright yellow that could be seen for miles as my husband and I drove past them while visiting ancient *castellos* and other monuments that dot the area. Of course, I highly recommend a visit for a full-sensory experience but you certainly don't need to travel to Europe to enjoy this stew because of the profusion of produce now available in local grocers all year-round.

1 tbsp	freshly squeezed lemon juice
4 to 5	baby or small artichokes
2 tsp	extra-virgin olive oil
1 cup	chopped spring or green onions
2	thin slices peameal/Canadian bacon, chopped (about 1.75 oz/50 g), (see tip)
7 oz	(200 g) lean ground veal
1½ cups	fresh or frozen young fava (broad beans), shelled (see tip)
1 cup	fresh green peas
20	asparagus spears, tough ends removed, chopped
5 cups	no-salt-added beef broth
1 tbsp	chopped fresh thyme
¼ tsp	sea salt

Freshly ground black pepper to taste

Whole-grain croutons or toasted bread*

MAKE AHEAD Boil artichokes the night before and refrigerate until ready to use.

➤ Bring a medium pot of water and lemon juice to boil. Clean artichokes by removing tough outer leaves until you reach the tender parts. Cut off any remaining tough tips with a serrated knife or kitchen shears. Slice artichokes in half, discard any hairy bits and quickly immerse into the pot of boiling water. Scald for about 3 to 4 minutes. Drain artichokes and chop into chunks; discard leaves that are tough to chop. Set aside.

➤ In a large pot, heat olive oil over medium-high heat. Add onions and cook until softened, about 1 to 2 minutes. Stir in bacon and ground veal. Break up veal into large pieces and continue to cook until no longer pink, about 3 to 4 minutes.

➤ Add reserved artichokes and remaining vegetables and stir for 3 minutes before pouring in broth. Add thyme, salt and pepper; cover, reduce heat to medium-low and simmer for 30 minutes. Ladle soup into bowls and serve hot with croutons.

⇆ VARIATION To make this soup creamier, carefully ladle half of the hot soup into the bowl of a food processor and purée until smooth. Stir back into pot and serve soup into bowls.

TIPS Fava beans have a rich, buttery texture that make them a must-have for this stew. Substitute lima beans or soybeans (edamame) for favas if you can't find them. Be sure to shell fava or any of the substitutes before adding them to this soup.
➤ Peameal or Canadian bacon, also known as cured pork loin, replaces pancetta to give it a similar taste without the abundance of saturated fat. You can substitute turkey bacon-style for peameal for similar benefits.

5-6 SERVINGS **GLUTEN-FREE*** REPLACE WITH GF BREAD **MAKE AHEAD**

PER SERVING(6) 211 CALORIES | 6 G TOTAL FAT (2 G SATURATED FAT) | 32 MG CHOLESTEROL | 328 MG SODIUM | 23 G CARBOHYDRATE | 9 G FIBER | 20 G PROTEIN

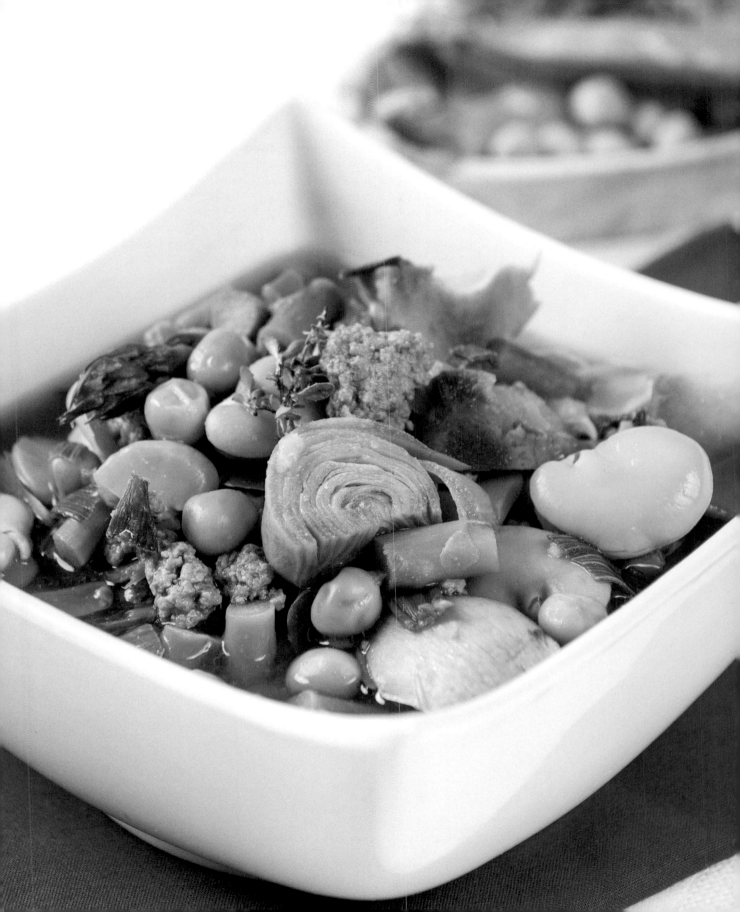

Summer Minestrone
Minestrone d'estate

I KNOW WHAT YOU'LL BE THINKING — August isn't the month when we normally crave soup. But when I lived at home, I couldn't wait for this time of year to taste this scrumptious soup that had its origins in my dad's vegetable garden. And neither could my sister — my mom attributes her chubby cheeks as a toddler to her voracious appetite for bowls of this minestrone. Every single vegetable came from the garden — I often thought we grew them just so we could enjoy this soup over and over again. Today, I still make it in the heat of summer using locally grown produce or from a visit to my parents' veggie patch — my dad, who's in his late 70s, still grows most of the same vegetables. Aromatic celery, hearty flat beans, fresh chard and ripe tomatoes...no wonder my kids are now the ones asking for bowlfuls every time I make it.

2 tsp	extra-virgin olive oil
1	onion, chopped
1	medium white potato (skin on), diced
2 cups	chopped celery with leaves
2 cups	chopped flat green beans
2 cups	chopped ripe tomatoes
7 cups	reduced-sodium vegetable broth
4 cups	chopped Swiss chard, stalks trimmed
2 tbsp	each: chopped fresh parsley and fresh basil
	Sea salt and freshly ground black pepper to taste
1½ cups	dry whole-grain or spelt ditale pasta (see tip)
	Freshly grated Parmigiano-Reggiano or Pecorino Romano cheese

➤ In a large pot, heat olive oil over medium-high heat. Add onion and cook until softened, about 1 to 2 minutes. Add potato, celery, beans and tomatoes; stir continuously until they start to soften, about 4 to 5 minutes. Add remaining ingredients except pasta and cheese and stir.

➤ Cover, reduce heat to medium and simmer for 25 minutes, stirring occasionally. Add pasta to soup and cook for 12 more minutes. Ladle soup into bowls and serve hot with freshly grated cheese.

TIP You can substitute elbow-shaped or any other short-cut pasta for ditale if you prefer, or make it gluten-free by choosing a brown rice or corn pasta. Adjust your cooking time to suit the pasta variety.

MAKE AHEAD The abundance of fresh vegetables does require some extra chopping to make this soup, but it's worth it. Chop up vegetables a day or two before. Or freeze soup (it freezes very well) without pasta; bring it to a boil on the day you're serving it and add pasta.

↻ LOW IN...CALORIES

Before you disregard celery as a stalk with all crunch and little nutrients consider this: it's a good source of insoluble fiber, up to 2 grams per cup, with very little calories and no fat. It also offers respectable amounts of folate, vitamins A, C and K, and calcium. Looking for a stress reliever? Phthalides, a group of phytochemicals found in celery, are known to lower the levels of stress hormones, which in turn can lower blood pressure.

 6 SERVINGS   GLUTEN-FREE SEE TIP   MEATLESS   MAKE AHEAD

PER SERVING 287 CALORIES | 5 G TOTAL FAT (1 G SATURATED FAT) | 0 MG CHOLESTEROL | 160 MG SODIUM | 50 G CARBOHYDRATE | 5 G FIBER | 14 G PROTEIN

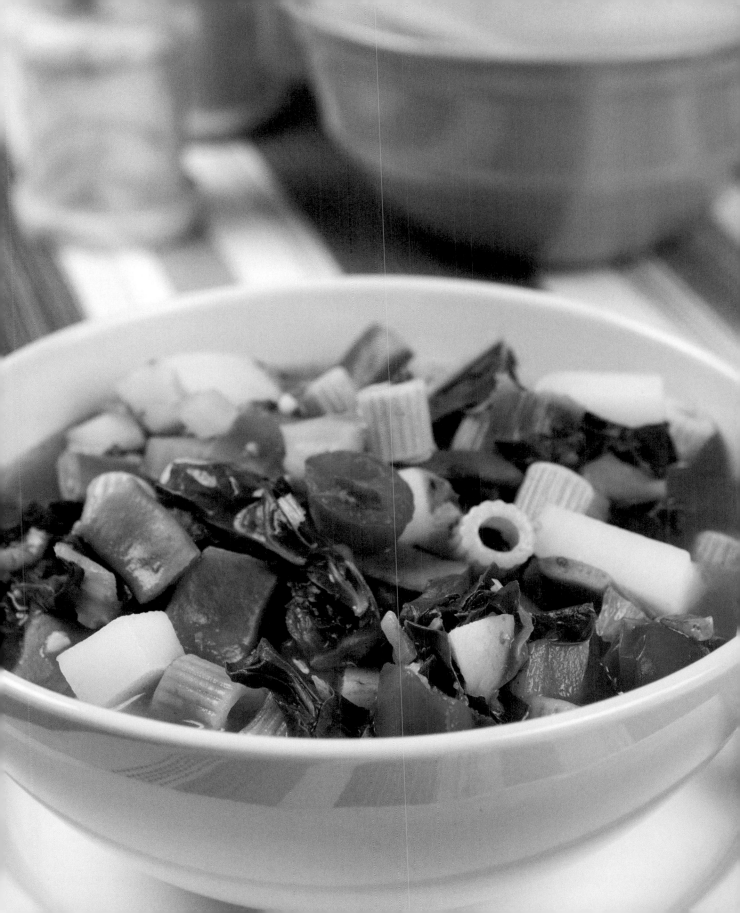

Classic Italian Chicken Soup

Brodo classico di pollo Italiano

DURING GRADE SCHOOL, MY SISTER AND I COULDN'T WAIT to race home at lunchtime and find a bowl of chicken soup on the table. Whether we sloshed through a torrential downpour or blustery snowy conditions, the wafting scent of this soup as we came through the door instantly took the chill away and spelled comfort. With the goodness of herb-infused chicken broth, chunks of chicken, fresh tomatoes and nourishing pastina, this soup does more than fill tummies — it feeds the soul, the brain and the heart.

1 tbsp	extra-virgin olive oil
1	onion, chopped
¼ cup	green onions
¾ cup	each: diced celery and diced carrots
7 cups	reduced-sodium chicken broth
2 cups	chopped ripe tomatoes (about 2 medium tomatoes)
1½ cups	diced rotisserie-style cooked chicken breast, skin removed
2	bay leaves
1 tbsp	minced fresh sage
	Sea salt and freshly ground black pepper to taste
½ cup	dry spelt orzo pastina* (see tip)
	Freshly grated Parmigiano-Reggiano cheese

➤ In a large pot, heat olive oil over medium-high heat. Add onions and cook until softened, about 1 to 2 minutes. Add celery and carrots and stir continuously until they start to soften, about 3 to 4 minutes. Stir in chicken broth, tomatoes, chicken, bay leaves, sage, salt and pepper.

➤ Reduce heat to medium, cover and simmer for 20 minutes, stirring occasionally. Add pastina to soup and cook until al dente, about 10 to 12 more minutes. Ladle soup into bowls and serve hot with freshly grated cheese.

TIP In place of chunky noodles that North Americans are accustomed to seeing in their chicken soup, smaller bits of noodles (pastina) take their place here. There is no end to the shape or variety of pastina — from star- or pearl-shaped nuggets to pastina made with better-for-you ingredients like spelt (used here), kamut, whole-grain or brown rice flours.

MAKE AHEAD Cook the chicken the day before or purchase it at your grocery store's take-out counter.

∩ HIGH IN...CARNOSINE

Mom's advice that homemade chicken soup is good for you is no myth. Studies have proven that the ultimate comfort food made with real chicken broth contains carnosine, an amino acid that blocks infection and inflammation caused by the cold virus. Furthering the healing, the potent herb sage contains a variety of aromatic oils, flavonoids and phenolic acids such as rosmarinic acid, an antioxidant that works quickly to reduce inflammation in the bronchial tubes.

6 SERVINGS   **40 MIN OR LESS**   **GLUTEN-FREE*** REPLACE WITH GF PASTA   **MAKE AHEAD**

PER SERVING 174 CALORIES | 6 G TOTAL FAT (1 G SATURATED FAT) | 42 MG CHOLESTEROL | 282 MG SODIUM | 12 G CARBOHYDRATE | 2 G FIBER | 21 G PROTEIN

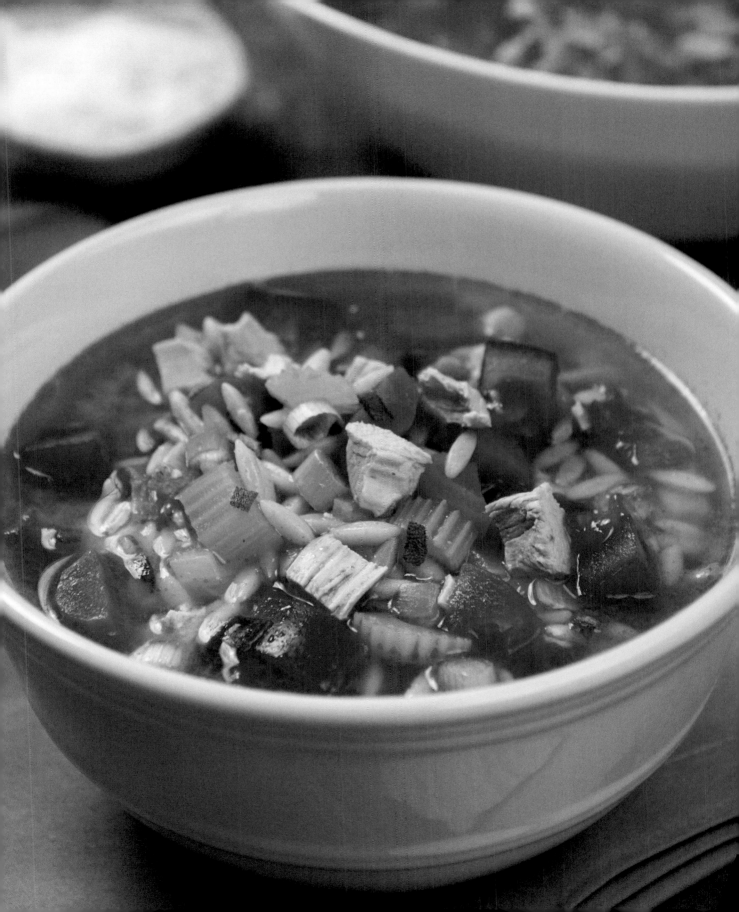

Roasted Tomato Soup

Pappa al pomodoro

WHEN IT'S TOMATO BOTTLING SEASON, you can expect to find a sea of bright ripening tomatoes over a tarp on the floor of my parents' garage. It's the last phase of ripening before the tomatoes become our year's worth of homemade tomato sauce. The plump, succulent tomatoes are also ideal to make this *pappa*, traditionally smothered over bread to make a thick porridge-like soup. Here, a crunchy crouton takes a minimal lead so you can enjoy the sweetness this soup offers all on its own.

12	large ripe plum tomatoes (Roma or San Marzano) or small-cluster tomatoes, about 3 lbs/1.4 kg
1	onion, cut into quarters
4	cloves garlic, sliced in half
1½ tbsp	extra-virgin olive oil + a little more for brushing
4	slices whole-grain bread* (about ¾ inch/2 cm thick)
½ tsp	dried oregano
1 cup	reduced-sodium vegetable broth
¼ cup	chopped fresh basil
½ tsp	sea salt
Freshly ground black pepper to taste	
⅓ cup	2% evaporated milk
Freshly cracked black pepper to taste	
Chopped fresh basil for serving	

➤ Preheat oven to 425°F.

➤ Trim tops of tomatoes and cut them in half lengthwise. Place in a large bowl along with onion wedges and garlic; toss with 1½ tbsp olive oil. Set tomatoes, onion and garlic in a single layer on a baking sheet. Place on the *middle* rack of preheated oven and cook for about 15 minutes, or until tomatoes are softened and wilted. Remove skins from tomatoes.

➤ While tomatoes are in the oven, place bread slices on a baking sheet and brush both sides lightly with olive oil. Sprinkle with a pinch of oregano on each slice. Place baking sheet in oven for 5 to 7 minutes, until bread is crispy.

➤ Add roasted tomatoes, onion and garlic, along with pan juices, to the bowl of a food processor and purée until tomatoes are smooth. Pour into a medium pot; add broth, basil, salt and pepper and bring to a gentle boil on medium heat for about 10 minutes. Stir in evaporated milk and heat through just before serving. Ladle soup into bowls and serve hot topped with 1 slice of toasted whole-grain bread. Sprinkle with more black pepper and chopped basil.

MAKE AHEAD Broil tomatoes and toast bread a day before using.

∩ HIGH IN...LYCOPENE

Tomatoes are an excellent source of lycopene, an antioxidant that is a powerful protector against prostate cancer, heart disease and skin damage from the sun's harmful rays. Cooking increases the concentration of lycopene in red foods like tomatoes.

4 SERVINGS 40 MIN OR LESS GLUTEN-FREE* REPLACE WITH GF BREAD MEATLESS MAKE AHEAD

PER SERVING 179 CALORIES | 7 G TOTAL FAT (1 G SATURATED FAT) | 3 MG CHOLESTEROL | 410 MG SODIUM | 25 G CARBOHYDRATE | 6 G FIBER | 8 G PROTEIN

Creamy Cauliflower Soup

Vellutata di cavolfiore

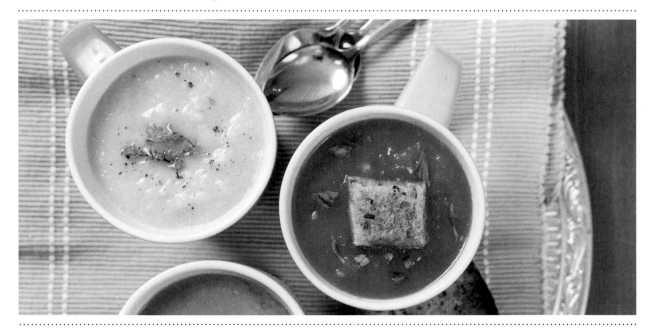

1	medium head cauliflower
1 tbsp	extra-virgin olive oil
1 tsp	light butter
2 cups	peeled, cubed Yukon Gold potatoes (about 2 medium potatoes)
1½ cups	chopped leeks (white parts only) or onions
2	cloves garlic, minced
1 cup	chopped celery hearts
5 cups	reduced-sodium vegetable broth
½ tsp	sea salt
Pinch	ground nutmeg
Freshly ground black pepper to taste	
2 tbsp	chopped fresh parsley
Freshly grated Parmigiano-Reggiano cheese (optional)	

➤ Remove and discard leaves and large stalks from cauliflower. Pull apart florets to make several fist-sized pieces. Cut pieces into smaller bite-sized chunks — you'll have about 6 cups. Set aside.

➤ In a large pot, heat olive oil and butter over medium-high heat. Add potatoes, leeks and garlic and cook for 2 to 3 minutes, stirring frequently. Toss in cauliflower and celery and cook for 1 to 2 more minutes, being careful not to brown the bottom of the pan or the soup will taste slightly charred. Pour vegetable broth into pot, stir and season with salt, nutmeg and pepper. Bring to a boil, then reduce heat to medium-low, cover and simmer for 20 minutes.

➤ Remove soup from heat and immerse a stick hand blender in pot to purée soup until smooth (or carefully transfer soup in batches to the bowl of a food processor and return soup to pot). Return pot to burner, stir and ladle soup into bowls. Serve hot with a sprinkle of parsley and grated cheese, if using.

6 SERVINGS   40 MIN OR LESS   GLUTEN-FREE   MEATLESS

PER SERVING 121 CALORIES | 3 G TOTAL FAT (1 G SATURATED FAT) | 1 MG CHOLESTEROL | 342 MG SODIUM | 21 G CARBOHYDRATE | 3 G FIBER | 4 G PROTEIN

Cabbage-Bread Soup with Beans & Vegetables
Ribollita

THE NAME "RIBOLLITA" MEANS "REBOILED" — an invitation to grab whatever lurks in the fridge and toss it into this hearty potage. In fact, it was once considered a peasant's meal for its cheap ingredients, easy preparation and nourishing properties. Because our fridge was always stocked with a variety of fresh vegetables — would you expect anything less from a grocery manager? — there were plenty of variations in Mom's ribollita, but it always included fresh greens, beans and potatoes. Once chunks of obligatory bread were piled high in the center of the table, we were all summoned to dinner and we all dug in.

1 cup	dried navy or cannellini beans, or 1 can (19 oz/540 mL) no-salt-added navy or cannellini beans
1 tbsp	extra-virgin olive oil
1 cup	chopped leeks
2	cloves garlic, minced
1 cup	sliced celery
1 cup	diced carrots
½ cup	diced mini white potatoes (skin on)
3 cups	shredded savoy cabbage (see tip)
3 cups	chopped collard greens, center stalks removed
1 cup	no-salt-added whole peeled tomatoes, drained and chopped
5 cups	reduced-sodium vegetable broth, divided
2	bay leaves
2 tbsp	chopped fresh rosemary
Pinch	sea salt
Freshly ground black pepper to taste	
2 cups	cubed day-old multigrain bread*
Extra-virgin olive oil (optional)	

➤ Soak beans overnight in enough water to cover them in a glass or ceramic bowl. Drain beans, rinse and drain again when ready to use. (If using canned beans, drain, rinse beans and add them into pot during last 15 minutes of cooking time.)

➤ In a large pot, heat oil over medium-high heat. Add leeks and garlic and cook until leeks are softened, about 2 minutes. Add celery, carrots and potatoes and stir continuously until they start to soften, about 2 to 3 minutes. Stir in cabbage, collard greens, peeled tomatoes, beans and half the broth; simmer for about 7 to 8 minutes. Add remaining ingredients, except bread and olive oil. Reduce heat to medium-low, cover and simmer for 30 minutes, stirring occasionally. Remove and discard bay leaves. Ladle soup into bowls and serve hot topped with bread pieces and a drizzle of olive oil, if desired. (Alternatively, place bread cubes at the bottom of soup bowl and ladle soup over top.)

TIP Don't confuse savoy cabbage for green cabbage. Savoy has softer curlier leaves with deep ridges that add a delicate texture to soups like this one.

⇆ VARIATION Swap vegetables like sweet potatoes or squash for white potatoes. Or try kale instead of collard greens.

∩ HIGH IN...PHYTONUTRIENTS

Both cabbage and collard greens belong to the family of winter greens known as brassicas. Together, they possess potent weapons in warding off life-threatening illness, such as cancer, heart disease and diabetes. They bring no shortage of nutrients to this soup, including a notable quantity of vitamins A and C, calcium, fiber, folate and protein.

  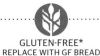

6 SERVINGS   **GLUTEN-FREE*** REPLACE WITH GF BREAD   **MEATLESS**

PER SERVING 191 CALORIES | 4 G TOTAL FAT (1 G SATURATED FAT) | 0 MG CHOLESTEROL | 218 MG SODIUM | 30 G CARBOHYDRATE | 9 G FIBER | 11 G PROTEIN

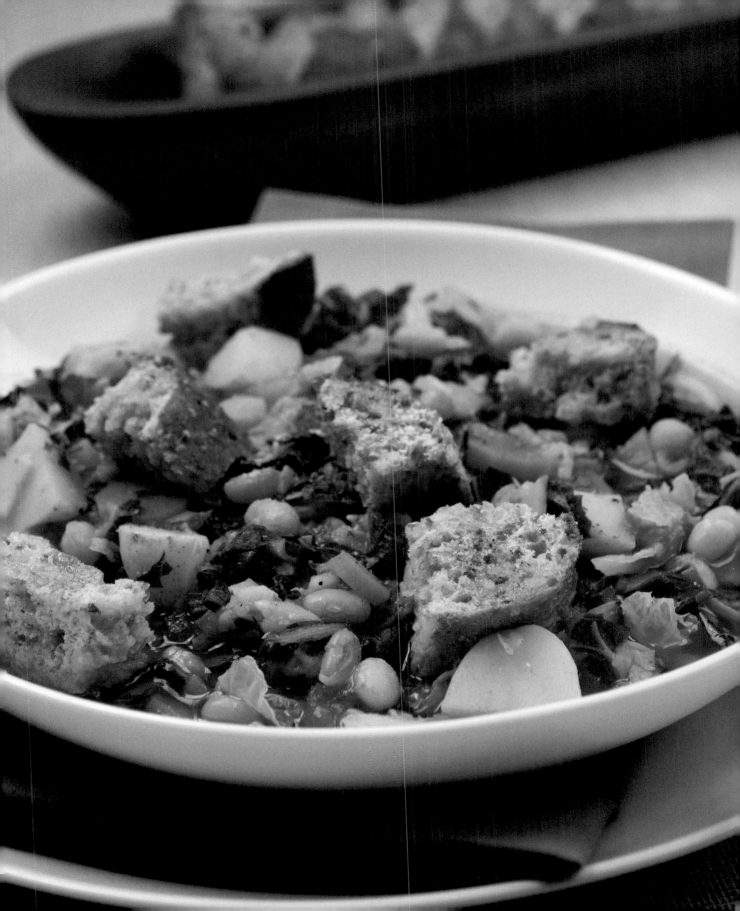

Creamy Chickpea–Squash Soup
Crema di ceci e zucca

I WAS 16 YEARS OLD WHEN I FIRST TASTED THIS UNFORGETTABLE SOUP. I remember it well because it was being served in the magnificent regal dining room of a Tuscan hotel during a tour of Italy I took with my parents and sister, a detour from the typical stay with relatives who lived in small towns. What was more memorable than the setting was this soup's robust flavor. Rich and creamy, it wasn't a typical dish I ate at home or considered part of Italian gastronomy. But I soon discovered that "cream" soups, particularly from the northern regions, have a significant presence in the cuisine, and for very good reason.

1½ cups	dried chickpeas (about 10.5 oz/300 g) or 2 cans (19 oz/ 540 mL each) no-salt-added chickpeas
2 tsp	extra-virgin olive oil
3	slices turkey bacon-style, chopped (2.8 oz/80 g)
1	onion, chopped
4	cloves garlic, minced
1½ cups	chopped celery with leaves (see tip)
2 cups	peeled, cubed butternut squash
7 cups	no-salt-added vegetable or chicken broth
2	sprigs fresh rosemary
½ tsp	sea salt
Freshly ground black pepper to taste	
¼ cup	2% evaporated milk
Extra-virgin olive oil and crushed red pepper flakes for garnish (optional)	

➤ Soak chickpeas overnight in enough water to cover them by several inches in a glass or ceramic bowl. Drain chickpeas, rinse and drain again when ready to use. (If using canned chickpeas, drain and rinse chickpeas just before preparing ingredients).

➤ In a large pot, heat olive oil over medium-high heat and add bacon. Stir continuously until bacon is lightly browned, about 1 to 2 minutes. Add onion, garlic and celery and cook until softened. Add chickpeas, squash, chicken broth, rosemary, salt and pepper; cover and bring to a boil. Reduce heat to medium and simmer until chickpeas are tender, about 45 minutes. (If using canned chickpeas, reduce cooking time to 20 minutes and follow the remaining instructions.) Remove and discard rosemary stems.

➤ Remove soup from heat and immerse a stick hand blender in pot to purée soup until smooth (or carefully transfer soup in batches to the bowl of a food processor and return soup to pot). Return pot to burner and stir in evaporated milk until fully incorporated. Ladle into bowls and serve hot with a drizzle of olive oil (rosemary-infused is even better!) and crushed red pepper flakes, if desired.

TIP Don't discard the celery tops. Not only do the leaves impart great flavor to this soup but also much more vitamins and minerals, including vitamin C and calcium, than its stalks (*for more information, see page 114*).

HIGH IN...BETA-CAROTENE (VITAMIN A)

Although not a typical ingredient in this rich soup, squash not only adds sweetness and creaminess but it also makes a big nutritional impact with loads of beta-carotene, which the body converts to vitamin A. Chickpeas offer a smaller amount of beta-carotene, and together they provide more than 40 percent of the recommended daily intake of vitamin A — it helps boost the immune system and support the health of eyes and skin. Also note this soup's high-fiber count at 9 grams a serving.

6 SERVINGS   GLUTEN-FREE

PER SERVING 169 CALORIES | 4 G TOTAL FAT (1 G SATURATED FAT) | 8 MG CHOLESTEROL | 461 MG SODIUM | 27 G CARBOHYDRATE | 5 G FIBER | 8 G PROTEIN

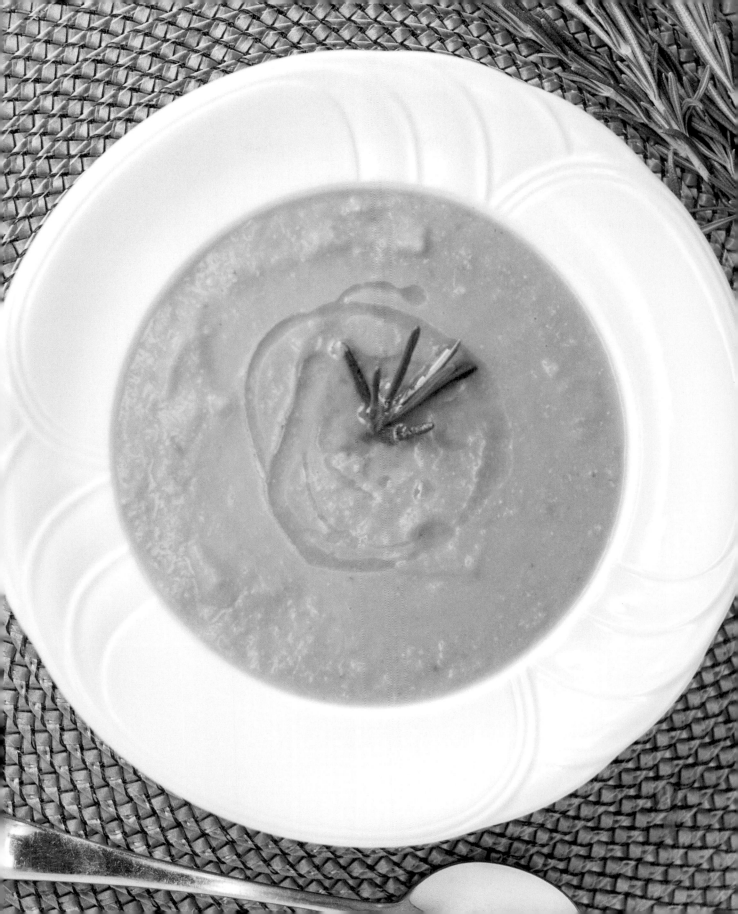

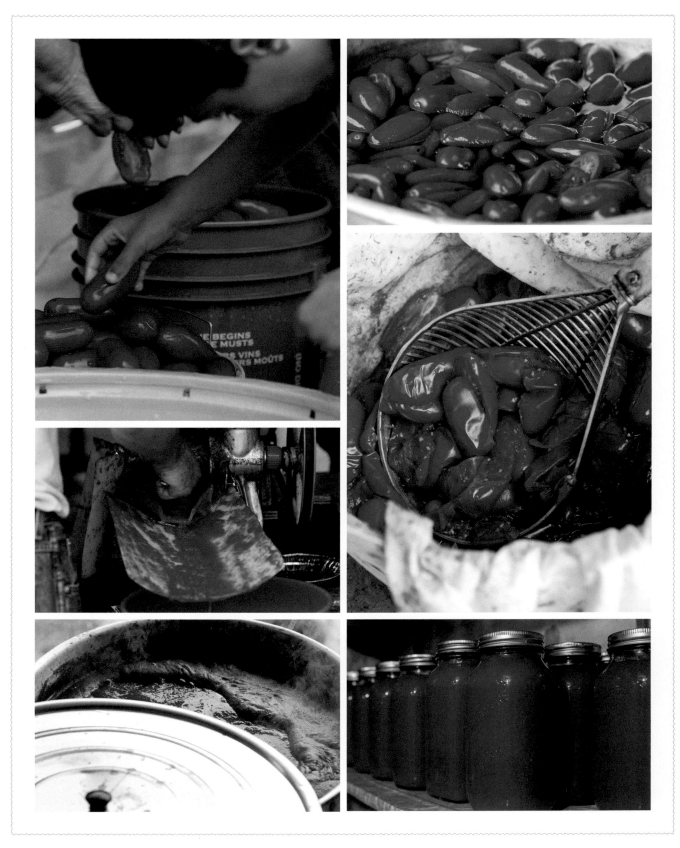

The Ritual
Making Homemade Tomato Sauce

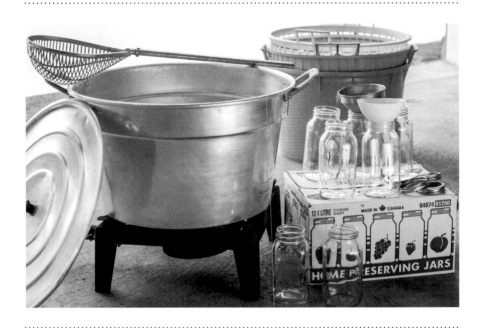

You know it's that time of year when my family is making homemade tomato sauce. The garage floor is covered in a sea of red, the aroma of simmering tomatoes lingers on the wind, and the garage is abuzz with the clanking of pots, the whir of the tomato-milling machine and the occasional hollering of orders. It's a time-honored tradition my family has followed ever since I was born and over several generations before me. It begins with a trip to a local farm, where my parents and I source the ripest, plumpest San Marzano or Roma tomatoes, depending on the year's crop. Once the tomatoes have ripened, they're ready for their day. And it's an early one, with punch-in at 7 a.m. to ensure there's enough time to tackle more than a dozen bushels of tomatoes between my parents and siblings. Mom preps the spotless garage — our makeshift factory — with stations: cutting, milling, cooking, filling, packing. We all take our places — even the kids pitch in for a short time until they realize the intensity of labor and slip away for more leisurely play. It's an exhausting day, but it's one we don't ever want to do without, despite the ease of buying puréed tomatoes, despite the rising costs of bottling, despite the time involved in making sauce from scratch. But what we really don't want to let go of is a ritual that brings our family together and nurtures our already close bond, not only because we worked as a team to make a prized staple in our everyday cooking but also because we made the basis for so many meals that will bring us together again and again.

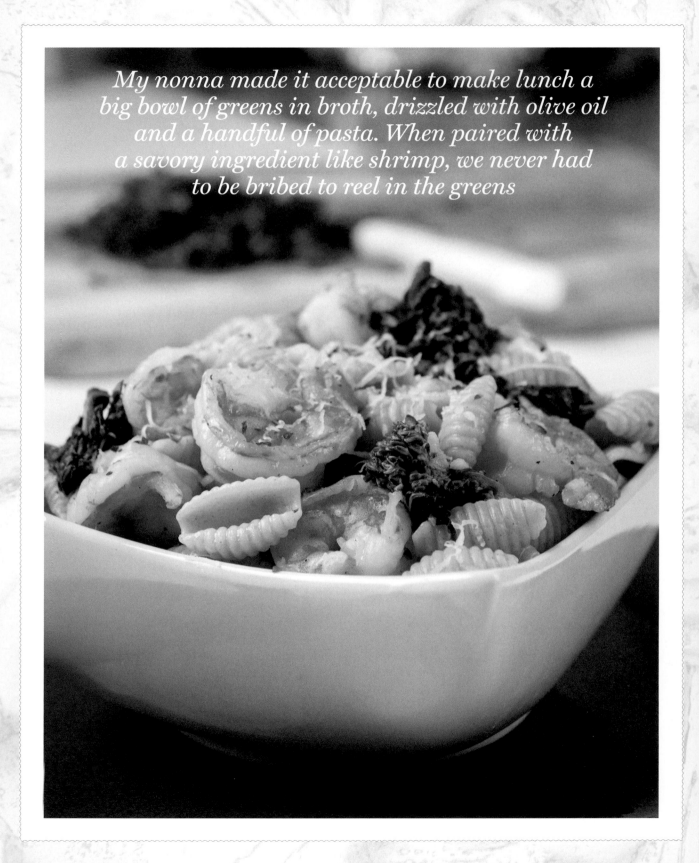

My nonna made it acceptable to make lunch a big bowl of greens in broth, drizzled with olive oil and a handful of pasta. When paired with a savory ingredient like shrimp, we never had to be bribed to reel in the greens

Pastas & Risottos

Pasta e Risotti

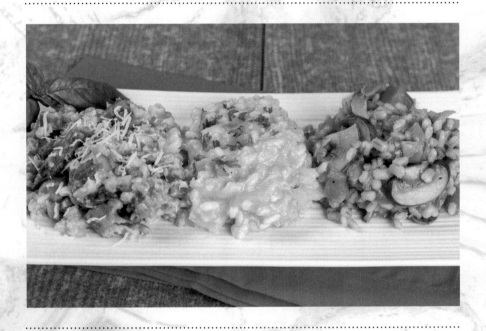

When my twin sister was diagnosed with Celiac disease, our whole family had to learn to cook creatively without gluten. So, until Ma mastered making her own alternative pasta and pizza, we leaned on what we knew best in our home-cooking repertoire — creamy risottos

Farfalle with Creamy Tuna & Red Pepper Sauce

Farfalle con crema di tonno e peperoni

MY VISITS TO ITALY ARE NOT COMPLETE without sharing a plate of pasta with my cousin Rita and her family. We've built many memories together, from sleepovers as young girls to nightly strolls in the town piazza to beach excursions. There are other good reasons for accepting a dinner invite from her: She's not only a fabulous cook but also surrounded by places and family whose culinary roots run deep — her in-laws founded one of the largest cheese manufacturers in Southern Italy; her sister-in-law runs a popular pizzeria; and her summer abode overlooks the Mediterranean Sea in a centuries-old seaport where fishermen have been bringing home their catches to make memorable dishes like this one. It combines tuna and tomato, among other unlikely combinations, to make a distinctively sweet-savory pasta sauce that takes me back to the time I spent with her.

13 oz	(375 g) whole wheat farfalle (bowtie) pasta*
1 tbsp	extra-virgin olive oil
1	onion, chopped
2 cups	diced red bell peppers (about 1 to 2 peppers)
1 can	(28 oz/796 mL) no-salt-added whole peeled tomatoes with liquid, chopped
½ tsp	sea salt
¼ tsp	granulated sugar
Pinch	ground nutmeg
Pinch	freshly ground black pepper
1 can	(6 oz/170 g) flaked light tuna (skipjack preferably) in water, drained
2 tsp	capers in brine, rinsed
3 to 4 tbsp	crumbled light goat's cheese (2 oz/56 g)
1 tbsp	chopped fresh parsley

➤ Bring a large pot of water to a boil. Cook pasta al dente according to package directions.

➤ In the meantime, heat olive oil over medium-high heat in a very large pot or deep non-stick skillet and add onion and peppers; cook until softened, about 5 to 6 minutes. Add peeled tomatoes with liquid, salt, sugar, nutmeg and black pepper; reduce heat to medium and cook for 7 to 8 minutes, stirring occasionally.

➤ Stir in tuna, capers and light goat's cheese until well combined and heated through.

➤ Reserve a couple ladles of pasta water. Drain pasta and toss well with tuna sauce. If pasta is a little dry, add some pasta water as you toss. Sprinkle pasta with parsley and serve immediately.

⌂ HIGH IN...VITAMIN C

With so many nutrients packed into this version of a stovetop tuna casserole, consider it a meal-in-one. The red peppers and tomatoes pack a wallop of vitamin C — providing more than 100 percent of the daily requirement in just one serving — while the tuna provides an excellent source of lean protein and B vitamins, anti-inflammatory omega-3s and antioxidant-rich selenium.

5-6 SERVINGS   30 MIN OR LESS   GLUTEN-FREE* REPLACE WITH GF PASTA   MEATLESS

PER SERVING(6) 355 CALORIES | 5 G TOTAL FAT (1 G SATURATED FAT) | 12 MG CHOLESTEROL | 279 MG SODIUM | 55 G CARBOHYDRATE | 8 G FIBER | 19 G PROTEIN

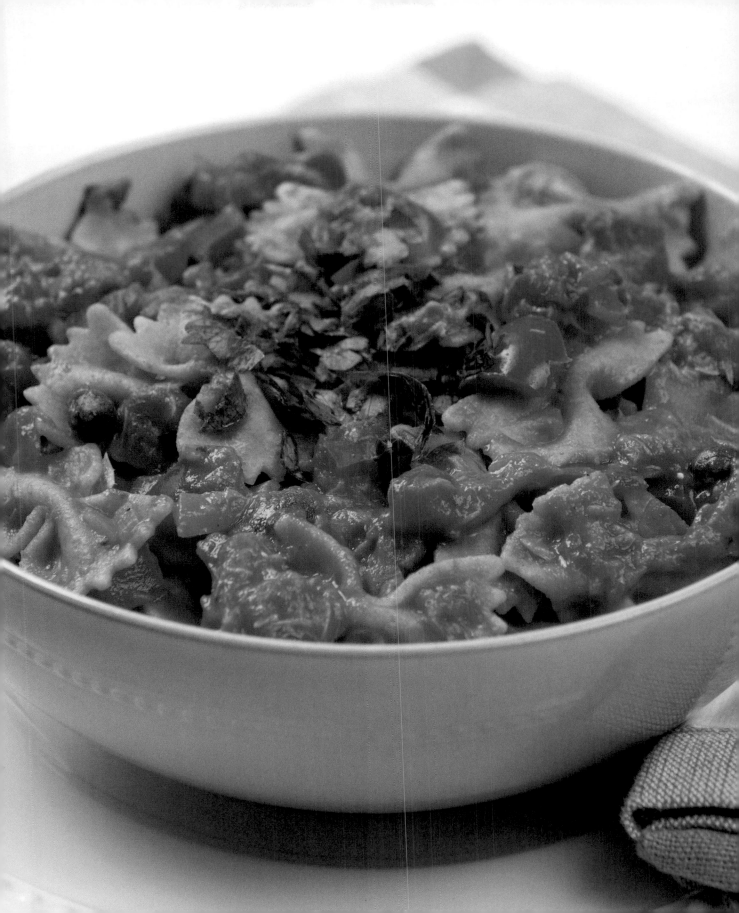

Pumpkin Gnocchi in a Sage Cream Sauce
Gnocchi di zucca in crema di salvia

GNOCCHI IS NOT A TRADITIONAL PASTA we handcraft in our family. But that never stops my dad from attempting new dishes — he's always been the experimenter in the kitchen like the curious (but, thankfully, not mad) scientist in the lab. I remember the first time I helped him make gnocchi from scratch — eagerly following his direction. Like every Sunday morning, Ma prepared a fragrant tomato-meat *sugo* while Dad and I twisted each morsel of dough on the tines of a fork. They were the best gnocchi I'd ever tasted. Make these with your special somebodies and I guarantee they'll be the best loved, too.

Gnocchi

¾ cup	100% whole durum wheat semolina flour (*see tip, page 236*)
½ cup	whole wheat flour
½ cup	potato starch
1 tsp	sea salt
¼ tsp	ground nutmeg
1 cup	canned pure pumpkin (*see tip, page 254*)
1 cup	part-skim ricotta cheese, well drained
1	egg, beaten
1 tbsp	freshly grated Parmigiano-Reggiano cheese

Sage Cream Sauce

1½ tbsp	light butter
2	cloves garlic, minced
2 tbsp	all-purpose unbleached flour
½ cup	1% milk
¾ cup	reduced-sodium vegetable or chicken broth
1 tsp	chopped fresh sage leaves
Pinch	sea salt
Pinch	ground nutmeg
Pinch	freshly ground black pepper
1 tbsp	crumbled light goat's cheese

MAKE AHEAD Prepare these gnocchi and freeze them in a freezer storage bag or container for up to three weeks.

➤ In a large bowl, combine flours, starch, salt and nutmeg. Set aside.

➤ Stir together pure pumpkin, ricotta, egg and cheese in another large bowl until well combined. Gradually add flour mixture and mix gently just until a dough forms. Avoid over-mixing.

➤ Place dough on a very well-floured surface and divide the dough into 5 equal pieces. Roll out each piece into a long rope about ¾ inch (2 cm) thick. Cut the gnocchi into about ½- to ¾-inch (1- to 2-cm) pieces, resembling little "pillows." Shape each gnocchi by either pressing it gently with your middle fingers over a gnocchi board or using the tines of a fork to give them ridges.

➤ Place gnocchi in single layer on baking sheet dusted with flour and freeze them for about 30 minutes before cooking them.

➤ Prepare sauce just before pasta is ready to cook. In a medium pot, melt butter over medium-high heat and add garlic. Stir for 1 minute and whisk in flour until it forms a paste. Add in milk, a little at a time, as mixture thickens. Whisk in broth, sage, salt, nutmeg and pepper. Bring sauce to a gentle boil and reduce heat to low. Whisk occasionally for 5 more minutes. Stir in goat's cheese; keep warm.

➤ To cook pasta, bring a large pot of salted water to a boil. Drop gnocchi into pot a few at a time and give them a gentle stir. Once pot comes to a boil again and all gnocchi rise to the top, let them boil for 3 or 4 more minutes. Drain them using a slotted spoon. Serve with a good drizzle of Sage Cream Sauce.

↺ LOW IN...CARBS

Traditionally made with white potatoes, gnocchi reign supreme in the pasta carbohydrate kingdom. But we've cut the carb count by about half in these gnocchi and instead crowned them queen for their massive hit of beta-carotene, all thanks to the addition of canned pure pumpkin.

5 SERVINGS   MEATLESS   MAKE AHEAD

PER SERVING 329 CALORIES | 7 G TOTAL FAT (4 G SATURATED FAT) | 57 MG CHOLESTEROL | 529 MG SODIUM | 53 G CARBOHYDRATE | 3 G FIBER | 13 G PROTEIN

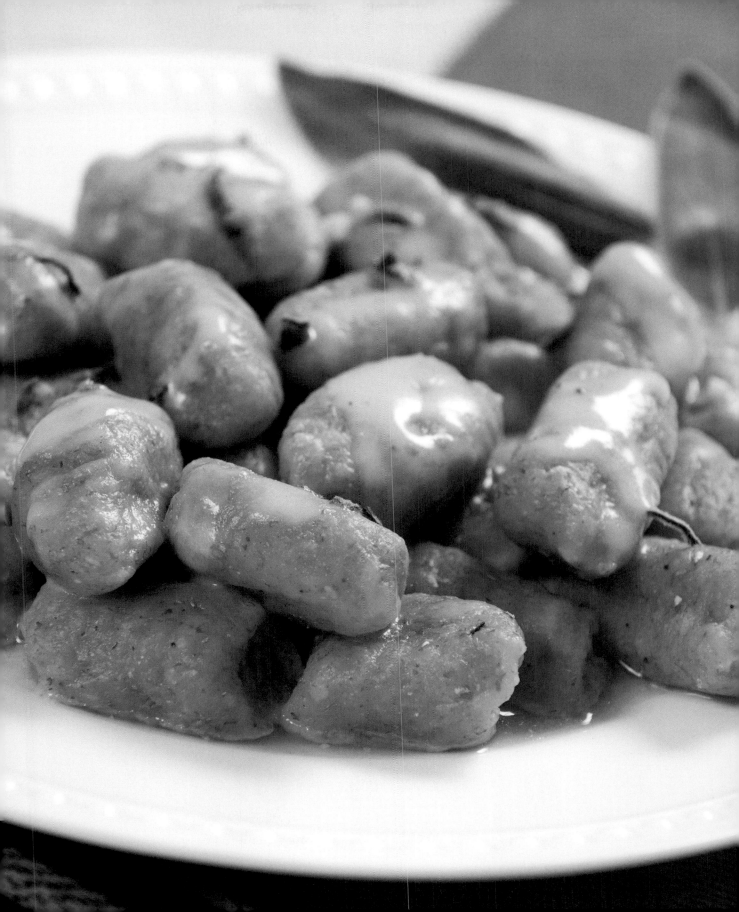

Gnocchetti with Rapini & Shrimp

Gnocchetti con rapini e gamberetti

WHEN I WAS YOUNG, "EATING OUR GREENS" meant filling our plates with lots of non-traditional dark, leafy greens, including rapini, also known as broccoli rabe. My darling nonna made it acceptable to make lunch a big bowl of greens in broth, drizzled with olive oil and a pinch of salt along with chunks of fresh bread for dunking or a handful of pasta thrown in for good measure. Delicious on its own, but when paired with a savory ingredient — here, it's shrimp — we never had to be bribed to reel in the greens. And when my mom upped the ante and tossed rapini in a buttery pasta, it was an even bigger catch.

1	large bunch rapini (see tip)
17.5 oz	(500 g) spelt or whole-grain gnocchetti or orecchiette pasta* (see tip)
2 tsp	extra-virgin olive oil
1 tbsp	light butter
4	cloves garlic, minced
1 lb	(454 g) frozen raw large shrimp, peeled, deveined and thawed (tails removed)
⅓ cup	dry white wine
⅔ cup	reduced-sodium vegetable or chicken broth, divided
2 tsp	cornstarch
¼ cup	minced fresh parsley
	Sea salt and freshly ground black pepper to taste
4 tbsp	freshly grated Asiago cheese
¼ tsp	crushed red pepper flakes

TIPS Rapini, sometimes labeled broccoli rabe, has dark green leaves with very small florets resembling broccoli.
➤ Gnocchetti, a dry pasta shaped like small gnocchi, are perfect for scooping up the buttery sauce. Orecchiette pasta also works well.

➤ Trim tough ends of rapini and discard. Cut tender portions into large pieces — you'll have about 7 cups. Cook rapini in a medium pot of boiling water until tender-crisp, about 2 to 3 minutes. Drain well and set aside.

➤ Bring a large pot of water to a boil and cook pasta al dente according to package direction.

➤ While pasta is cooking, heat olive oil and butter over medium-high heat in a deep non-stick skillet. Add garlic and cook until lightly browned, about 2 minutes; add shrimp and cook, stirring frequently, until shrimp starts to turn pink, about 2 minutes. Pour in wine and all broth except 2 tbsp. Cook until shrimp turn pink. Toss in parboiled rapini. Combine reserved 2 tbsp of broth with cornstarch and add to mixture, stirring until well combined and broth thickens a little. Add parsley and season with salt and pepper.

➤ Reserve a couple ladles of pasta water and drain pasta. Place it in a large shallow serving bowl. Pour shrimp mixture over drained pasta and toss gently. Add reserved pasta water if pasta is a little dry. Sprinkle with grated Asiago and crushed red pepper flakes and serve.

⌂ HIGH IN...PROTEIN

Shrimp, which takes the place of sausage here, has often been blacklisted for the wrong reasons yet you rarely hear about all its health benefits. As a carb-free food, shrimp takes what can normally be a high-carb dish and turns it into an impressive nutritious meal, with more than half of the daily protein requirement per serving. If weight control is an issue, take note: Shrimp is also a terrific source of zinc and iodine, both of which can help the body regulate how it consumes energy, stores fat and controls cravings.

6 SERVINGS   **30 MIN OR LESS**   **GLUTEN-FREE***
REPLACE WITH GF PASTA   **MEATLESS**

PER SERVING 494 CALORIES | 11 G TOTAL FAT (4 G SATURATED FAT) | 127 MG CHOLESTEROL | 280 MG SODIUM | 64 G CARBOHYDRATE | 5 G FIBER | 31 G PROTEIN

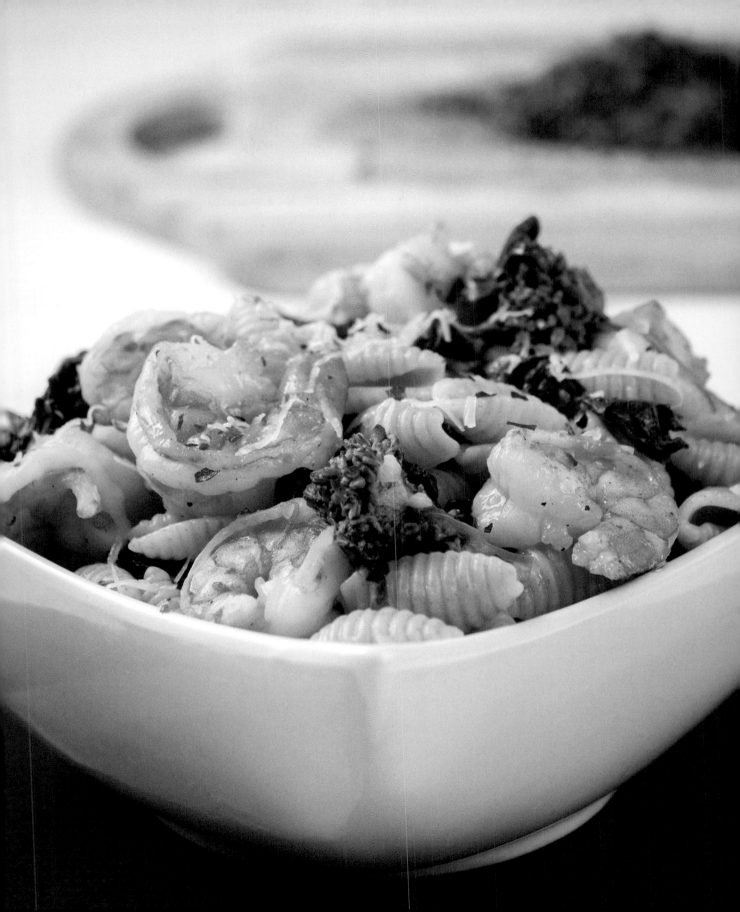

Baked Spinach–Ricotta Rotolo in Béchamel–Pesto Sauce

Rotolo di spinaci e ricotta alla besciamella

YOU KNOW YOU'VE STUMBLED UPON A GOOD THING when friends and family ask over and over again for a recipe. Then again, you really can't go wrong when you bring together creamy béchamel sauce, aromatic sweet basil pesto and creamy ricotta — it's a win-win-win combo. I've had lots of practice to get it right — I've been making the dish since my teens as a special-occasion lasagna when cousins visit from out of town and as a rotolo (pasta roll-up) like this one. Here, I've assembled it in individual bundles for an easy weeknight dinner.

Filling

2 tsp	extra-virgin olive oil
2	cloves garlic, minced
7 cups	packed baby spinach leaves, coarsely chopped (about 8 oz/225 g)
1 tub	(1 lb/475 g) part-skim ricotta cheese, drained
1	egg white
1 tbsp	each: chopped fresh parsley and chopped fresh basil
¼ cup	packed shredded part-skim mozzarella cheese (1 oz/28 g)
Pinch	each: ground nutmeg and sea salt

Freshly ground black pepper to taste

6	sheets fresh whole-grain lasagne sheets (13 oz/360 g, each about 4.5 x 9 inch/11 x 23 cm), (see tip)
¼ cup	reduced-sodium vegetable or chicken broth

Sauce

1	recipe Béchamel Sauce (see page 16)
2 tbsp	basil pesto (see Basil Pesto Genovese recipe, page 18) or use store-bought basil

➤ To make the filling, heat olive oil over medium-high heat in a large pot and cook garlic until lightly browned, about 1 to 2 minutes. Add dry spinach leaves, toss and cook until wilted. Drain well and squeeze out liquid. Let cool. Combine spinach with ricotta, egg white, fresh herbs, mozzarella, nutmeg, salt and pepper until well combined. Divide up filling into 6 equal portions.

➤ To prepare sauce, follow directions as per recipe. Stir in basil pesto until well combined. Keep warm until ready to use.

➤ Preheat oven to 350°F.

➤ To assemble the rotolo, blanch lasagne sheets in a pot of boiling water for 2 to 3 minutes to make them pliable and easier to work with. Drain, run under cold water, drain again. Working on a clean, flat surface, take one sheet and spread one portion of ricotta-spinach mixture evenly over lasagne sheet, leaving 1 inch (2.5 cm) on all sides. Starting from one end, roll sheet tightly. Lightly coat a 9 x 13-inch baking pan with cooking spray, add broth and place rotolo pieces seam side down as they're assembled. Repeat with remaining lasagne sheets. You'll have 6 rotolo.

➤ Pour béchamel-pesto sauce over top and bottom of rotolos to cover them completely and reserve some of the sauce for serving. Cover pan tightly with foil paper and bake in a preheated oven for 30 to 35 minutes. Let cool for 5 minutes before cutting and serving.

➤ To serve, cut each rotolo into 4 pieces; serve 3 pieces per serving and drizzle with extra béchamel sauce and grated cheese, if desired.

TIP Use fresh lasagne sheets like the ones from Olivieri, available in the refrigerated section of your grocery store, to make smaller bundles.

8 SERVINGS   MEATLESS

PER SERVING 304 CALORIES | 11 G TOTAL FAT (6 G SATURATED FAT) | 39 MG CHOLESTEROL | 322 MG SODIUM | 35 G CARBOHYDRATE | 4 G FIBER | 17 G PROTEIN

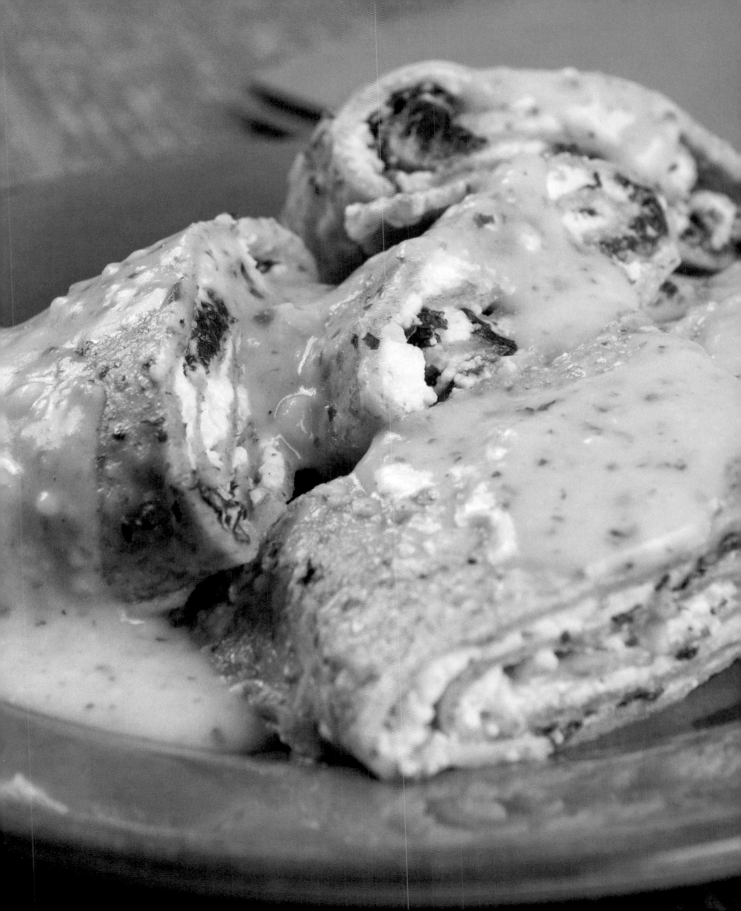

Baked Rigatoni Casserole with Roasted Eggplant & Toasted Breadcrumbs

Rigatoni con melanzane e mollica

SUMMER ROAD TRIPS to New Jersey and New York have always been highlights of my youth. The rolling countryside in upstate New York, the rocky precipices along Pennsylvania's interstates, the architectural gems — it's a picturesque drive that merits attention. What stands out most from those trips, of course, is spending time with family — I have many cousins who live there, even a cousin Vinny! During our stays, the table was always a feast for the eyes, courtesy of my cousins and their ever-expanding families. There were platters of fresh buffalo mozzarella with fresh-picked tomatoes and basil, fish salads, veal cutlets and pastas with homemade sauces, like this pasta bake my cousin Lena and her mother have been making for decades.

1	large eggplant (about 1 lb/ 454 g), cut into large chunks
2 tsp	sea salt
2 tsp	extra-virgin olive oil
⅓ cup	toasted whole wheat dry breadcrumbs, divided (see tip)
2 tbsp	cornmeal
16 oz	(454 g) whole-grain rigatoni pasta
4 cups	prepared tomato pasta sauce (*See Basic Pasta Tomato Sauce, page 10*)
1 cup	cubed light bocconcini or part-skim mozzarella (about 4.5 oz/130 g)
2	hard-boiled eggs, sliced and halved
2 tbsp	chopped fresh basil
1 tbsp	freshly grated Parmigiano-Reggiano cheese
½ tsp	dried oregano

MAKE AHEAD Prepare recipe the night before, leaving the toppings (remaining breadcrumbs, Parmigiano-Reggiano cheese, basil and oregano) to be added just before you pop it into the oven.

➤ Preheat oven to broil setting. In a large bowl, combine eggplant and salt. Let sit for 15 minutes to draw out bitterness. Rinse and pat dry. Toss well with olive oil and place on baking sheet. Broil on upper rack for 20 minutes, turning in between, until they're lightly browned. Set aside. Reset oven to 350°F.

➤ Coat a deep 9 x 13-inch glass or ceramic baking dish with cooking spray and sprinkle half of the toasted breadcrumbs along the bottom and sides of dish. Repeat with all of cornmeal.

➤ Bring a large pot of water to a boil and cook pasta al dente according to package directions. Drain pasta and toss with 3 cups of tomato pasta sauce. Ladle half the pasta into the greased baking dish to create one layer. Add half the broiled eggplant, bocconcini, egg slices, basil and remaining 1 cup sauce. Add the rest of the pasta and repeat layer: eggplant, bocconcini, egg slices and basil. Top with remaining breadcrumbs, grated cheese and oregano.

➤ Bake in preheated oven for 20 minutes. Let sit for 5 minutes before serving.

TIP Toast whole wheat breadcrumbs in a non-stick skillet on medium heat and stir frequently for 5 minutes until golden brown.

↻ LOW IN...FAT

While this pasta bake typically includes cured meats like salami or mortadella, I've left them out to cut down on the saturated fats and make this dish meatless. Slowly broiling eggplants instead of deep-frying them gives them a creamy texture without oily residue left behind.

 6 SERVINGS

 MEATLESS
 MAKE AHEAD

PER SERVING 448 CALORIES | 9 G TOTAL FAT (3 G SATURATED FAT) | 73 MG CHOLESTEROL | 328 MG SODIUM | 77 G CARBOHYDRATE | 11 G FIBER | 21 G PROTEIN

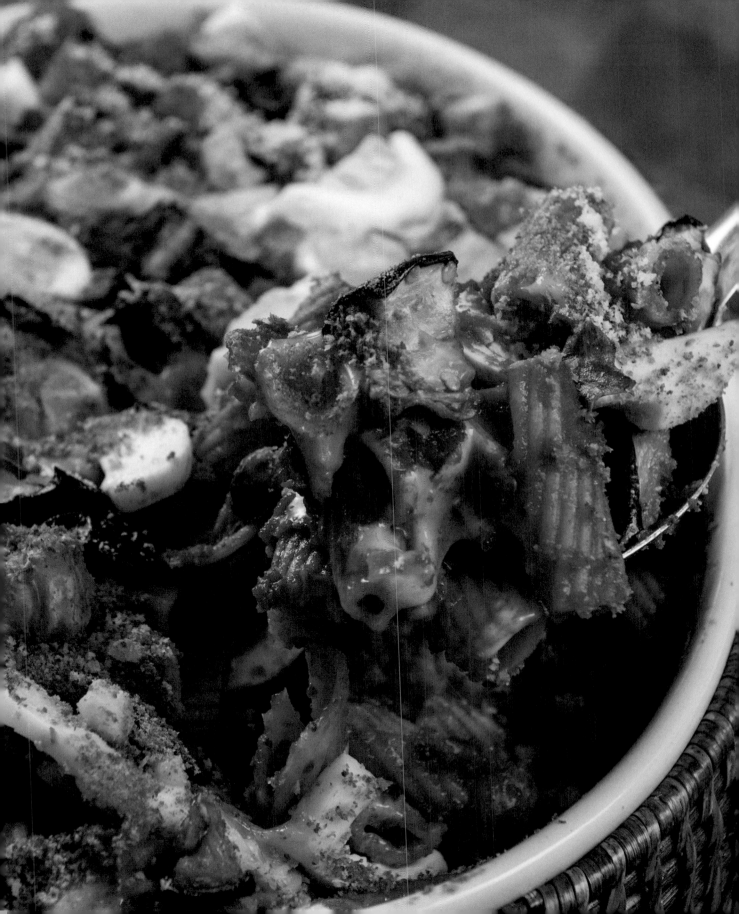

Linguine with Sardines & Fennel

Linguine con sarde e finocchio

WHEN WE WERE BORED of the same old meals, my parents always had a few cheats tucked away in the pantry. This pasta dish was one of them and we always looked forward to it. I say the pantry, even though this dish includes fresh ingredients, because back then fresh fennel wasn't readily available, so they resorted to prepared tins with sardines, fennel and currants imported from Italy. It was also my first connection to uniquely Sicilian cuisine, which often combines savory, salty and sweet in the same mouthful.

1	small fennel bulb with fronds (see tip)
1 pkg	($^1/_{230}$ oz/0.125 g) pure ground saffron
¾ cup	hot water
13 oz	(375 g) whole-grain or spelt linguine pasta*
3 tbsp	breadcrumbs*
2 tsp	extra-virgin olive oil
2	cloves garlic, minced
½ cup	chopped onion
¼ cup	white wine
2 cans	(4 oz/106 g each) sardines in water, drained
3	anchovy fillets in olive oil, rinsed, padded dry and minced
2 tbsp	dried currants or golden raisins, soaked in water and drained
	Sea salt and freshly ground black pepper to taste
1 tbsp	pine nuts, toasted

TIP Find a bulb with as many fronds as possible. They add tremendous flavor to this dish. Tender wild shoots with many fronds are better if you can find them. If so, replace fennel bulb with about 2 cups of chopped fennel shoots.

➤ Remove the fronds from the fennel bulb, coarsely chop and set aside. Remove stalks and the inner core at the top of fennel bulb; discard. Thinly slice bulb. It will probably yield more than you need, but just use 2 cups. Add saffron to hot water, stir and reserve.

➤ Bring a pot of water to a boil and cook pasta al dente according to package directions.

➤ Add breadcrumbs to a large non-stick skillet and toast on medium heat. Keep an eye on them as you stir occasionally for 3 minutes, until crumbs are golden brown. Transfer to a bowl and set aside.

➤ Wipe down the skillet with a paper towel. Add olive oil and heat over medium-high heat. Add garlic and cook until lightly golden, about 2 minutes. Add onions and fennel slices; cook until vegetables begin to brown, about 5 to 6 minutes. Stir in wine and reserved saffron broth; add sardines and simmer until all vegetables have softened. Add anchovy pieces, currants, salt and pepper. Reduce heat to medium-low and let simmer for another 2 minutes.

➤ Drain pasta, reserving a couple ladles of pasta water. Transfer pasta to skillet and gently toss with sardine-fennel sauce, adding the remaining pasta water, if needed. Add reserved fronds. Serve each dish topped evenly with toasted breadcrumbs and pine nuts.

⌂ HIGH IN...VITAMIN D

The sardine is one of the most nutrient-rich foods, with an impressive amount of vitamins, minerals, enzymes and protein. As a small fish that's eaten whole, its soft bones make it a rich source of bone-boosting vitamin D and calcium. Per serving, it has significantly more vitamin D than a glass of milk. While both sardines and anchovies used here are fatty fish sources, they come in the form of heart-healthy omega-3 fatty acids that lower triglycerides and blood pressure.

 4-5 SERVINGS

 30 MIN OR LESS

 GLUTEN-FREE*
REPLACE WITH GF PASTA & BREADCRUMBS

 MEATLESS

PER SERVING(5) 400 CALORIES | 7 G TOTAL FAT (1 G SATURATED FAT) | 19 MG CHOLESTEROL | 231 MG SODIUM | 68 G CARBOHYDRATE | 10 G FIBER | 17 G PROTEIN

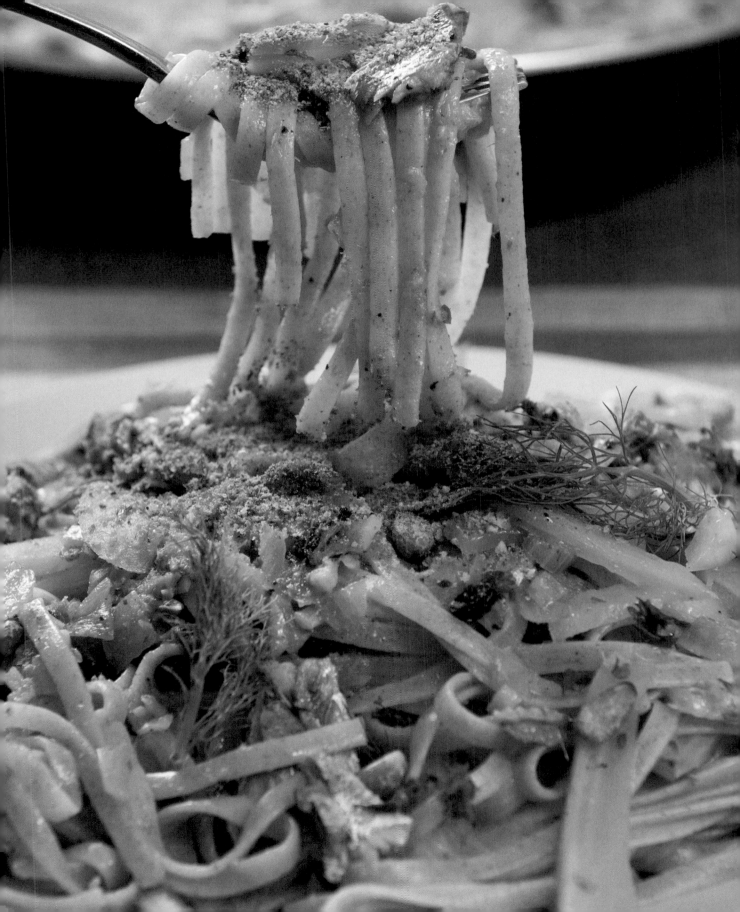

Penne in Red Pepper–Tomato Vodka Sauce
Penne alla vodka

WHEN I FIRST MET MY HUSBAND more than 20 years ago (let's just say I was 2 at the time), I learned quickly that Penne alla Vodka was one of his favorite pasta dishes. The traditional recipe of penne pasta doused in a rich barely-tomato-cream sauce (strike 1) and flavored with fatty pancetta (strike 2) might have helped me find a way to get closer to his heart through his stomach but I was afraid I could be leading him down heart attack lane if I continued to cook it that way. The odds were stacked against me, but I was determined to develop a recipe that was healthier without him noticing. Well? Ever since, he asks me to make it all the time — my version, that is!

2 tsp	extra-virgin olive oil
1	onion, chopped
2	cloves garlic, chopped
1 cup	canned no-salt-added whole peeled tomatoes
1 cup	roasted red peppers (see tip)
1½ cups	no-salt-added tomato purée (passata)
⅓ cup	reduced-sodium chicken broth
¼ cup	vodka
2	slices turkey bacon-style (1.8 oz/52 g), thinly sliced
2	bay leaves
	Sea salt and freshly ground black pepper to taste
16 oz	(454 g) whole-grain or brown rice penne pasta*
1 tbsp	light butter
1 tbsp	all-purpose flour or corn flour*
1 cup	1% milk
Pinch	sea salt
¼ cup	chopped fresh basil
2 tbsp	freshly grated Asiago cheese
Pinch	crushed red pepper flakes

MAKE AHEAD Prepare the sauce up to three days before. Keep refrigerated.

➤ In a medium pot, heat olive oil over medium-high heat. Add onion and garlic and cook until onions are softened, about 2 minutes.

➤ In a food processor, pulse peeled tomatoes and roasted red peppers until puréed and add to pot. Stir chicken broth, vodka, turkey bacon, bay leaves, salt and pepper into pot. Let simmer, covered, on low heat, stirring occasionally, for 45 minutes. Remove and discard bay leaves.

➤ Bring a large pot of water to a boil and cook pasta al dente according to package directions.

➤ While pasta is cooking, prepare a cream, béchamel-style sauce. Heat butter on medium-high heat in a small pot. Slowly whisk in flour until it becomes a paste. Slowly add in milk, whisking continuously for 1 minute. Let it come to a very slow simmer, add salt and cook for 3 to 4 more minutes, whisking as sauce thickens. Just before pasta is finished cooking, stir cream sauce into vodka sauce, combining well. Add basil and adjust seasoning if desired.

➤ Drain pasta, toss with sauce and serve with grated Asiago cheese and crushed red pepper flakes.

TIP For this recipe, grill about 3 to 4 Sheppard or red bell peppers on medium-low heat, turning frequently, until skins are slightly charred. Place peppers quickly into a paper bag — the steam will help blister the skin so it can be easily peeled away.

⟲ LOW IN...FAT

You might think that dropping the rich table cream most recipes demand will make this dish bland, but it's not the case. Low-calorie roasted red peppers add a creamy, smoky flavor with no saturated fat but a great deal of vitamin C.

 6 SERVINGS
 30 MIN OR LESS
 GLUTEN-FREE* REPLACE WITH GF PASTA & FLOUR

 MAKE AHEAD

PER SERVING 434 CALORIES | 7 G TOTAL FAT (1 G SATURATED FAT) | 10 MG CHOLESTEROL | 209 MG SODIUM | 74 G CARBOHYDRATE | 12 G FIBER | 16 G PROTEIN

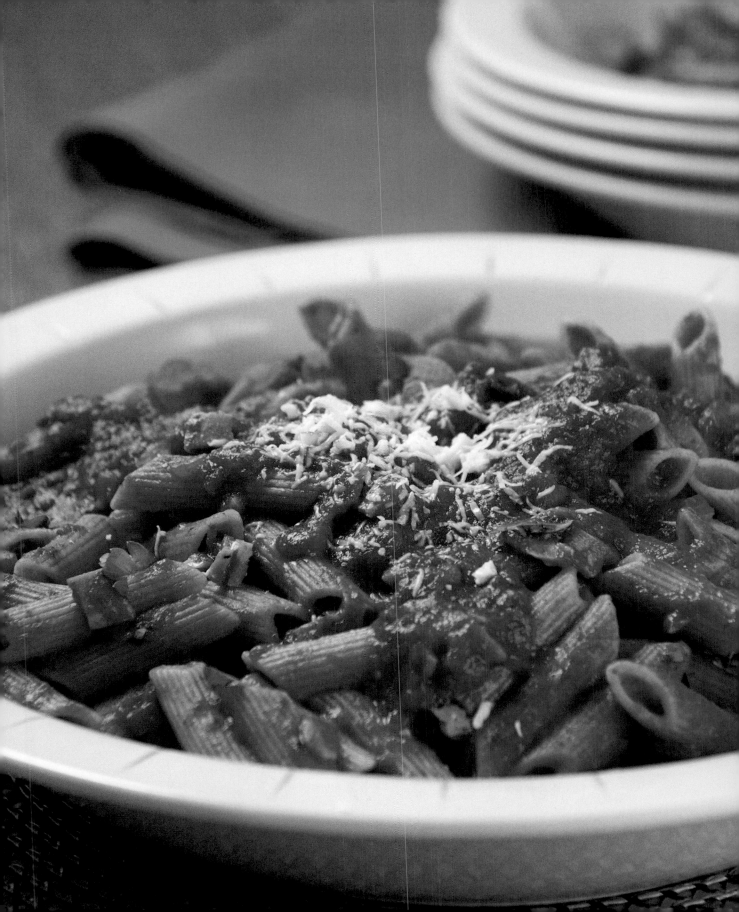

Linguine Puttanesca
Linguine alla puttanesca

THERE'S BEEN MUCH DEBATE ABOUT THE ORIGINS of the Puttanesca sauce, popularized in the 1960s in Italy, but one thing is certain — translated to English, "*alla puttanesca*" means "prostitute-style." Hmm, food for thought, although it's probably not a discussion you'll want to have at the dinner table. Thankfully, it's not the sensational title that draws our family to this dish; rather, it's the incredible ease in preparing the dish — some of my at-the-ready pantry staples include diced tomatoes, capers and the black olives used here. And, for those who are served this meal, well, you could say it uncovers a blending of flavors that's almost too sinful to enjoy.

13 oz	(375 g) whole-grain or spelt linguine pasta*
2 tsp	extra-virgin olive oil
4	cloves garlic, minced
1½ cups	halved ripe cherry tomatoes
1 can	(28 oz/796 mL) no-salt-added San Marzano whole peeled tomatoes, chopped (reserve liquid or purée for another use)
½ cup	reduced-sodium vegetable broth
¼ cup	chopped fresh parsley
2 tbsp	green olive slices, rinsed
2 tsp	capers in brine, rinsed and patted dry
2	anchovy fillets in olive oil, rinsed, patted dry and minced (optional)
¼ tsp	crushed red pepper flakes
4 tsp	freshly grated Parmigiano-Reggiano cheese

➤ Bring a large pot of water to a boil. Cook pasta al dente according to package directions.

➤ In the meantime, heat olive oil over medium-high heat in a very large saucepan or deep non-stick skillet. Add garlic and cherry tomatoes and cook, stirring frequently, until tomatoes soften, about 2 to 3 minutes. Stir in peeled tomatoes and vegetable broth. Cook for 5 to 6 more minutes. Add parsley, green olives, capers, anchovies, if using, and crushed red pepper flakes, tossing until well combined.

➤ Drain pasta and toss well with half the Puttanesca sauce. Divide linguine evenly over four pasta plates, ladle remaining sauce evenly over pasta and sprinkle each with 1 tsp grated cheese.

↻ LOW ON...THE GLYCEMIC INDEX

White pasta that is cooked until soft is known to raise blood sugar levels rapidly, making it a food with a high GI on the Glycemic Index. However, you can lower pasta's GI rating and, therefore, slow down how quickly the digestive system breaks it down into sugar by cooking it "al dente," which means "to the tooth" or "to the bite." Follow package directions to get a perfectly cooked al dente pasta.

  4 SERVINGS

 30 MIN OR LESS

 GLUTEN-FREE*
REPLACE WITH GF PASTA

 MEATLESS

PER SERVING 446 CALORIES | 6 G TOTAL FAT (1 G SATURATED FAT) | 3 MG CHOLESTEROL | 274 MG SODIUM | 87 G CARBOHYDRATE | 7 G FIBER | 16 G PROTEIN

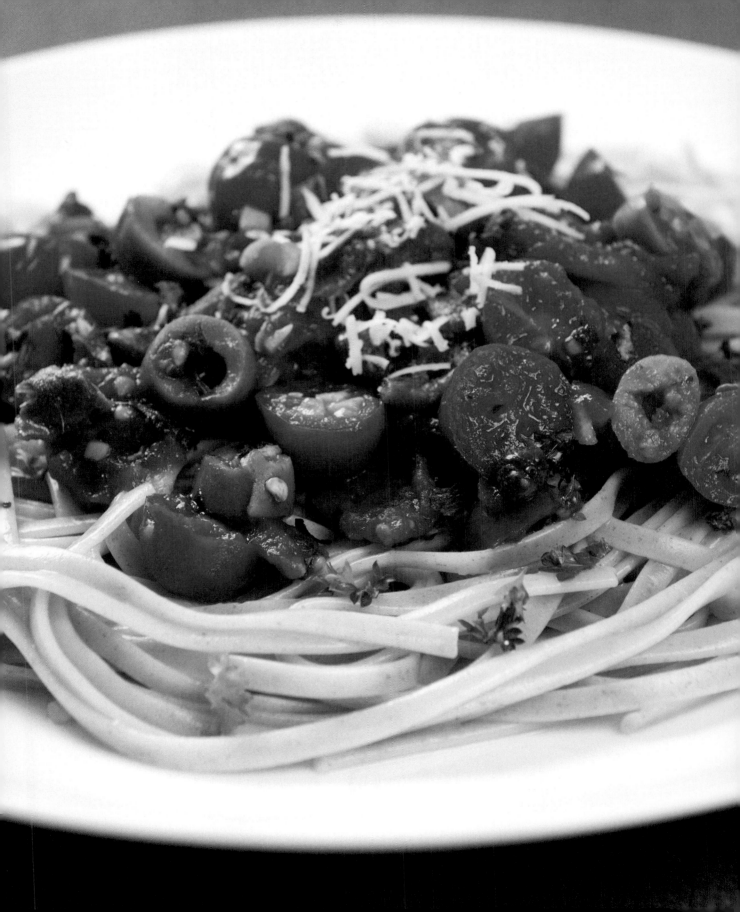

Baked Fusilli with Tomato-Meat Sauce & Ricotta

Fusilli al forno con ragù e ricotta

MY MOTHER-IN-LAW IS PROOF that even though her family emigrated several generations ago, the family and food of Italy are still entrenched in her life and culture. Her prowess in the kitchen, which has been shaped by her mother, Calabrian mother-in-law and nonnas, is evident in the many dishes she makes, including her lasagna with a rich Bolognese-type meat sauce and a creamy ricotta cheese center. It's now the basis for my equally loved pasta bake that, unlike many lasagnas, doesn't have to wait until the weekend to be made or enjoyed.

1 tsp	extra-virgin olive oil
10.5 oz	(300 g) lean ground turkey
2	cloves garlic, minced
½ cup	chopped onions
¼ tsp	fennel seeds
4 tbsp	no-salt-added tomato paste
1 cup	water
4 cups	no-salt-added tomato purée (passata)
2	bay leaves
¼ tsp	sea salt

Freshly ground black pepper to taste

16 oz	(454 g) whole-grain fusilli or gemelli pasta*
1 cup	part-skim ricotta cheese, drained
2 tbsp	freshly grated Parmigiano-Reggiano cheese

Freshly ground black pepper to taste

2 tbsp	shredded part-skim mozzarella
1 tbsp	chopped fresh basil

MAKE AHEAD Prepare meat sauce one or two days before and refrigerate until ready to use in recipe.

➤ In a deep non-stick skillet or medium pot, heat olive oil over medium-high heat. Add ground turkey and cook for 4 to 5 minutes, stirring often and breaking it up into smaller chunks. Add garlic, onions and fennel seeds; cook for 2 minutes more until onions are softened.

➤ Stir in tomato paste and water. Bring to a boil and stir in tomato purée, bay leaves, salt and pepper. Reduce heat to medium and simmer for 25 minutes, stirring occasionally. Remove and discard bay leaves.

➤ Preheat oven to 350°F.

➤ Bring a large pot of water to a boil and cook pasta al dente according to package directions (don't overcook).

➤ While pasta is cooking, prepare the ricotta filling. Combine ricotta, Parmigiano-Reggiano cheeses and black pepper in a medium bowl.

➤ Coat a deep 9 x 13-inch glass or ceramic baking dish with cooking spray. Add a ladle of meat sauce to the bottom of dish and spread out evenly.

➤ Drain pasta and toss with about 4 ladles of tomato pasta sauce. Ladle half of the pasta into the greased baking dish to create one layer. Drop half the ricotta mixture by heaping teaspoons over pasta layer. Add the rest of the pasta and top with remaining meat sauce, ricotta mixture, mozzarella and basil. Bake in preheated oven for 20 minutes. Let stand for 5 minutes before serving.

6 SERVINGS

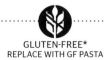
GLUTEN-FREE*
REPLACE WITH GF PASTA

MAKE AHEAD

PER SERVING 479 CALORIES | 9 G TOTAL FAT (4 G SATURATED FAT) | 45 MG CHOLESTEROL | 348 MG SODIUM | 77 G CARBOHYDRATE | 10 G FIBER | 29 G PROTEIN

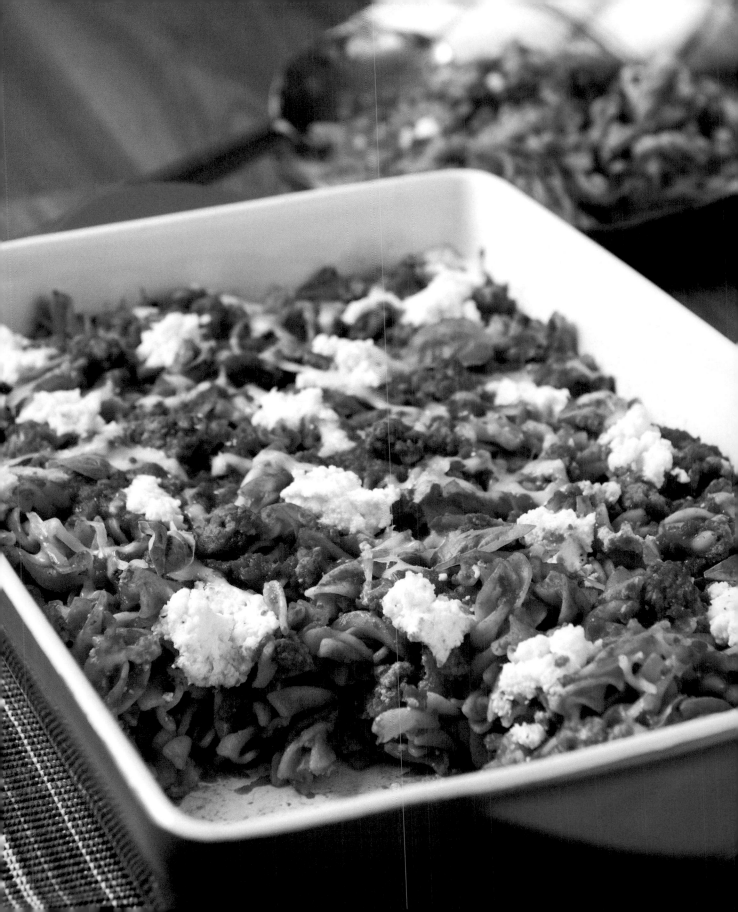

Pappardelle in a Wild Mushroom Sauce

Pappardelle ai funghi

WHEN MY FRIEND HILARY FIRST TASTED A PLATE of Pappardelle ai Funghi while visiting friends who were living the quintessential country lifestyle in Tuscany, she says it felt like she had won the lottery. Her hosts, who were phenomenal cooks in their own right (picture freshly baked fruit crostata, stuffed green peppers and homemade pasta in pesto), took a break from their kitchen and brought their guests to a nondescript eatery along the highway. Feeling adventurous, Hilary ordered Pappardelle al Cinghiale e Funghi (wide noodle pasta with wild boar sausage and mushrooms). "It was outstanding," she recalls of the experience. To recreate a similar dish (without the boar) *and* get the same reaction, I enlisted Hilary as my official taste tester for this recipe to make it as delicious as the way she remembers it.

1 oz	(28 g) dried porcini mushrooms
2 cups	boiled water
16 oz	(454 g) whole-grain pappardelle or tagliatelle or fresh whole-grain fettuccine pasta* (see tip)
2 tsp	extra-virgin olive oil
2 tsp	light butter
½ cup	chopped onions
2	cloves garlic, chopped
2 pkg	(16 oz/454 g) cremini or white button mushrooms, very thinly sliced
½ cup	white wine
½ cup	no-salt-added vegetable broth
3 tbsp	light (5%) sour cream
2 tbsp	chopped fresh parsley
¼ tsp	sea salt
Freshly ground black pepper to taste	
2 tbsp	freshly grated Parmigiano-Reggiano cheese

⇄ VARIATION Give this dish more depth by using a homemade chicken or turkey stock instead of a vegetable stock.

➤ To reconstitute dried porcini, soak them in boiled water for 15 minutes. Remove mushrooms from water (reserve liquid) and gently rinse them under warm water repeatedly, using your thumbs, until all the grit and sand have been removed. Drain mushrooms and slice thinly. Strain the dark water through a fine mesh sieve or coffee filter to remove grit. Discard water at the bottom of bowl with grit. You'll have about 1¾ cups of water left after removing mushrooms. Set aside mushrooms and water.

➤ Bring a large pot of water to a boil and cook pasta al dente according to package directions.

➤ In the meantime, heat olive oil and butter over medium-high heat in a large, deep non-stick skillet. Add onions and garlic and cook until onions are softened, about 1 to 2 minutes.

➤ Add reserved porcini mushrooms, cremini mushrooms and wine to skillet. Stir continuously until mushrooms are softened, about 3 to 4 minutes. Pour in reserved mushroom water and vegetable broth; bring to a gentle simmer. Whisk in sour cream. Stir in parsley, salt and pepper.

➤ Drain pasta, add to mushroom sauce and toss until well coated. Serve with freshly grated cheese.

TIP Pappardelle are broad, flat noodles resembling ribbons. If you can't find a whole-grain version, try whole-grain tagliatelle or fresh lasagna sheets cut into medallion strips.

5-6 SERVINGS 30 MIN OR LESS GLUTEN-FREE* REPLACE WITH GF PASTA MEATLESS

PER SERVING(6) 342 CALORIES | 6 G TOTAL FAT (2 G SATURATED FAT) | 7 MG CHOLESTEROL | 151 MG SODIUM | 57 G CARBOHYDRATE | 7 G FIBER | 14 G PROTEIN

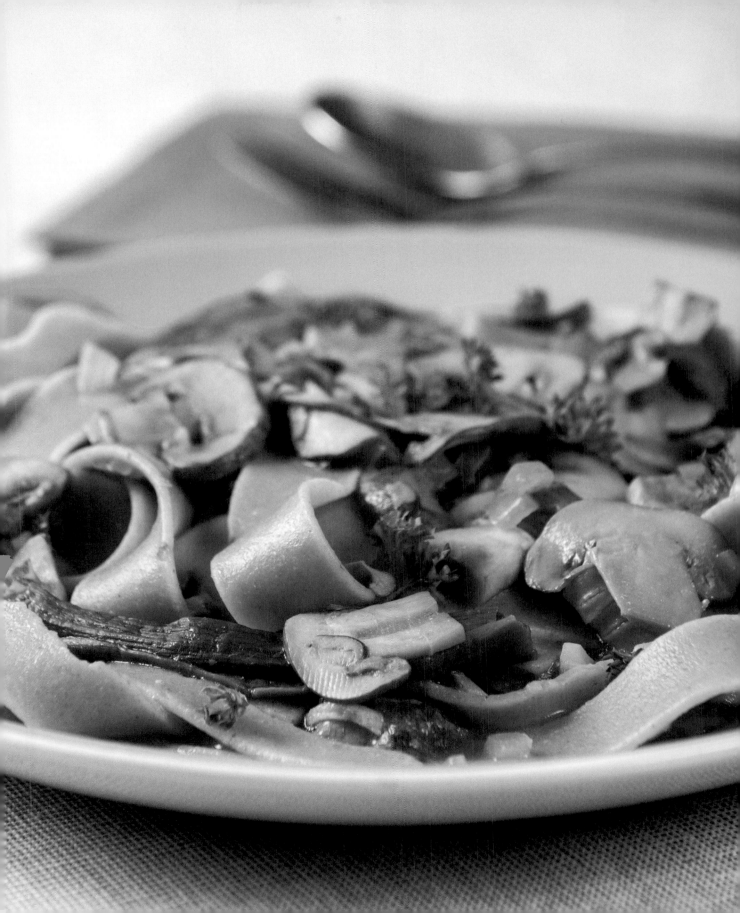

Cavatappi in a Creamy Salmon Sauce
Cavatappi al salmone

THE ABUNDANCE OF SALMON IN OUR RIVERS AND OCEANS makes the fish a common North American seafood delight. Salmon's versatility makes it a favorite in other cuisines, too. Native Italians love to toss it into pasta. So does my sister's family who can't get enough of salmon and are always looking for ways to add it into their meals — grilled, broiled, tossed in a salad, even raw in sushi. This recipe gets their undivided attention.

12 oz	(340 g) vegetable cavatappi pasta* (see tip)
12 oz	(340 g) boneless, skinless salmon fillet (see tip)
	Sea salt and freshly ground black pepper to taste
1 tsp	extra-virgin olive oil
½ cup	white wine
½ cup	chopped green onions
4 tbsp	light cream cheese
1½ tbsp	no-salt-added tomato paste
1 cup	1% milk
Pinch	ground nutmeg
	Sea salt and freshly ground black pepper to taste
2 tbsp	chopped fresh parsley

TIPS You can also use a brown rice short-shaped pasta for this dish but my kids love the corkscrew shape of cavatappi. I use a high-fiber durum wheat pasta made with dehydrated vegetables.
➤ To remove the skin from a salmon fillet, carefully position a sharp knife between the flesh and the skin of the fish; use your free hand to gently pull off the skin while holding down the flesh with the flat side of the knife.

➤ Bring a large pot of water to a boil. Cook pasta al dente according to package directions.

➤ Cut salmon into two or three large pieces. Season with salt and pepper.

➤ In a large non-stick skillet, heat olive oil over medium-high heat. Add salmon fillets and cook for 3 to 4 minutes on each side, until fish is easily flaked at the edges with a fork. Break up the large pieces into smaller bite-sized pieces. Don't worry if the middle sections are still not fully cooked; they'll cook further in the sauce and you don't want to dry them out. Pour in wine and add green onions; cook until onions are softened, about 1 to 2 minutes. Reduce heat to medium-low. Stir in cream cheese, tomato paste and milk until well incorporated and simmer for 2 more minutes. Add nutmeg, salt and pepper. Keep warm.

➤ Drain pasta and toss in salmon sauce until well coated. Serve sprinkled with parsley.

⌂ HIGH IN...OMEGA-3 FATTY ACIDS

Next to anchovies, salmon (the wild type specifically) has the highest concentration of omega-3 fatty acids of any fish source. In fact, it has two of the most crucial types of omega 3s — eicosapentaenoic acid (EPA) and docosahexaenoic (DHA), which are credited with lowering the risk of certain cancers, heart disease, hypertension, rheumatoid arthritis and depression. In this dish, one serving offers about 1,500 milligrams of omega-3s. Salmon is also high in protein, potassium and a range of B vitamins — all of which are contributors to a healthy cardiovascular system. Opt for wild-caught salmon versus farmed salmon, which can have considerably more fat and may not be environmentally friendly.

 4 SERVINGS   30 MIN OR LESS   GLUTEN-FREE* REPLACE WITH GF PASTA   MEATLESS

PER SERVING 504 CALORIES | 9 G TOTAL FAT (3 G SATURATED FAT) | 53 MG CHOLESTEROL | 174 MG SODIUM | 70 G CARBOHYDRATE | 5 G FIBER | 29 G PROTEIN

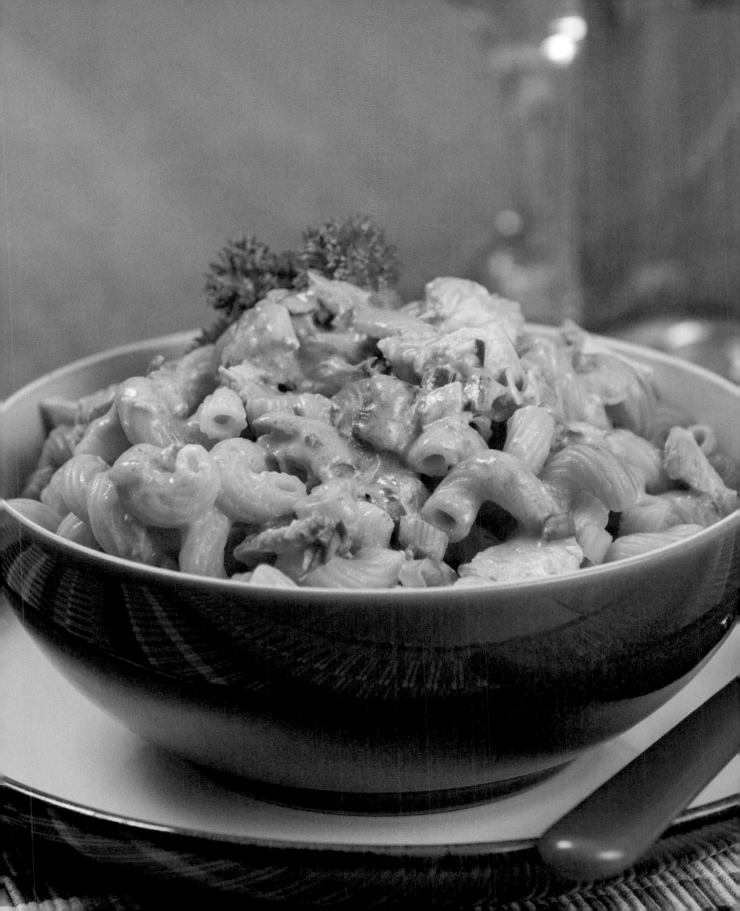

Macaroni with Ricotta & Cherry Tomatoes

Macaroni con ricotta e pomodorini

THERE IS HARDLY A PASTA DISH THAT MY KIDS SAY NO TO, ALTHOUGH I ADMIT, sometimes they pick out their least favorite veggies if the recipe calls for them. But if I had to label a classic with guaranteed appeal, it's this one, a sort-of equivalent to the fast mac and cheese my mom also made when we were kids as a quick lunch during school days (remember those days when we went home for lunch?). With a little bit of everything — healthy carbs, protein and vitamins — it scores as the ideal dish for devouring before running to soccer practice.

13 oz	(375 g) whole-grain macaroni or elbow pasta*
2 cups	cherry or grape tomatoes
2 tsp	extra-virgin olive oil
1	clove garlic, minced
½ tsp	Italian herb seasoning
¼ tsp + pinch sea salt	
1¼ cups	part-skim ricotta cheese (see tip)
1	egg white
2 tbsp	freshly grated Parmigiano-Reggiano cheese
2 tbsp	minced fresh basil
¼ tsp	ground nutmeg
¼ tsp	freshly ground black pepper

➤ Preheat oven to broil setting.

➤ Bring a large pot of water to a boil and cook pasta al dente according to package directions.

➤ In the meantime in a large bowl, coat cherry tomatoes with olive oil, garlic, Italian herb seasoning and pinch of salt.

➤ Line a baking sheet with foil paper, coated with cooking spray, and spread out seasoned tomatoes in a single layer. Cook 6 inches under broil element just until skins begin to break, about 4 to 5 minutes, stirring halfway through cooking. Set aside.

➤ Place ricotta in a medium bowl and use a fork to break apart any lumps. Stir in egg white, cheese, basil, nutmeg and ¼ tsp salt.

➤ Drain pasta, reserving a ladle of pasta water, and add pasta and reserved water back into pot over hot burner. Add in ricotta mixture and stir until pasta is well coated. Gently toss in broiled tomatoes and add black pepper. Serve hot with more grated cheese if desired.

TIP Choose a smooth ricotta for a creamier texture, or pulse in a food processor until desired consistency.

⇆ VARIATION Throw in a couple handfuls of fresh baby spinach leaves just before you stir in the ricotta.

    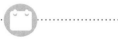

4 SERVINGS | 30 MIN OR LESS | GLUTEN-FREE* REPLACE WITH GF PASTA | MEATLESS

PER SERVING 476 CALORIES | 9 G TOTAL FAT (4 G SATURATED FAT) | 12 MG CHOLESTEROL | 262 MG SODIUM | 69 G CARBOHYDRATE | 4 G FIBER | 29 G PROTEIN

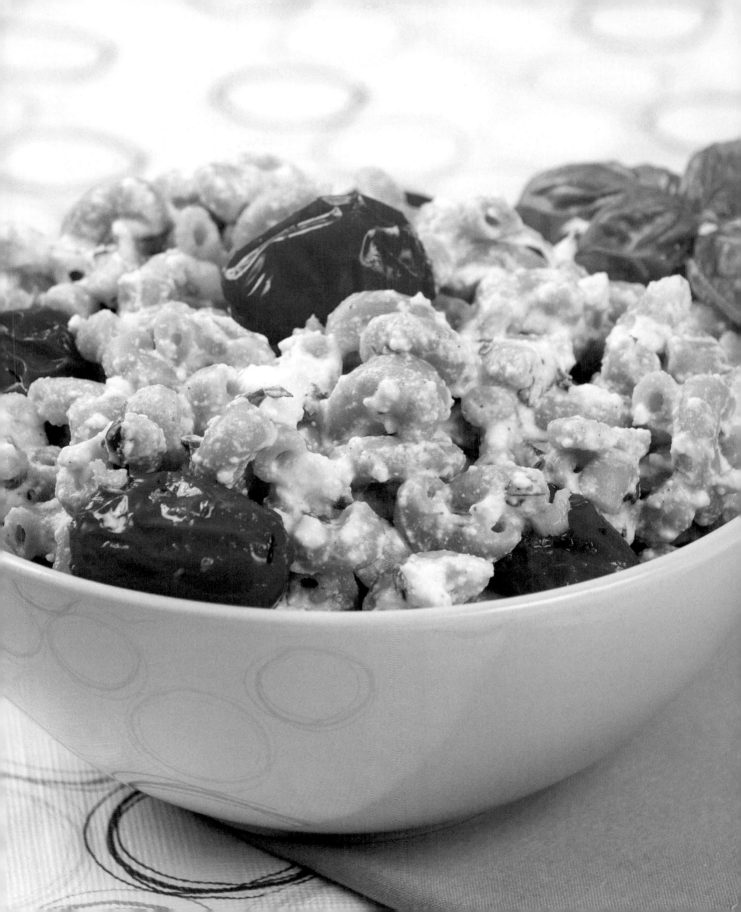

Mom's Lasagna
Lasagne della mamma

IT GOES WITHOUT SAYING THAT THIS IS *THE* DISH you can find being served at most of our family gatherings and has been since my mother left her native Sicily in 1961. As a little girl, I would wake up early on a Sunday morning to turn the handle on the pasta machine and churn out nearly see-through sheets of fresh pasta. They were then carefully transferred to a tablecloth to dry before being crafted into an eight-layer-high lasagna that resembled the leaning Tower of Pisa after landing on the dish. I'm no architect and neither are most passionate cooks (except for my friend Nancy) so I rely on thicker, store-bought fresh pasta for my lasagna for an easier and healthier alternative. Although my version doesn't have the height of my mom's iconic dish, it has the same unique taste that comes from combining sweet peas, boiled eggs, fresh tomato sauce, ground veal, fresh herbs — and lots of love.

1 tsp	extra-virgin olive oil
10.5 oz	(300 g) lean ground veal
½ cup	chopped onions
1	clove garlic, minced
¼ tsp	sea salt
Freshly ground black pepper to taste	
4 cups	prepared pasta sauce (*see recipe, page 10*)
1¼ cups	frozen green peas
6	sheets fresh whole-grain lasagne sheets like Olivieri (13 oz/360 g, each about 4.5 x 9 inch/11 x 23 cm)
2	hard-boiled eggs, finely chopped or grated
2 cups	packed shredded part-skim mozzarella (8 oz/225 g)
2 tbsp	freshly grated Parmigiano-Reggiano cheese

TIP You'll find fresh lasagne noodles in the refrigerated section of your grocery store. You can also use 12 uncooked dry lasagne noodles for this recipe. Replace 2 fresh lasagne sheets with 4 dry noodles.

MAKE AHEAD Prepare the sauce up to three or four days before assembling lasagna. You can boil your eggs the day before and refrigerate until ready to use.

➤ In a large pot, heat olive oil over medium-high heat. Add veal and cook for 5 minutes, stirring often and breaking chunks up into smaller pieces. Add onions and garlic and cook until onions are softened, about 2 minutes. Season with salt and pepper. Add prepared pasta sauce and peas to pot; simmer on low heat while preparing lasagna.

➤ Preheat oven to 350°F.

➤ To assemble the lasagna, blanch lasagne sheets in a pot of boiling water for 2 to 3 minutes.

➤ Coat an 8 x 12-inch baking pan with cooking spray. Spread about 1 cup of sauce evenly over bottom of pan. Place 2 lasagne sheets in pan and cover with 1 cup sauce, half the chopped eggs and one-third of the mozzarella. Repeat layer: 2 lasagne sheets, 1 cup sauce, half the chopped eggs and one-third of the mozzarella. Top with 2 lasagne sheets, 1 cup sauce and the remaining one-third mozzarella. Sprinkle with grated cheese.

➤ Cover tightly with foil paper and bake in preheated oven for 30 minutes. Set oven to broil setting. Remove foil and place the pan on the *middle* oven rack to broil for 3 to 4 minutes. Allow lasagna to cool for 5 minutes before cutting into 9 equal pieces before serving.

⌂ HIGH IN...PHYTONUTRIENTS

The phytonutrients in green peas make a big impact on health. Diets high in coumestrol and saponins (a sizable amount in just one of these servings), have been shown to ward off the risk of stomach cancer by as much as 50 percent. Other disease-fighting compounds like phenolic acids and flavonols act as impressive antioxidant and anti-inflammatory agents.

9 SERVINGS

MAKE AHEAD

PER SERVING 299 CALORIES | 9 G TOTAL FAT (4 G SATURATED FAT) | 98 MG CHOLESTEROL | 328 MG SODIUM | 36 G CARBOHYDRATE | 5 G FIBER | 19 G PROTEIN

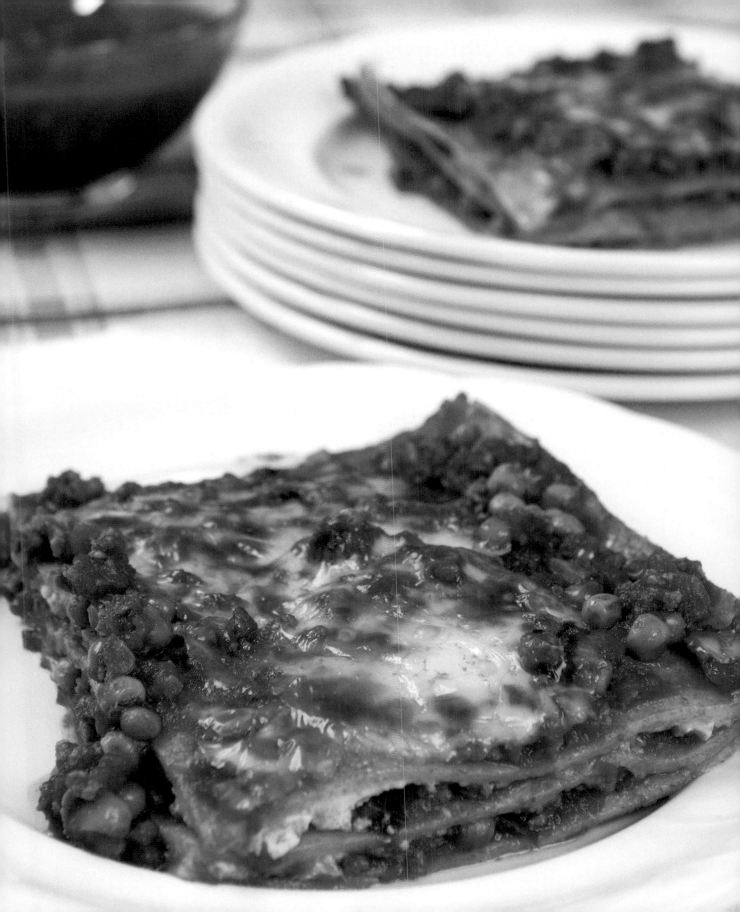

Asparagus Farro Risotto
Risotto di farro agli asparagi

WHEN MY TWIN SISTER was diagnosed with Celiac disease more than 20 years ago, our whole family had to learn to cook creatively without gluten. That was a huge feat for an Italian family whose main staples were pasta and bread. At the time, boxed gluten-free pastas were scarce — I made regular trips to the children's hospital, one of the few places in the city that sold gluten-free pastas. So, until Ma mastered making her own alternative pasta and pizza, we leaned on what we knew best and what tasted best in our home-cooking repertoire — risottos, traditionally made with high-starch Arborio rice and accompanied with either fragrant spices, vegetables or seafood. I've adapted what I learned then to make risottos with other healthy grains (not all gluten-free). The result: rich, creamy dishes with no compromise on taste or texture.

1	bunch asparagus, about 20 medium spears
3½ cups	reduced-sodium vegetable or chicken broth
2 tsp	extra-virgin olive oil
2 tsp	light butter
1	onion, chopped
1	clove garlic, chopped
1½ cups	semi-pearled farro (*see tip, page 210*)
½ cup	white wine
2 tbsp	crumbled light goat's cheese (1 oz/28 g)
2 tbsp	each: chopped fresh parsley and fresh basil
	Sea salt and freshly ground black pepper to taste
	Freshly grated Parmigiano-Reggiano cheese for serving (optional)

⇆ VARIATION Make this a spring-vegetable risotto with the addition of fresh peas and/or zucchini.

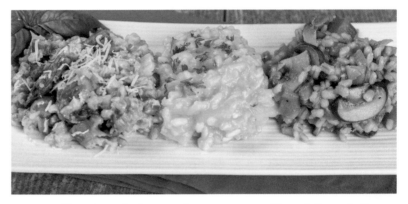

➤ Snap off tough ends from each asparagus stalk and discard. Cut asparagus into ¾-inch (2-cm) pieces and set aside.

➤ In a medium pot, heat broth over medium heat and keep hot.

➤ In a large pot, heat olive oil and butter over medium-high heat. Add onion and garlic and cook until onions are softened, about 1 to 2 minutes. Add farro and stir continuously to coat well, about 1 minute. Add wine and cook until almost completely absorbed, stirring continuously. Reduce heat to medium-low. Add half of the cut asparagus.

➤ Add hot broth slowly, one ladle at a time to allow liquid to be absorbed before adding more. Stir continuously for about 20 to 25 minutes or until farro is al dente and chewy. Add remaining asparagus about halfway through cooking.

➤ Stir in goat's cheese, parsley and basil. Serve hot with black pepper and a sprinkle of freshly grated cheese, if desired.

4 SERVINGS

40 MIN OR LESS

MEATLESS

PER SERVING 396 CALORIES | 7 G TOTAL FAT (2 G SATURATED FAT) | 5 MG CHOLESTEROL | 102 MG SODIUM | 60 G CARBOHYDRATE | 8 G FIBER | 16 G PROTEIN

Saffron Risotto
Risotto alla Milanese

5 cups	reduced-sodium vegetable broth
¼ tsp	pure ground saffron (see tip)
¾ cup	canned no-salt-added cannellini beans, drained and rinsed
2 tsp	each: extra-virgin olive oil and light butter
1	onion, chopped
1½ cups	arborio or carnaroli rice
½ cup	brown arborio or short-grain brown rice
½ cup	dry white wine
2 tbsp	freshly grated Parmigiano-Reggiano cheese
1 tbsp	each: chopped fresh parsley and fresh basil

Freshly ground black pepper to taste

➤ In a medium pot, heat broth over medium heat until hot. Sprinkle in saffron, stir and lower heat. Add 2 tbsp of broth along with navy beans to food processor and purée until the mixture forms a paste.

➤ In a large pot, heat olive oil and butter over medium-high heat. Add onion; cook until softened, about 2 minutes. Add rices and stir until well coated. Pour in wine and stir until almost fully absorbed. Reduce heat to low. Over the next 20 minutes, ladle in hot broth a little at a time, stirring regularly, until well absorbed. Before adding in the final ladle, stir in puréed beans until well incorporated. Remove risotto from heat, sprinkle with cheese and serve topped with fresh herbs and black pepper.

TIP To get ¼ tsp of saffron, use 2 pkg (each 0.125 g).

⌂ HIGH IN...FIBER

While the arborio rice used in the saffron risotto doesn't have the same amount of fiber as a brown rice, thin-skinned cannellini beans add a sizable dose of cholesterol-lowering soluble fiber. Both barley and farro have more than four times the amount of fiber in arborio rice and more than double the amount in brown rice.

 4-5 SERVINGS   30 MIN OR LESS   GLUTEN-FREE   MEATLESS

PER SERVING(5) 275 CALORIES | 5 G TOTAL FAT (2 G SATURATED FAT) | 9 MG CHOLESTEROL | 125 MG SODIUM | 44 G CARBOHYDRATE | 5 G FIBER | 8 G PROTEIN

Wild Mushroom Barley Risotto
Risotto d'orzo ai funghi porcini

0.5 oz	(14 g) dried porcini mushrooms
3 cups	reduced-sodium vegetable or chicken broth
1 tsp	each: extra-virgin olive oil and light butter
2	cloves garlic, minced
½ cup	chopped onions
1 cup	pearl barley
2 cups	peeled, cubed eggplant
1 pkg	(8 oz/227 g) cremini or white button or oyster mushrooms, thinly sliced, divided
¼ cup	white wine
¼ tsp	sea salt
4 tbsp	freshly grated Asiago cheese
3 tbsp	chopped fresh basil

Freshly ground black pepper to taste

➤ Reconstitute porcini mushrooms by soaking in 1½ cups boiled water for 10 minutes. Remove mushrooms from water (reserve water) and rinse them under warm water, using your thumbs, until all the grit has been removed. Drain and chop; set mushrooms aside. Strain mushroom water through a fine mesh sieve to remove grit. Combine mushroom water (discard grit at the bottom of bowl) with broth.

➤ In a large pot, heat olive oil and butter over medium-high heat. Add garlic and onions and cook until onions are softened, about 1 minute. Add barley and stir until well coated. Stir in eggplant, half the cremini mushrooms, wine and salt; cook for 1 to 2 more minutes, until wine is almost absorbed. Reduce heat to medium-low.

➤ Add a ladle of broth at a time to large pot until liquid is absorbed. Cook for about 20 to 25 minutes or until barley is al dente, stirring occasionally. Add remaining mushrooms about halfway through cooking. Stir in cheese, basil and pepper. Serve.

 4 SERVINGS   40 MIN OR LESS   MEATLESS

PER SERVING 325 CALORIES | 8 G TOTAL FAT (4 G SATURATED FAT) | 15 MG CHOLESTEROL | 383 MG SODIUM | 50 G CARBOHYDRATE | 10 G FIBER | 14 G PROTEIN

Spaghetti Carbonara with Zucchini Threads

Spaghetti alla carbonara con zucchine

I HAVE A CONFESSION — my husband almost always prefers a red sauce on his pasta, so making a pasta dish without it can be a tricky proposition. These recipes seem to be the exception. I owe my comfort level when combining veggies with pasta to my family history — in part, you might say it's good genes that had my siblings and I eating our veggies from early on, but I think the bigger influence has been my dad's practice of coming home from work at the grocery store with bags of both conventional and unusual vegetables to tinker with in the kitchen. When he got home, he'd pile up the grocery bags on the landing and we'd each grab one and drag it to the kitchen where produce would get its spotlight, either in a popular pairing, like the cauliflower and broccoli dish (right), or solo, added to a traditional recipe like Spaghetti Carbonara.

13 oz	(375 g) whole-grain or brown rice spaghetti*
2	large slices peameal/Canadian bacon (about 3.5 oz/100 g)
3	cloves garlic, chopped
¾ cup	reduced-sodium chicken broth
3	large eggs
¼ cup	light (5%) sour cream
4 tbsp	freshly grated Parmigiano-Reggiano cheese
1 tbsp	light butter, melted
½ tsp	freshly cracked black pepper
¼ tsp	sea salt
1	small zucchini, cut into matchsticks (julienne)
2 tbsp	minced fresh parsley for garnish

Crushed red pepper flakes (optional)

⇆ **VARIATION** Substitute 5 asparagus stalks for 1 small zucchini. Snap ends off asparagus and cut into matchsticks. Follow the same directions.

➤ Bring a large pot of water to a boil and cook spaghetti al dente according to package directions.

➤ In the meantime, coat a non-stick skillet with cooking spray, heat over medium-high heat and add bacon slices. Cook peameal bacon about 2 minutes on each side. Remove from pan, chop cooked bacon into small cubes, add back to skillet and cook with garlic until browned, about 2 more minutes. Remove from skillet and reserve. You want to keep the bacon crisp as you'll be adding it in at the very end. Pour chicken broth into skillet and cook just until heated through. Set aside and keep hot.

➤ In a large bowl, whisk together eggs until silky. Add sour cream, grated cheese, melted butter, pepper, salt and hot broth and whisk thoroughly. (The hot broth tempers the eggs so they don't clump up when you pour them over the pasta.)

➤ During the last 3 minutes of the pasta's cooking time, add zucchini to the pasta pot. Drain pasta and zucchini and return them to pot. Reduce heat to low and return pot to burner. Pour egg mixture over cooked pasta and toss very quickly to coat evenly. Add bacon and garlic and toss for 1 more minute. Sprinkle with parsley and crushed red pepper flakes, if using. Serve immediately.

↻ LOW IN...FAT

A carbonara dish prepared with pancetta, table cream and extra eggs dumps 7 grams more fat and double the amount of saturated fat than this recipe. Peameal (also known as Canadian bacon) is much leaner than its Italian counterpart.

5 SERVINGS

30 MIN OR LESS

GLUTEN-FREE*
REPLACE WITH GF PASTA

PER SERVING 399 CALORIES | 10 G TOTAL FAT (4 G SATURATED FAT) | 133 MG CHOLESTEROL | 395 MG SODIUM | 60 G CARBOHYDRATE | 6 G FIBER | 22 G PROTEIN

Rotini with Broccoli, Cauliflower & Sun-Dried Tomatoes

Rotini con broccoli, cavolfiore e pomodori secchi

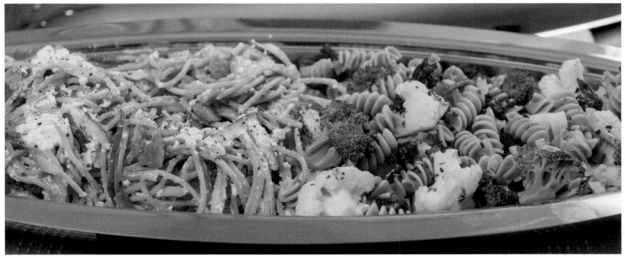

2 cups	chopped broccoli
2 cups	chopped cauliflower
13 oz	(375 g) whole-grain or brown rice rotini pasta*
2 tbsp	extra-virgin olive oil, divided
½ cup	chopped onions
2	cloves garlic, minced
½ cup	reduced-sodium vegetable or chicken broth
1 cup	sun-dried tomatoes, reconstituted and cut into strips (3 oz/85 g)
4 tbsp	chopped fresh basil
2 tbsp	freshly grated Parmigiano-Reggiano cheese
Sea salt to taste	
Pinch	crushed red pepper flakes

➤ Trim tough ends from broccoli and cauliflower. Cut tender portions into bite-sized pieces. In a medium pot, cook broccoli and caulflower in boiling water until tender-crisp, about 2 to 3 minutes. Drain well and set aside.

➤ Bring a large pot of water to a boil and cook rotini al dente according to package directions. (You can use the same water you used to boil the broccoli and cauliflower for more flavour. Be sure to top it up so it's enough for the pasta to cook.)

➤ In a large non-stick skillet, heat 1 tbsp oil over medium-high heat. Add onions and garlic and cook until onions are softened, about 2 minutes. Add parboiled broccoli and cauliflower, broth and sun-dried tomatoes until well combined and heated through.

➤ Drain pasta, bring pasta and broccoli-cauli mixture to pot, mixing well. Add remaining olive oil, basil, grated cheese and season with salt and crushed red pepper flakes. Serve immediately with extra grated cheese, if desired.

 4-5 SERVINGS   30 MIN OR LESS   GLUTEN-FREE* USE GF PASTA   MEATLESS

PER SERVING(5) 374 CALORIES | 8 G TOTAL FAT (2 G SATURATED FAT) | 2 MG CHOLESTEROL | 250 MG SODIUM | 68 G CARBOHYDRATE | 9 G FIBER | 16 G PROTEIN

White Lasagna with Asparagus & Ham

Lasagne bianche con asparagi e prosciutto cotto

WHEN LASAGNA WAS ON THE MENU and mom was short on time, we would make a trip to the nearby fresh noodle store. (Yes, we were lucky to have one in our neighborhood!) As we waited in line, we could see long layers of semolina pasta sheets come off the industrial rollers, to be cut into all sorts of shapes. The lasagne sheets were custom cut and ready to be smothered in a homemade sauce. With so much convenience, I learned to make lasagna of all types, including this lasagna *bianca* — it's both a convenient meal that tucks fresh ingredients in between cheesy layers and boasts an elegant presentation, whether for a weeknight meal or a dinner party.

1	large bunch asparagus, about 25 spears
1 tsp	extra-virgin olive oil
3	cloves garlic, minced
Sea salt and freshly ground black pepper to taste	
6 slices	reduced-sodium extra-lean deli-style prosciutto cotto or ham (4 oz/110 g)
16	dry lasagne noodles (about 12.5 oz/350 g)
1½ cups	packed shredded part-skim mozzarella (6 oz/170 g)
2 tbsp	freshly grated Parmigiano-Reggiano cheese

Sauce

1	recipe Béchamel Sauce (*see page 16*)
¼ cup	reduced-sodium chicken broth
1 tbsp	chopped fresh basil

➤ Snap off tough ends from each asparagus stalk and cut into long pieces, about 3 pieces per stalk. In a large non-stick skillet, heat olive oil on medium-high heat. Add garlic and cook for 1 minute. Add asparagus, salt and pepper and cook until asparagus is bright green and tender-crisp, about 2 to 3 minutes. Set aside. Cut ham into cubes, about 1 x 1-inch (2.5 x 2.5-cm) pieces.

➤ Prepare Béchamel Sauce, as per directions in recipe. Stir chicken broth and basil into sauce. Keep warm.

➤ Preheat oven to 350°F.

➤ To prepare lasagna, blanch lasagne sheets in a pot of boiling water for 2 to 3 minutes. Drain and let sit in cold water. Lightly coat a 9 x 13-inch baking pan with cooking spray. Spread ½ cup of sauce over the bottom of the baking pan. Lay 4 lasagne sheets (trim pasta to fit) in pan and spread ¼ cup of sauce over noodles. Top with one-quarter of the chopped ham, one-third of the asparagus and one-quarter of the mozzarella. Repeat layers two more times: 4 lasagne sheets, ¼ cup of sauce, one-quarter of the chopped ham, one-third of the asparagus and one-quarter of the mozzarella. Place final layer: 4 lasagne sheets, remaining sauce, ham and mozzarella.

➤ Cover lasagna with parchment paper (so cheese doesn't stick), then wrap tightly with foil paper and bake in preheated oven for 30 minutes. Reset oven to broil setting. Remove foil and parchment and place the pan on the *middle* oven rack to broil for 3 to 4 minutes. Let stand for 5 minutes before cutting into 9 equal pieces before serving.

⇆ **VARIATION** Make this a meatless lasagna by substituting ½ cup of thinly sliced grilled portobello mushrooms for the ham and replacing chicken broth with vegetable broth.

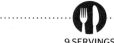

9 SERVINGS

MEATLESS (SEE VARIATION)

PER SERVING 303 CALORIES | 9 G TOTAL FAT (5 G SATURATED FAT) | 30 MG CHOLESTEROL | 386 MG SODIUM | 39 G CARBOHYDRATE | 5 G FIBER | 17 G PROTEIN

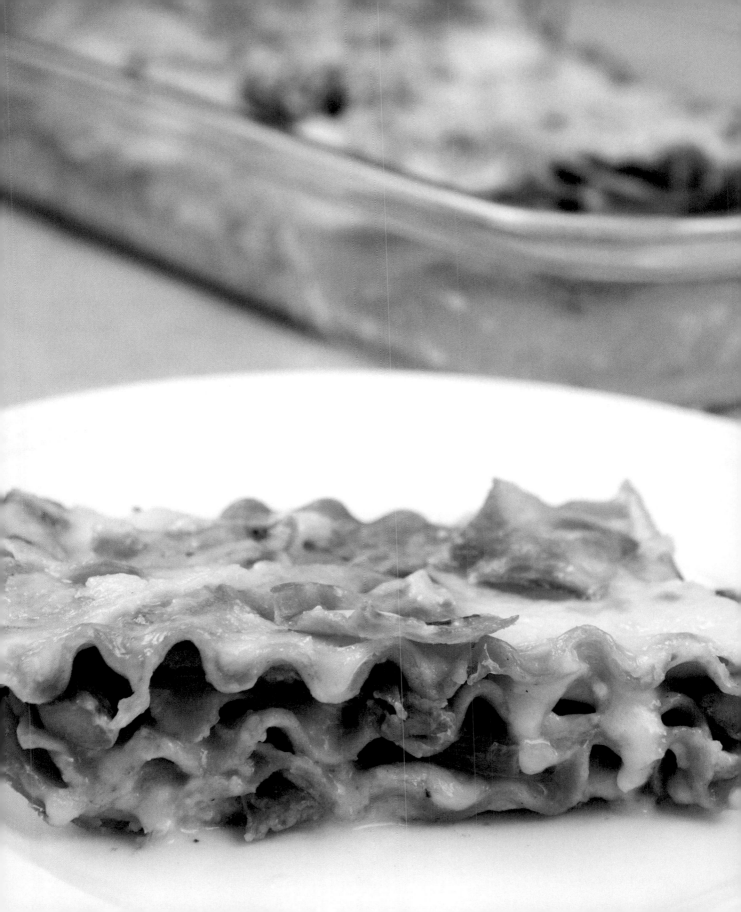

Fettuccine with Trapanese Pesto

Fettuccine con pesto alla Trapanese

ADDING FRAGRANT INGREDIENTS TO TRADITIONAL AROMATIC BASIL PESTO can only make it better. At least that's what the people of Trapani thought when crewmen from the northern region of Liguria brought their signature basil pesto into the port city in Sicily centuries ago. The Trapanesi quickly adopted it and added their own local ingredients — tomatoes and almonds — to make their own delectable version. I've taken their lead and made the recipe my own by bolstering this flavorful pesto with arugula for a peppery note and added health benefits. My family likes that history has repeated itself, and I'm grateful to have one more super-easy meal in my culinary bag of tricks.

¼ cup	slivered almonds
2 cups	ripe grape or cherry tomatoes, about (10.5 oz/ 300 g)
½ cup	packed fresh basil leaves
¼ cup	packed baby arugula leaves
1 tbsp	extra-virgin olive oil
3 tbsp	freshly grated Pecorino Romano cheese (see tip)
2	cloves garlic, coarsely chopped
¼ tsp	sea salt
Freshly ground black pepper to taste	
13 oz	(375 g) whole-grain fettuccine pasta*

➤ Preheat oven to 350°F. Place almonds on a baking sheet and toast in oven for 7 to 8 minutes, until lightly golden.

➤ In the meantime, bring a large pot of water to a boil. Add cherry tomatoes and scald for 2 to 3 minutes or just until skins begin to break. Use a strainer to scoop out tomatoes and let drain in a colander.

➤ Place tomatoes, almonds, basil, arugula, olive oil, grated cheese, garlic, salt and pepper into the bowl of a food processor and whirl until smooth.

➤ Bring a pot of water back to a boil and cook pasta al dente according to package directions. Drain pasta, reserving a couple ladles of pasta water. Toss with pesto and some pasta water, if pasta is dry, and serve.

TIP I use Pecorino Romano, made with sheep's milk, in this dish for its sharper taste.

4-5 SERVINGS

30 MIN OR LESS

GLUTEN-FREE*
REPLACE WITH GF PASTA

MEATLESS

PER SERVING(5) 352 CALORIES | 8 G TOTAL FAT (2 G SATURATED FAT) | 4 MG CHOLESTEROL | 163 MG SODIUM | 58 G CARBOHYDRATE | 9 G FIBER | 13 G PROTEIN

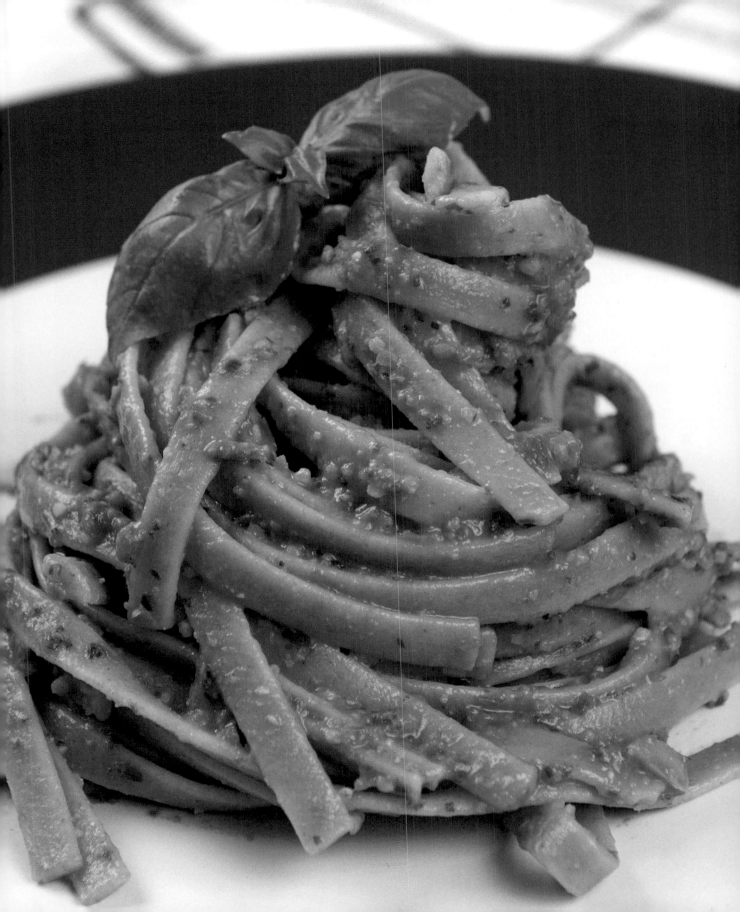

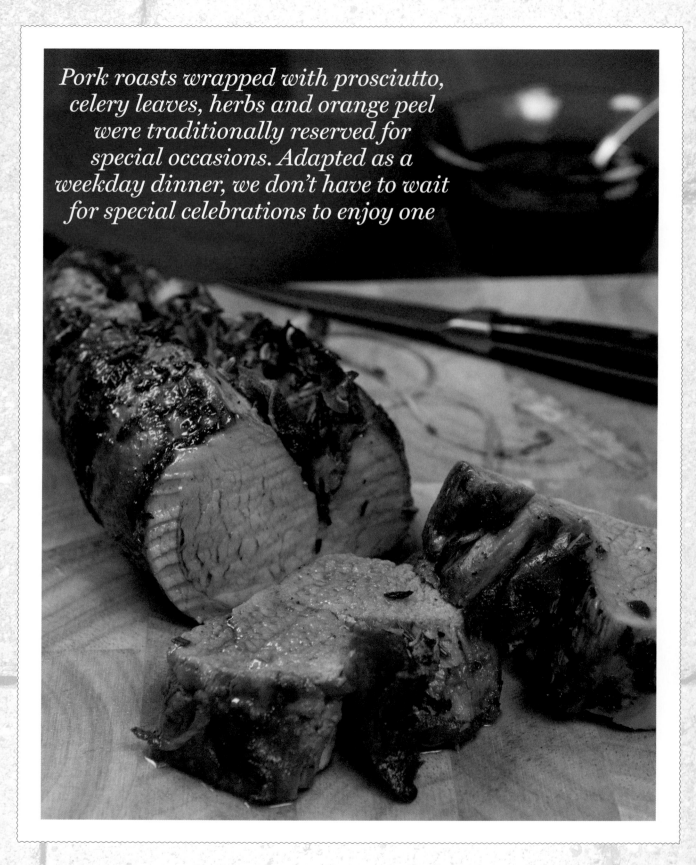

Pork roasts wrapped with prosciutto, celery leaves, herbs and orange peel were traditionally reserved for special occasions. Adapted as a weekday dinner, we don't have to wait for special celebrations to enjoy one

Meats, Fish & Meatless Mains

Carni, pesce e secondi vegetariani

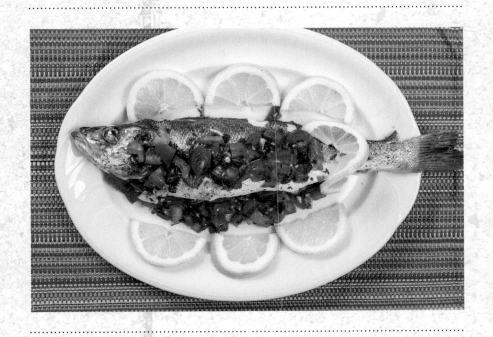

Freshly squeezed lemon, capers and anchovies have always been part of my culinary lexicon

Chicken Cacciatore
Pollo alla cacciatora

THIS HEARTY ONE-SKILLET DISH features a mix of ingredients once whipped up to feed hungry hunters who brought home the day's catch along with whatever ingredients they could scrounge up in the woods, hence the word *cacciatore*, meaning "hunter." I like to let my own little hunters — the kids — pull out their own vegetable treasures from the fridge to either substitute or add to this dish.

8	boneless skinless chicken thighs (about 1¼ lbs/565 g)
Sea salt and freshly ground black pepper to taste	
2 tsp	extra-virgin olive oil
1	onion, diced
2	cloves garlic, minced
2 cups	quartered white button mushrooms
½ cup	dry white wine or beer
2 cups	canned no-salt-added diced tomatoes with juice
2 tbsp	no-salt-added tomato paste
¾ cup	reduced-sodium chicken broth
1 tsp	Italian herb seasoning
¼ cup	pitted black olives, rinsed and drained (see tip)
1 tbsp	capers in brine, rinsed and patted dry
1 tbsp	each: chopped fresh parsley and fresh basil

➤ Trim excess fat from chicken thighs. Season pieces with salt and pepper. In a large non-stick skillet, heat olive oil over high heat and sear pieces until browned, about 2 to 3 minutes per side. Remove from skillet, set aside and keep warm.

➤ Reduce heat to medium-high. Add onion, garlic and mushrooms to skillet, stirring to incorporate any pan scrapings while vegetables soften, about 2 minutes. Add wine and let simmer until liquid is reduced to about half. Stir in diced tomatoes with juice, tomato paste, broth and Italian herb seasoning. Bring to a gentle boil.

➤ Return the cooked chicken pieces to the pan, submerging them in tomato-mushroom mixture. Sprinkle in olives, cover and simmer for 20 minutes on medium heat. Add capers and fresh herbs and cook for 1 more minute before serving.

➤ Transfer chicken to a serving platter and spoon sauce over chicken pieces. Serve with plain pasta, rice or crusty bread.

TIPS I like the taste of dry-cured black olives (rinsed well) in this dish. To release their pits, place olives on a cutting board and gently pound them (a ceramic cup works!).
➤ The chunky, flavorful sauce makes it ideal for dunking with bread or covering pasta or rice.

↻ LOW IN...**FAT**

This traditional dish is typically prepared with a variety of both white and dark chicken pieces. Here, juicier skinless chicken thighs are a healthier alternative — with only 9 grams of fat per piece, they offer more nutrients than white meat alone, including more iron and zinc, and less fat than skinned pieces. Skinned thighs, legs and wings can add up to four or five times more fat than skinless thighs.

  4 SERVINGS   **30 MIN OR LESS**   **GLUTEN-FREE**

PER SERVING 261 CALORIES I 11 G TOTAL FAT (2 G SATURATED FAT) I 120 MG CHOLESTEROL I 278 MG SODIUM I 14 G CARBOHYDRATE I 3 G FIBER I 21 G PROTEIN

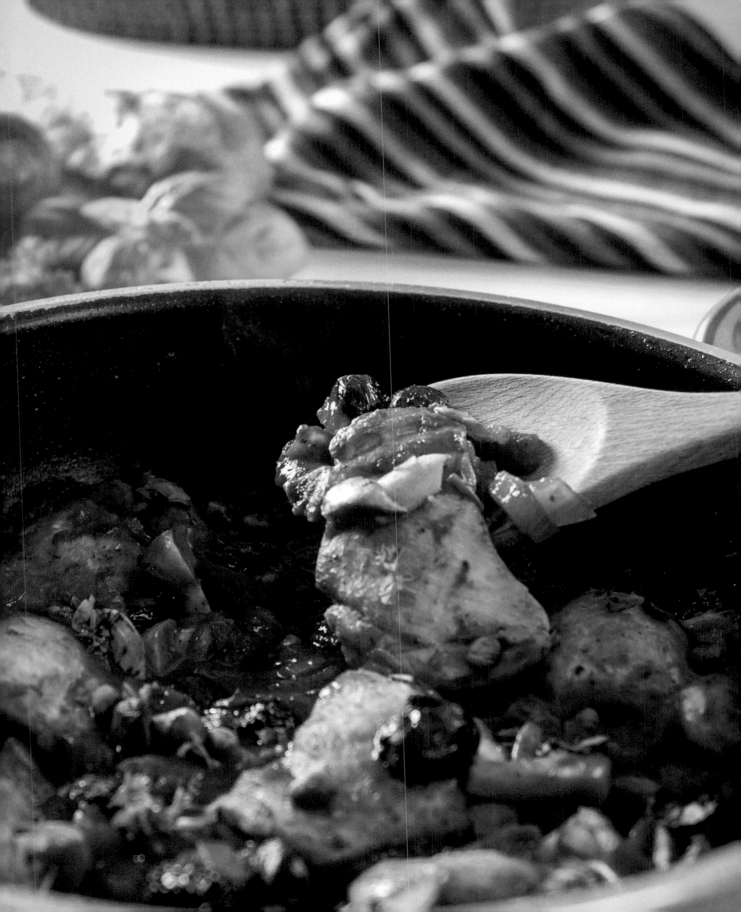

Chicken Marsala

Pollo al marsala

IF YOU'VE NEVER COOKED WITH MARSALA, you're in for a sweet surprise. I've enjoyed the fortified wine — which hails from the city of Marsala on the sun-drenched island of Sicily — in everything from saucy meat dishes to decadent desserts to my mom's morning "protein" shakes (don't ask!). The point is, its distinctively sweet taste makes it a perfect pairing in sauces with meats. And this one is no exception.

4	skinless boneless chicken breasts (about 1½ lbs/680 g or about 6 oz each)
Sea salt and freshly ground black pepper to taste	
1 tsp	high-oleic sunflower or safflower oil
2 tsp	light butter
2 cups	chopped leeks
¾ cup	Marsala wine (see tip)
¾ cup	no-salt-added chicken broth
¼ tsp	sea salt
1 tbsp	cornstarch
3 tbsp	light (5%) cream
½ tsp	Italian herb seasoning

➤ Butterfly cut chicken breasts in half horizontally so you have 8 thin cuts of chicken breast. With a mallet, gently pound the breast meat and season with salt and pepper.

➤ In a very large non-stick skillet, heat oil on high heat. Sear chicken breasts until lightly browned, about 2 to 3 minutes per side. (Cook in batches if your pan isn't large enough.) Remove and keep warm.

➤ Using the same pan, heat butter over medium heat until melted. Add leeks, scraping up pan drippings, and cook for 2 minutes. Stir in marsala and simmer until slightly reduced, about 2 more minutes. Add chicken broth and salt and return chicken pieces to pan, scooping some of the leeks on top of breasts. Simmer for 5 minutes.

➤ Whisk cornstarch with light cream until cornstarch is dissolved. Pour evenly into pan, sprinkle in Italian herb seasoning and turn chicken pieces while stirring the sauce. Reduce heat to low and let simmer for 2 more minutes or until chicken is tender and no longer pink in the center. Serve hot with whole-grain pasta or brown rice and a salad.

TIP Marsala is similar to port, Madeira or sherry and comes in two main varieties. Use a dry variety in savory dishes like this one. Reserve sweet Marsala for dessert recipes.

⌂ HIGH IN...VITAMIN K

Like other members of the allium family of vegetables — onions, garlic, scallions — leeks are an excellent source of vitamin K, which helps to regulate cholesterol levels in the blood and increase bone density. While the body makes its own resources, the bacteria in your intestines that make vitamin K can become depleted in some instances. One serving of this recipe offers 25 percent of the daily recommended value of vitamin K.

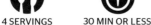

4 SERVINGS   30 MIN OR LESS   GLUTEN-FREE

PER SERVING 289 CALORIES | 7 G TOTAL FAT (3 G SATURATED FAT) | 78 MG CHOLESTEROL | 221 MG SODIUM | 16 G CARBOHYDRATE | 1 G FIBER | 29 G PROTEIN

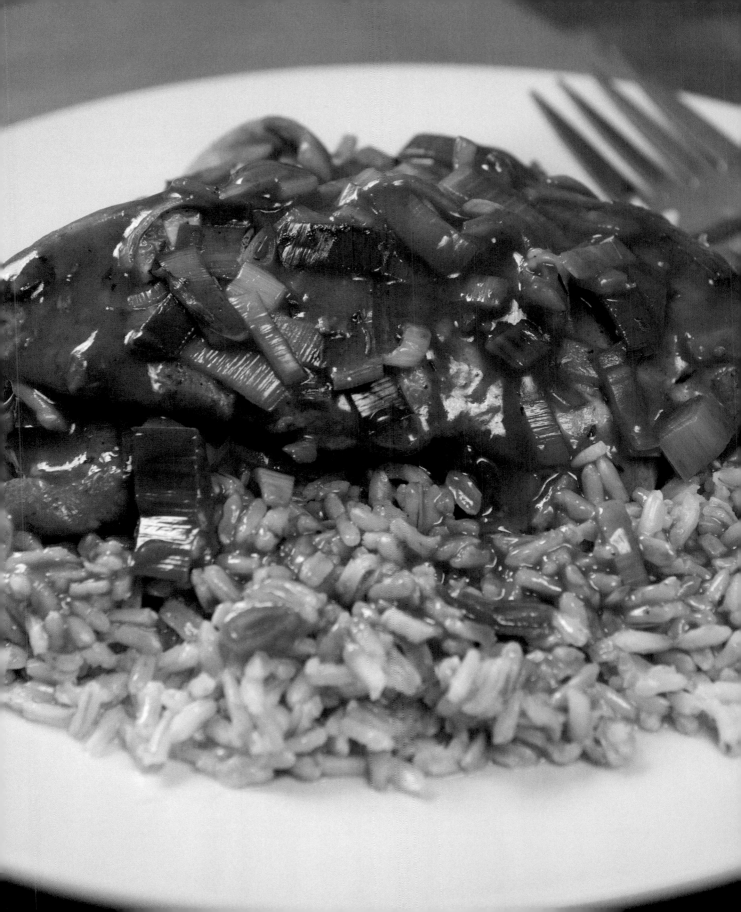

Turkey Saltimbocca
Saltimbocca di tacchino

THIS IS NO TYPICAL TURKEY DINNER, not that my family minds the traditional fare and all the fixings, but that's a labour of love that takes hours to cook, while this dish is prepared to "jump in your mouth" as its name suggests. This skillet meal — using turkey instead of veal as the main star — does a brief dance in the pan and lands in your plate in a flash. That's what I call having your turkey and eating it, too, within minutes.

4 to 6	very thin slices prosciutto (about 1.5 oz/35 g)
4 to 6	turkey scallopini cutlets (1 lb/454 g total), (see tip)
8 to 12	fresh sage leaves
2 tsp	extra-virgin olive oil, divided
2 tsp	light butter, divided
¼ cup	white wine
½ tsp	cornstarch
¼ cup	no-salt-added chicken broth

Sea salt and freshly ground black pepper to taste

➤ On a clean working surface, gently press a piece of prosciutto on top of each turkey cutlet. Lay a couple of sage leaves in the center of each cutlet and secure them by weaving a toothpick in and out of the cutlet.

➤ You'll be cooking the cutlets in two batches. In a large non-stick skillet, heat half the olive oil and butter over medium heat. Place 2 to 3 of the cutlets in the pan, prosciutto-side down, and cook until prosciutto is crispy and slightly browned, about 3 to 4 minutes. Turn cutlet over and cook just until no longer pink, about 2 minutes. Don't overcook or they'll be tough. Transfer cutlets to a serving dish, remove toothpicks (be careful, they're hot!) and keep warm while preparing other cutlets and sauce. Repeat with remaining cutlets.

➤ In the same skillet, heat the white wine on medium heat for 2 minutes, scraping up the bits at the bottom of the pan. In a cup, whisk together the cornstarch and broth and pour into skillet with wine. Season with salt and pepper. Whisk sauce until smooth and bubbly. Pour sauce over turkey cutlets and serve. There's a reason why this recipe is called "saltimbocca" — you'll want to eat it up within minutes of coming out of the pan.

TIP If you're having trouble finding scallopini at the meat counter, buy turkey breasts, cut them into thin slices (about ¼ inch/0.5 cm thick) and gently pound them with a mallet.

⇆ VARIATION Add some antioxidant oomph by tossing in one or two handfuls of frozen mixed vegetables (peas and carrots are perfect) at the same time you stir in the chicken broth to make the accompanying sauce.

⌒ HIGH IN...LEAN PROTEIN

A single serving of turkey breast, which is used to make these scallopini, contains about 25 grams of protein and only 1 gram of fat and 110 calories, making it a rich source of high-quality lean protein. It also offers about 50 percent of the recommended daily intake of protein for adults.

4 SERVINGS   30 MIN OR LESS   GLUTEN-FREE

PER SERVING 184 CALORIES | 5 G TOTAL FAT (1 G SATURATED FAT) | 85 MG CHOLESTEROL | 258 MG SODIUM | 1 G CARBOHYDRATE | 0 G FIBER | 31 G PROTEIN

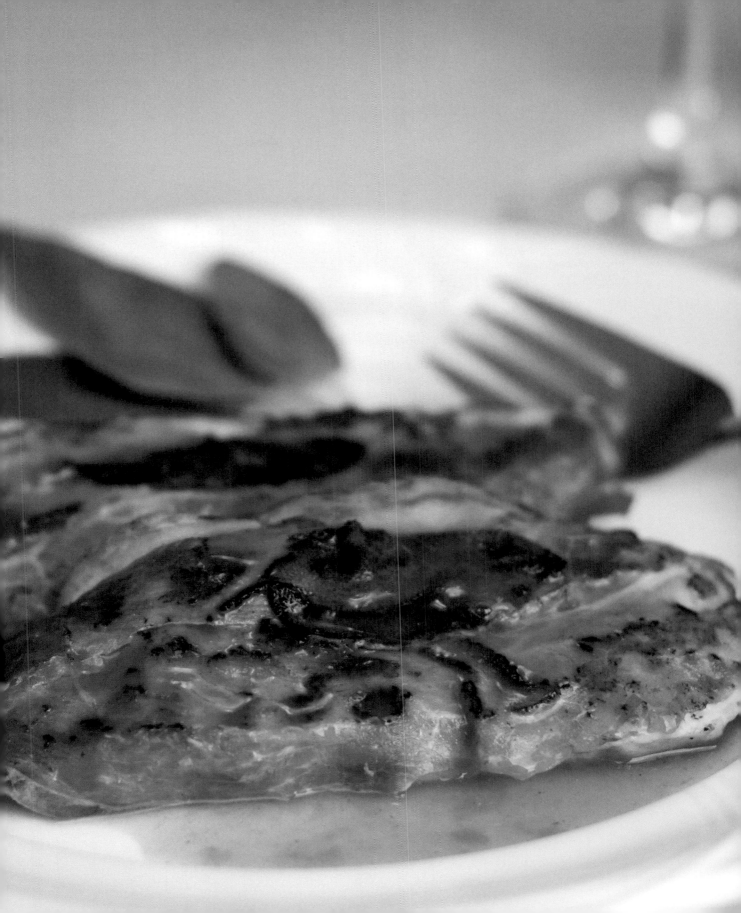

Chicken Breasts with Quinoa Stuffing
Pollo ripieno con quinoa

MY MOM DOESN'T MAKE JUST *ORDINARY* ROAST CHICKEN — her seasoned bread stuffing is always a hit and there's never enough, especially when all the grandkids dig in. I've adapted her recipe by turning it on its head with quinoa, and by using individual chicken breasts that cook faster than a whole chicken. And, yes, my kids all dig into the stuffing first.

4	bone-in skin-on chicken breast halves (about 2.5 lbs/ 1.1 kg)
	Sea salt and freshly ground black pepper to taste

Stuffing

2 tsp	extra-virgin olive oil
2	cloves garlic, minced
½ cup	chopped onions
⅓ cup	finely chopped peeled apples (I like Gala apples)
2 cups	cooked quinoa, well drained and fluffed
1	egg
¼ cup	chopped fresh parsley
2 tbsp	freshly grated Parmigiano-Reggiano cheese
½ tsp	Italian herb seasoning
½ tsp	sea salt
	Freshly ground black pepper to taste
¼ cup	no-salt-added chicken broth
¼ cup	white wine

Rub

1 tbsp	extra-virgin olive oil
2 tsp	chopped fresh rosemary
1	clove garlic, pressed or minced
¼ tsp	ground paprika

➤ Preheat oven to 350°F. Remove excess fat from chicken breasts, being careful not to tear the skin. Pat skin dry and season with salt and pepper.

➤ In a medium non-stick skillet, heat olive oil over medium-high heat. Add garlic and onions and cook until onions are softened, about 1 to 2 minutes. Stir in chopped apples and cook for another 3 to 4 minutes, until apples soften.

➤ In a medium bowl, combine quinoa, apple mixture, egg, parsley, cheese, Italian herb seasoning, salt and pepper. Set aside.

➤ To stuff each breast, take about ½ cup of quinoa stuffing and carefully tuck it under the skin, being careful to keep the skin intact so it "houses" the stuffing while cooking.

➤ To make the rub, combine olive oil, rosemary, garlic and paprika in a small bowl. Rub over the skin and exposed meat of chicken breasts.

➤ Arrange stuffed breasts in a greased roasting pan. Combine chicken broth and white wine and reserve; pour on the bottom of pan halfway through cooking. Cook for 40 to 45 minutes or until juices run clear when chicken is pierced with a fork. Serve stuffed chicken with pan juices.

MAKE AHEAD Prepare the stuffing one to two days ahead. Mix all the ingredients, except the egg, in a bowl, cover tightly and store in the refrigerator until ready to use. Combine the egg just before using.

⌂ HIGH IN...COENZYME Q10

Chicken breast is a moderate source of the coenzyme Q10, a powerful antioxidant that protects the body's cells from oxidation. As our bodies age, our natural supply of coQ10 decreases. In order for the body to synthesize coQ10, it needs an adequate amount of other nutrients, especially vitamin B6, which is also plentiful in chicken.

 4 SERVINGS   **GLUTEN-FREE**   **MAKE AHEAD**

PER SERVING (without skin) 401 CALORIES | 10 G TOTAL FAT (2 G SATURATED FAT) | 168 MG CHOLESTEROL | 395 MG SODIUM | 19 G CARBOHYDRATE | 3 G FIBER | 53 G PROTEIN

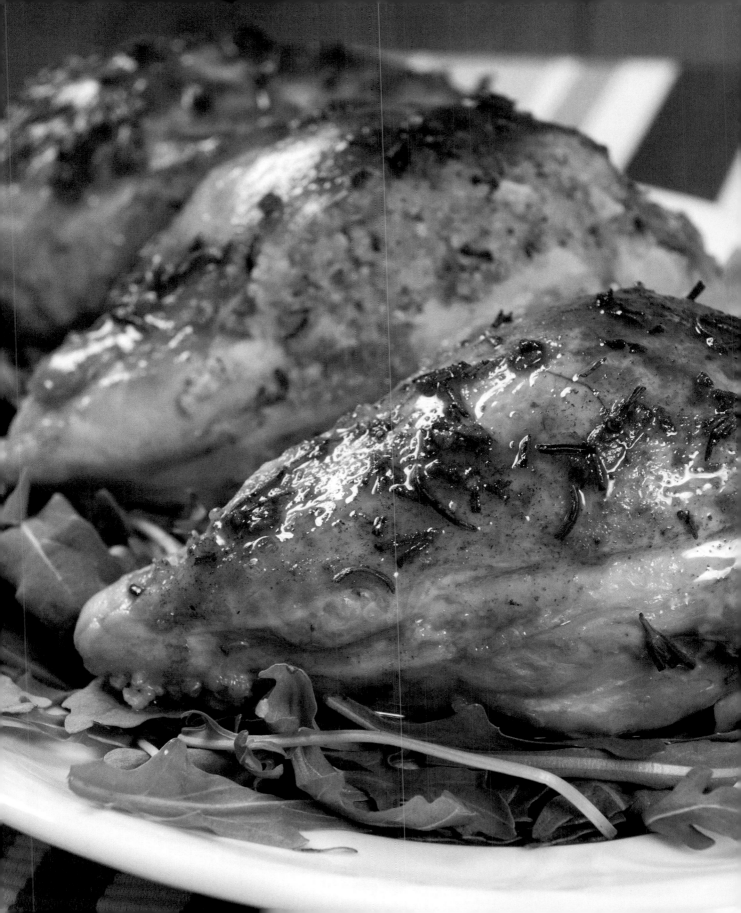

Eggplant Parmigiana with Quinoa
Melanzane alla parmigiana con quinoa

WHEN I DID AN INFORMAL POLL of favorite Italian dishes, this one came out on top. Its ooey-gooey goodness caps my list, too. In fact, my girlfriends told me it would be impossible to replicate its sumptuous taste if I didn't coat the eggplants in a heavy batter and deep fry them before layering them with loads of mozzarella, just like all the Italian nonnas I know do. Well...let's just say, I've got free lattes for the next year!

2 to 3	large eggplants, preferably Rosa Bianca/Sicilian variety (about 2.5 lbs/1.1 kg), (see tip)
2 tsp	sea salt
1 cup	uncooked quinoa (see tip)
2 tbsp	freshly grated Parmigiano-Reggiano cheese
⅓ cup	1% milk
2 tsp	extra-virgin olive oil
2½ cups	prepared tomato sauce (*see recipe for Basic Pasta Tomato Sauce, page 10*)
1 cup	packed shredded part-skim mozzarella cheese (4 oz/113 g)
4 tbsp	chopped fresh basil
1 tbsp	chopped fresh parsley
Sea salt and freshly ground black pepper to taste	

MAKE AHEAD Prepare this casserole-style dish the night before, refrigerate and bake it just before serving. The tomato sauce can be made up to one week before.

TIPS The tender white flesh of the Rosa Bianca eggplant, also known as the Sicilian eggplant, is the ideal variety to use for this dish. You'll recognize it for its violet and white-streaked skin and rounder body. It also has less seeds, which makes it less bitter-tasting.
➤ Choose a quinoa that's been pre-rinsed, since it needs to be dry before grinding. Rinsing removes the natural-occuring saponins that coat seeds and leave behind a bitter taste.

➤ Peel eggplants and trim ends. Cut into ¾-inch (2-cm) round slices and salt immediately on both sides. Let sit in a colander for 20 minutes to let them "sweat" and draw out bitterness. Pat dry. Preheat oven to broil setting.

➤ Add quinoa to the bowl of a food processor and whirl for several minutes until at least half of the quinoa reaches a flour consistency. Some of the quinoa will be intact, but that's fine because you'll want some texture here. Combine quinoa and grated cheese in a pie plate or shallow bowl. Add milk in another pie plate or shallow bowl. Dip both sides of eggplant slices in milk, then press gently into quinoa crumb mixture until sides are well coated.

➤ Place eggplant slices in a single layer on a large baking sheet coated with cooking spray. Coat tops with cooking spray for 3 to 4 seconds (broil eggplants in two batches). Place in preheated oven on upper rack about 6 inches from broil element. Broil until eggplants turn golden, about 10 to 12 minutes, turning them halfway through cooking. Reduce oven temperature to 350°F.

➤ To assemble, add olive oil and ⅓ of tomato sauce evenly into the bottom of a 9 x 13-inch baking pan. Nestle one layer of grilled eggplants into sauce, cutting a couple of eggplants to fill in spaces. Add ⅓ of tomato sauce, ½ of grated mozzarella and ½ of basil. Repeat with another layer. Top with parsley and black pepper. Cover pan with foil paper and bake in preheated oven for 20 to 25 minutes; remove foil for last 5 minutes of cooking. Let stand 5 minutes before serving.

↻ LOW IN...FAT

Not only does this Parmigiana have up to three times less fat than the classic preparation but its quinoa coating offers more protein and more fiber to this gluten-free main.

6 SERVINGS

GLUTEN-FREE

MEATLESS

MAKE AHEAD

PER SERVING 230 CALORIES I 7 G TOTAL FAT (3 G SATURATED FAT) I 13 MG CHOLESTEROL I 420 MG SODIUM I 40 G CARBOHYDRATE I 11 G FIBER I 11 G PROTEIN

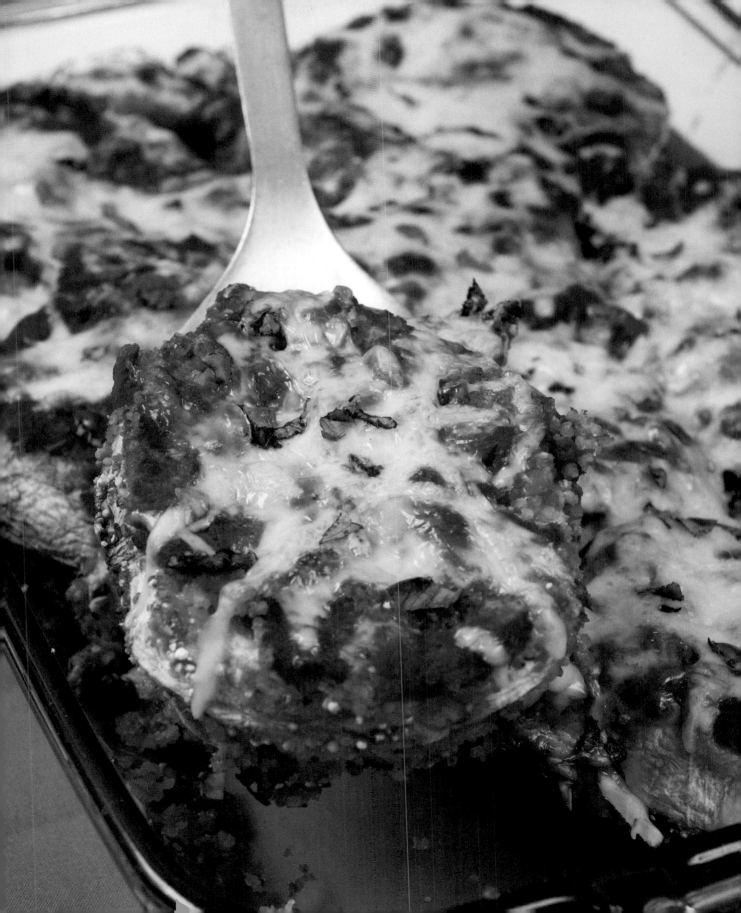

Italian-Style Meatloaf
Polpettone Italiano

THE QUINTESSENTIAL NORTH AMERICAN CLASSIC has always had a place on our dinner table but, of course, crafted *alla Italiana* like this recipe. My dad loves his meatloaf with a couple of hard-boiled eggs stuffed in its center for more interest in every slice — and you can do that here, too. This recipe is so well loved that it's become a favorite go-to among family and friends alike.

Meatloaf

½ cup	chopped onions
¼ cup	each: coarsely chopped carrots, celery and red bell peppers
2	cloves garlic, minced
10.5 oz	(300 g) extra-lean ground beef
10.5 oz	(300 g) lean ground turkey
1	egg
1	egg white
½ cup	oat bran or quick-cooking oats*
½ cup	mashed cooked sweet potato or canned pure pumpkin
¼ cup	minced fresh parsley
2 tbsp	minced fresh basil
2 tbsp	freshly grated Parmigiano-Reggiano cheese
½ tsp	sea salt

Freshly ground black pepper to taste

Sauce

1 tsp	extra-virgin olive oil
1 tbsp	no-salt-added tomato paste
1 tbsp	water
½ tsp	dried oregano
1 cup	chopped ripe tomatoes

⇆ **VARIATION** Need a little more green in your diet? Replace the mashed sweet potato with a handful or two of steamed spinach.

➤ Preheat oven to 375°F.

➤ Add onions, carrots, celery, peppers and garlic to the bowl of a food processor and pulse a few times until finely minced.

➤ Combine remaining meatloaf ingredients, from beef through black pepper, in a very large bowl. Add minced vegetable mixture. Mix well, using your hands, until all ingredients are well combined.

➤ On a clean surface, gently shape the meat into a rectangular log (about 4 x 9 inches/10 x 23 cm) with your hands. Coat a non-stick broiler pan with cooking spray. Add about 2 cups of water to the bottom basin of the pan. Transfer meatloaf to top rack of greased broiler pan.

➤ Prepare sauce by mixing olive oil with tomato paste, water and oregano. Use your hands to spread the seasoned tomato paste on the top and sides of loaf. Top loaf with chopped tomatoes.

➤ Cook in preheated oven for about 40 to 45 minutes or until juices run clear when cutting into loaf. Let meatloaf stand for 5 minutes before slicing and serving.

MAKE AHEAD Prepare the sweet potato a day ahead. Peel one large sweet potato, boil in water until tender, drain and mash. Store in the refrigerator until you're ready to use it. Cut prep time even further by chopping the veggies and refrigerating them before pulsing in food processor.

↻ LOW IN...FAT

The lean meats and wallop of antioxidant-rich veggies aren't the only things keeping this meatloaf on the low end of the fat scale. The cooking method — placing the loaf on a broiler pan — allows fatty juices to run off into the basin pan while searing the loaf's exterior to lock flavors inside. The addition of oats guarantees a super-moist meatloaf.

6 SERVINGS **GLUTEN-FREE*** CHECK LABELS **MAKE AHEAD**

PER SERVING 208 CALORIES | 8 G TOTAL FAT (3 G SATURATED FAT) | 85 MG CHOLESTEROL | 286 MG SODIUM | 13 G CARBOHYDRATE | 3 G FIBER | 21 G PROTEIN

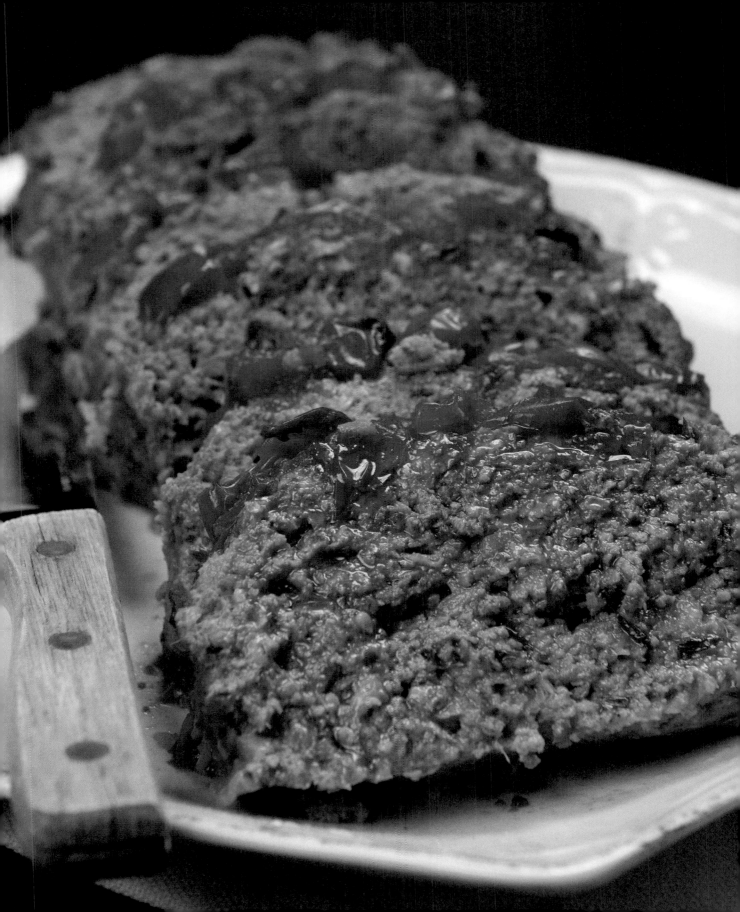

Roasted Fennel Sausages with Grilled Vegetables

Salsiccia di finocchio al forno con verdure grigliate

FOR ME, SAUSAGES just aren't the same without a hint of fennel. It goes back to the days when I watched my parents blend a profusion of herbs and spices into their own homemade sausages, a winter tradition widely practiced among Italians as an economical way to stock their freezers and feed their families. With this one-pan wonder, I've got something else besides taste keeping the kids at the table — the kaleidoscope of vegetables adds brilliant color to the dish.

4 tbsp	balsamic vinegar, divided
4	large lean pork fennel (Italian) sausages* (100 g/3.5 oz each), (see tip)
1	small red onion, cut into large wedges
1	red bell or Sheppard pepper, seeded and cut into large wedges
1	yellow bell pepper, seeded and cut into large wedges
8	mini red potatoes, halved or quartered, or 2 medium red potatoes (skin on), chopped into bite-sized pieces
2 tsp	extra-virgin olive oil
1 tbsp	fresh thyme or 1 tsp dried thyme
3	bay leaves
Sea salt and freshly ground black pepper to taste	

➤ Preheat oven to 400°F. Coat an extra-large baking pan with cooking spray. Drizzle 2 tbsp balsamic vinegar into pan. Lay sausages in pan about 1 inch (2.5 cm) apart.

➤ In a large bowl, combine cut vegetables and add olive oil, remaining balsamic vinegar, thyme, bay leaves, salt and pepper. Toss until vegetables are well coated. Pour into pan, fitting pieces into spaces around sausages. Cover pan with foil paper and cook for 25 minutes in preheated oven. Turn sausages over and stir vegetables, reduce heat to 375°F and cook, uncovered, for another 30 minutes.

➤ Discard bay leaves. Place sausages on a serving platter and keep warm. Set the oven to the broil setting and grill remaining vegetables in pan on *middle* oven rack for 4 to 5 minutes before adding to serving platter.

TIP If you can't find lean Italian sausages, choose lean pork sausages and add 1 tsp of fennel seeds to the baking pan.

↻ LOW IN...FAT

Using lean pork sausage cuts the fat by almost 50 percent. For example, one regular link of pork sausage has 235 calories with 21 grams of fat (8 grams saturated fat).

4 SERVINGS   GLUTEN-FREE*
                    CHECK INGREDIENTS

PER SERVING 259 CALORIES | 12 G TOTAL FAT (4 G SATURATED FAT) | 55 MG CHOLESTEROL | 436 MG SODIUM | 17 G CARBOHYDRATE | 2 G FIBER | 20 G PROTEIN

Skillet Turkey Sausage with Rapini & Sage

Salsiccia di tacchino in padella con rapini e salvia

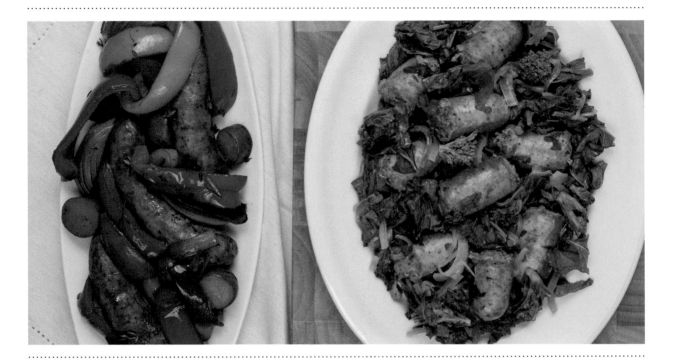

1	small bunch rapini (broccoli rabe)
1 tbsp	canola oil
4	lean turkey sausages* (3.5 oz/100 g each)
½ cup	sliced red onions
½ cup	white wine
2 tbsp	chopped fresh sage leaves
½ cup	no-salt-added chicken broth
	Sea salt and freshly ground black pepper to taste
Pinch	crushed red pepper flakes (optional)

➤ Trim stalks from rapini and chop leaves and florets into 2-inch (5 cm) chunks (you'll have about 5 to 6 packed cups). Set aside.

➤ In a large skillet, heat oil over medium-high heat. Sear sausages on all sides, turning frequently, about 4 to 5 minutes. Cut each sausage into three to four equal pieces. Reduce heat to medium and stir in red onions; cook for 1 minute. Add wine and sage; cover and cook until wine is absorbed. Add chicken broth and cook for 7 to 8 more minutes. Scatter rapini pieces over sausages, toss, cover and cook until rapini is wilted, about 3 to 4 minutes. Season with salt, pepper and crushed red pepper flakes, if using.

TIP Store-bought turkey sausage can sometimes be well salted so avoid adding more salt until rapini has had time to absorb all the flavors.

4 SERVINGS   30 MIN OR LESS   GLUTEN-FREE*
CHECK INGREDIENTS

PER SERVING 217 CALORIES | 12 G TOTAL FAT (2 G SATURATED FAT) | 49 MG CHOLESTEROL | 480 MG SODIUM | 4 G CARBOHYDRATE | 1 G FIBER | 19 G PROTEIN

Grilled European Sea Bass

Spigola alla griglia

IF THERE'S ONE THING THAT TIME-HONORED TRADITIONAL COOKING has taught me over the years it's that the simplest, freshest ingredients can create the most flavorful and enjoyable meal. This is certainly true for this recipe, which starts with a mild, flaky fish and adds unpretentious ingredients that are always on hand. Mom's font of knowledge in the kitchen has shown me that giving dishes the dressed-down treatment usually brings in the best catch.

2	1-lb (454 g) whole European sea bass with head and tail intact, cleaned and scaled (see tip)
	Sea salt and freshly ground black pepper to taste
2 cups	chopped ripe tomatoes
4	cloves garlic, minced
1 cup	chopped fresh parsley
1 tbsp	extra-virgin olive oil
2 tbsp	white wine
¼ tsp	Italian herb seasoning

➤ Preheat grill to medium heat. Prepare a packet with foil paper to house each fish; double up a large sheet of foil long enough to hold each fish when folded over.

➤ Rinse fish and pat dry with paper towel. Transfer to a clean working surface and put them on their sides. Carefully run a knife down the center of each fish, from the head to the tail, without cutting through to the spine. Sprinkle fish with salt and pepper. Transfer each fish to individual foil paper.

➤ Combine tomatoes, garlic, parsley and olive oil in a medium bowl. Fill each fish cavity with tomato-parsley mixture; top fish with any remaining mixture. Drizzle fish with wine and sprinkle with Italian herb seasoning. Fold foil over at sides and ends; pinch seams together to make an enclosed packet.

➤ Place on preheated greased grill, seam sides up. Cook until fish is flaked with a fork, about 10 minutes. Open up packages and serve hot.

TIP With firm flesh and few bones, a whole fish like sea bass is a great option for the grill. Keep the head and tail intact for a moist result.

⇄ VARIATION For a complete meal, add two more packages of foil on the grill while the sea bass is cooking. Include chopped sweet potatoes (seasoned with olive oil, nutmeg and sea salt) in one and asparagus (drizzled with olive oil, minced garlic and sea salt) in the other.

4 SERVINGS   **30 MIN OR LESS**   **GLUTEN-FREE**   **MEATLESS**

PER SERVING 202 CALORIES | 7 G TOTAL FAT (1 G SATURATED FAT) | 62 MG CHOLESTEROL | 108 MG SODIUM | 5 G CARBOHYDRATE | 1 G FIBER | 29 G PROTEIN

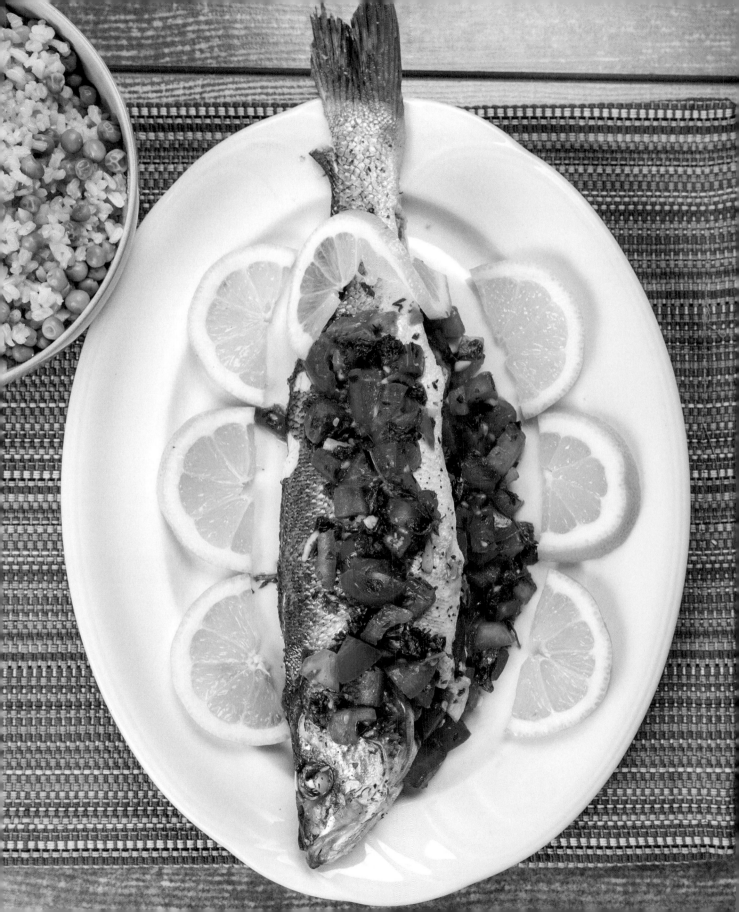

Walnut-Crusted Cod with Raisins

Baccalà in crosta di noci con uvetta

WHEN YOU GROW UP ON THE SAME STREET AS YOUR BEST FRIEND, you're bound to share some meals together and you're inevitably going to share some recipes. This gem is from my bestie Anna, whose mother has been making this recipe since she was a little girl living in Italy's Molise region. As soon as this fragrant dish came out of the oven, Anna proudly ran across the street to my house to deliver a sample tasting. Of course, it didn't last long, so I learned to make it on my own. This version uses a topping much like a crumble to keep the fillets juicy and moist.

1½ lbs	(680 g) fresh thick cod fillet
¼ cup	spelt or whole wheat dry breadcrumbs
2 tbsp	golden raisins
¼ cup	walnut pieces, finely chopped
1 tbsp	freshly grated Parmigiano-Reggiano cheese
1 tbsp	extra-virgin olive oil
	Sea salt and freshly ground black pepper to taste
¼ cup	white wine
12	small black olives (like Gaeta variety) in brine, rinsed and drained
3 tbsp	chopped fresh parsley

➤ Cut cod fillet into four pieces. Preheat oven to 350°F.

➤ In a small non-stick skillet, add breadcrumbs and toast on medium-low heat, stirring frequently until lightly golden, about 3 to 4 minutes. In the meantime, soak raisins in hot water for 10 minutes. Drain and set aside.

➤ In a small bowl, combine breadcrumbs, walnut pieces and cheese. Drizzle olive oil over mixture and toss until mixture is moist and crumbly.

➤ Coat a 9 x 9-inch baking dish with cooking spray. Season cod pieces lightly with salt and pepper and place in baking dish in a single layer. Drizzle with white wine.

➤ Spoon breadcrumb-walnut mixture evenly over piece of fish and gently press down. Scatter raisins and olives around cod. Bake until fish is opaque in the center and flakes easily with a fork, about 15 minutes. Reset oven to broil setting and cook fish for about 1 to 2 minutes until topping is golden brown. Top with parsley and serve.

🎧 HIGH IN...OMEGA-3 FATTY ACIDS

While you might question the amount of fat in this dish, keep in mind that most of it comes from the good-for-you walnuts. Among the nut family, walnuts have the highest concentration of a type of essential omega-3s called alpha linolenic acid (ALA). Essential omega-3s help to reduce inflammation, lower blood pressure and even boost brain function. About 20 percent of our dietary ALA is converted to other omega-3 fats, EPA and DHA, which are only found in animal foods like cod. Walnuts also increase the amount of HDL (good) cholesterol and lower the LDL (bad) cholesterol levels in blood when eaten in moderation.

4 SERVINGS   30 MIN OR LESS   MEATLESS

PER SERVING 277 CALORIES | 11 G TOTAL FAT (1 G SATURATED FAT) | 64 MG CHOLESTEROL | 250 MG SODIUM | 13 G CARBOHYDRATE | 2 G FIBER | 29 G PROTEIN

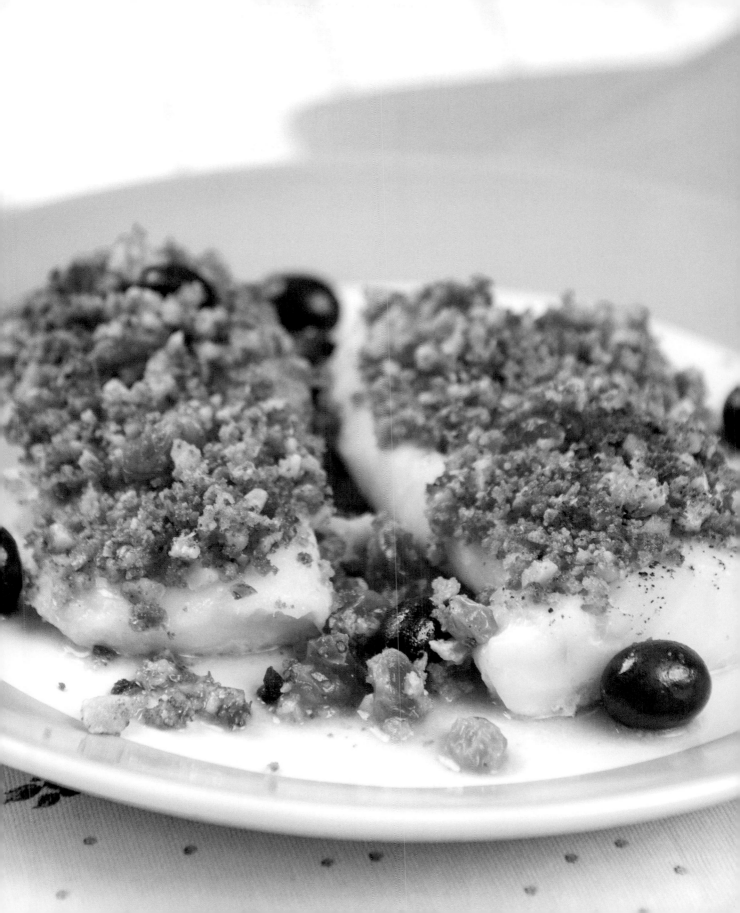

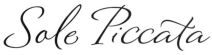

Sole Piccata

Sogliola alla piccata

FRESHLY SQUEEZED LEMON, capers and anchovies have always been part of my culinary lexicon. Sure, these ingredients — which often form the basis for the buttery Piccata sauce typically smothered on chicken or veal — were available on the surrounding Mediterranean lands in which my parents and their ancestors were raised. What makes them so appealing to fillets like this, however, are their subtle hits of sour and salt.

32 to 40	brown rice crackers (2 oz/ 60 g), (see tip)
Freshly ground black pepper to taste	
8	boneless skinless sole fillets (about 14 oz/400 g), (see tip)
⅓ cup	white wine
2 tbsp	freshly squeezed lemon juice
1 tbsp	extra-virgin olive oil
1 tbsp	light butter, melted
2	anchovy fillets in olive oil, rinsed, patted dry and minced
2	cloves garlic, minced
2 tsp	capers in brine, rinsed and patted dry
2 tbsp	chopped fresh parsley

➤ Preheat oven to 350°F. Spray a large baking pan with cooking spray.

➤ Place rice crackers in the bowl of a food processor and pulse until they reach a breadcrumb consistency. You'll have about ½ cup.

➤ Place crumbs in a shallow bowl or pie plate. Season sole fillets with black pepper and press lightly into crumbs one at a time, coating both sides. Place fillets side by side in baking pan without overlapping them.

➤ In a small bowl, combine white wine, lemon juice, olive oil, butter, anchovy pieces, garlic, capers and parsley and drizzle evenly over sole fillets.

➤ Bake for 12 to 15 minutes (not more or fish will be dry) until sole flakes easily with a fork. Serve hot.

TIPS I like to use Brown Rice Crisps by Want-Want or Mary's Organic Crackers, and for a nutty flavor, Blue Diamond's low-sodium Nut-Thins, either in the Almond or Pecan flavor.

➤ If you're using frozen sole fillets, make sure they're well thawed and drained before cooking.

☺ LOW IN...FAT

What's so great about sole is its low-fat content (only 1 gram of fat in every 3.5-ounce serving) and its high-protein count. A serving has 14 grams of protein, which is equivalent to about 3 ounces of chicken breast, almost 2 ounces of lean ground beef or 1 cup of red kidney beans.

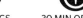

4 SERVINGS   **30 MIN OR LESS**   **GLUTEN-FREE**   **MEATLESS**

PER SERVING 238 CALORIES | 8 G TOTAL FAT (2 G SATURATED FAT) | 64 MG CHOLESTEROL | 282 MG SODIUM | 13 G CARBOHYDRATE | 1 G FIBER | 23 G PROTEIN

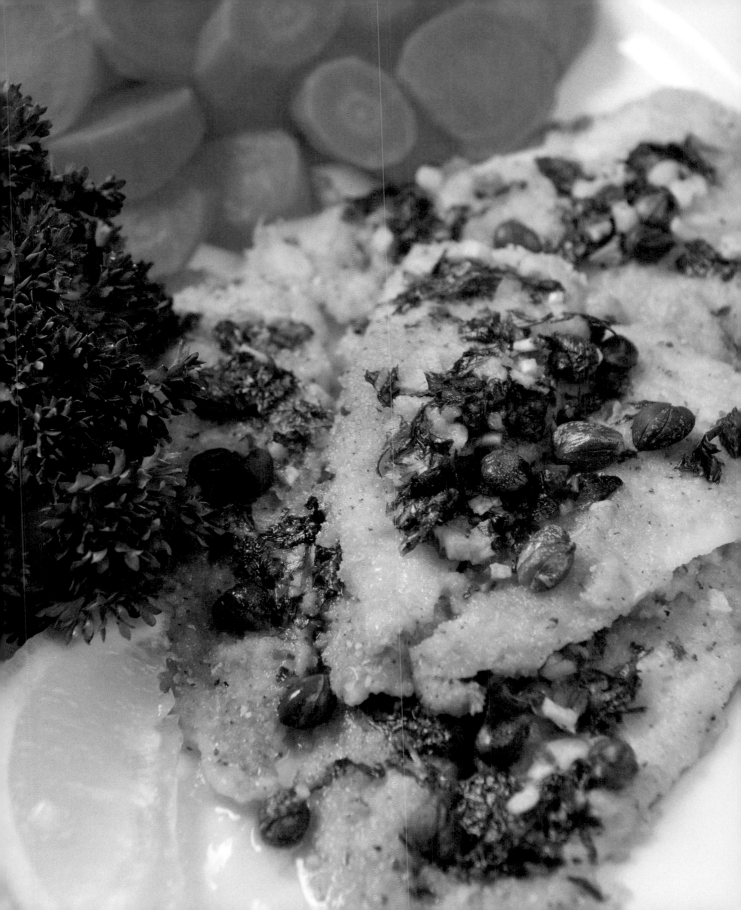

Eggs in Stewed Tomatoes & Garlic Spinach à la Florentine

Uova al pomodoro e spinaci alla Fiorentina

FEEDING A FAMILY OF FIVE on the pay of a grocery store manager and seamstress was tough even decades ago, so peasant-type dishes would sometimes grace the table. But we never knew it digging into this super-easy dish that not only blends great flavors and textures but also delivers a nutrient-packed meal on a shoestring budget.

Florentine Garlic Spinach

2 tsp	extra-virgin olive oil
1 tsp	light butter
4	cloves garlic, thinly sliced
6 cups	packed baby spinach leaves (7 oz/210 g)
¼ tsp	sea salt
Pinch	ground nutmeg

Eggs in Stewed Tomatoes

1 tsp	extra-virgin olive oil
½ cup	chopped onions
2 cups	chopped ripe tomatoes
½ cup	no-salt-added tomato purée (passata)
2 tbsp	chopped fresh basil
4	large eggs
Sea salt and freshly ground black pepper to taste	

➤ In a large non-stick skillet, heat olive oil and butter over medium-high heat. Add garlic and cook until lightly golden, about 3 to 4 minutes. Add spinach leaves and season with salt and nutmeg. Cook until spinach is wilted. Transfer to a serving platter and keep warm.

➤ Using the same skillet, heat olive oil over medium-high heat. Add onions and cook until softened. Add tomatoes and tomato purée and cook until tomatoes begin to break apart, about 2 to 3 minutes. Stir in basil and make 4 spots in sauce to drop in eggs. Reduce heat to medium. Carefully drop eggs over tomatoes (à la sunny-side up) but not touching each other.

➤ Lightly season eggs with salt and pepper and cover skillet tightly with a lid until egg yolks set, about 3 to 4 minutes.

➤ Spoon eggs and tomato sauce carefully over spinach and serve immediately.

🎧 HIGH IN...COMPLETE PROTEIN

Eggs are one of those foods that we can take for granted because they're rarely the star of a recipe, but they're loaded with high-quality and inexpensive protein, vitamins and minerals, including iron, vitamins A, B12, D and E, folate and iron, as well as disease-fighting nutrients. While the yolk has a significant dose of cholesterol, scientists have recently discovered that it's not dietary cholesterol like that found in eggs that raises blood cholesterol, but rather trans and saturated fats. Another benefit to eating eggs? They'll keep you feeling full longer.

 4 SERVINGS

 30 MIN OR LESS

 GLUTEN-FREE

 MEATLESS

PER SERVING 146 CALORIES | 8 G TOTAL FAT (2 G SATURATED FAT) | 183 MG CHOLESTEROL | 326 MG SODIUM | 11 G CARBOHYDRATE | 3 G FIBER | 9 G PROTEIN

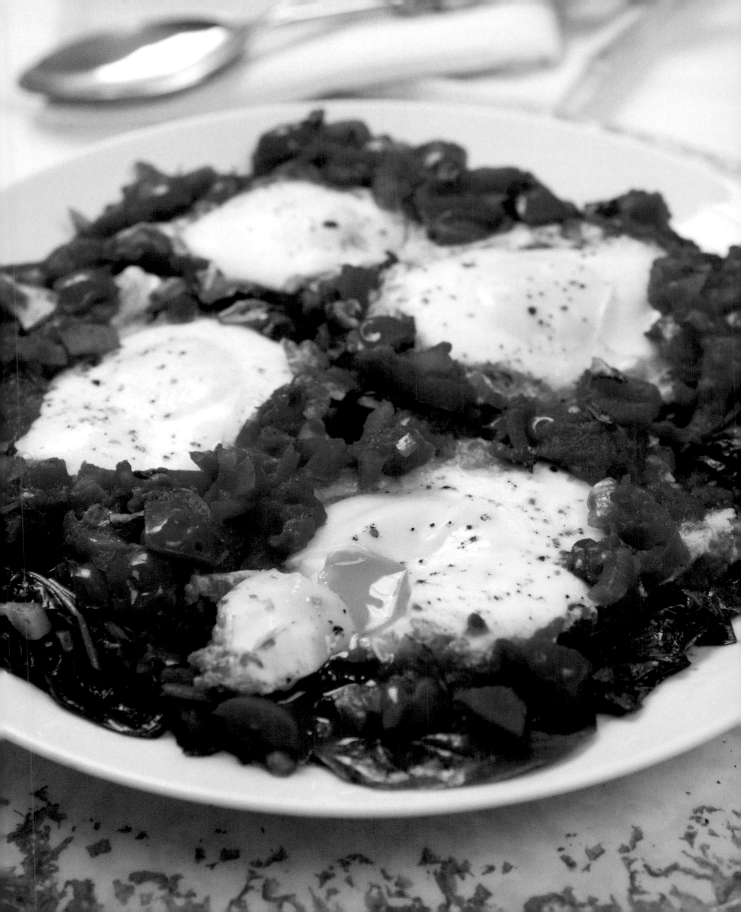

Herb-Bread-Stuffed Squid
Calamari ripieni di pane ed erbe

SQUID HAS ALWAYS MADE IT TO OUR HOLIDAY TABLE. Unlike the crispy-coated calamari rings that typically grace antipasti platters, it's my mom's specialty of stuffed squid that gives meaning to the meal. Like filling a piping bag with frosting, she packs a garlicky herbed stuffing into the squid tubes, then nestles them into a pan where they plump up to perfection while they bake.

6	medium squid tubes (about 6 inches/30 cm, 14 oz/400 g total), cleaned
2½ cups	cubed whole-grain bread (crusts removed)
¼ cup	1% milk
2	egg whites
½ cup	chopped fresh parsley
¼ cup	minced celery
3 tbsp	freshly grated Parmigiano-Reggiano cheese
1 tsp	capers in brine, rinsed, patted dry and chopped
3	cloves garlic, crushed or minced
½ tsp	Italian herb seasoning
¼ cup	white wine
1 cup	canned no-salt-added diced tomatoes, drained
2 tsp	extra-virgin olive oil
Sea salt and freshly ground black pepper to taste	

➤ Preheat oven to 350°F.

➤ Remove fins and tentacles of squid (reserve for another dish). Wash and pat squid tubes dry.

➤ In a large bowl, toss cubed bread with milk until absorbed. Add egg whites, parsley, celery, cheese, capers, garlic and Italian herb seasoning. Combine well (use your hands to work in ingredients and press together).

➤ Stuff squid tubes with 3 to 4 tbsp of stuffing each. Tubes won't be completely filled but they'll expand during baking. Close up tube openings with a toothpick.

➤ Coat a large baking pan with cooking spray. Pour in white wine. Place squid tubes in a single row and top with diced tomatoes; drizzle with olive oil. Season squid with salt and pepper.

➤ Bake in preheated oven for about 40 minutes, until squid is tender. Remove toothpicks and serve hot, either left whole or cut into round pieces.

MAKE AHEAD Prepare the bread stuffing a day before. Refrigerate until ready to use.

℧ LOW IN...FAT

Batterless, no-fry squid are actually low in fat and calories. Here, they start off as having fewer than 70 calories and only 1 gram of fat (and virtually no saturated fat) before being stuffed with an equally low-fat stuffing. Like shrimp, squid is high in cholesterol, but researchers have shown that because it's low in saturated fats, it does not impact blood cholesterol if eaten in moderation.

6 SERVINGS · MEATLESS · MAKE AHEAD

PER SERVING 341 CALORIES | 6 G TOTAL FAT (2 G SATURATED FAT) | 149 MG CHOLESTEROL | 432 MG SODIUM | 45 G CARBOHYDRATE | 9 G FIBER | 23 G PROTEIN

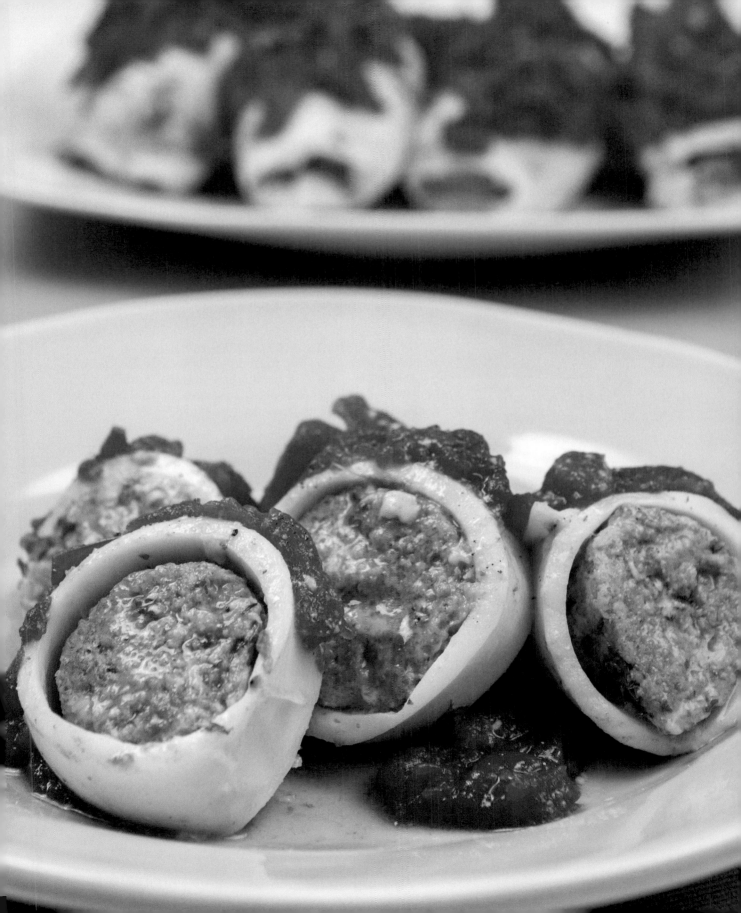

Sicilian Chicken Roll-Ups
Farsu farsumagru

I'VE ALWAYS FOUND THE MULTITUDE of Italian dialects to be poetic, each with its own rhythm and tongue-twisting phrases. I couldn't resist putting my own spin on this cleverly titled recipe using Sicilian vernacular — the original title *farsumagru* means "falsely lean" for its decadently rich ingredients of steak rolled with pork sausage and cured meats. But I'm adding the "false" (*farsu*) to this farsumagru because I'm a sucker not only for wordplay but also for healthy adaptations. Here, chicken breast rolls up with a delicious stuffing that'll have the entire family reciting this poetic title time and time again.

6	boneless skinless chicken breasts (about 1½ lbs/680 g)
¼ tsp	sea salt
Freshly ground black pepper to taste	

Stuffing

1	turkey sausage*, casing removed (about 3.5 oz/100 g)
1	clove garlic, minced
2	green onions, chopped
1 cup	packed chopped baby spinach leaves
½ cup	frozen green peas, thawed
2 tbsp	minced fresh parsley
2	slices reduced-sodium extra-lean deli-style prosciutto cotto or ham (2 oz/56 g), cut in thirds
3	thin slices light provolone cheese (1.5 oz/45 g), cut in half
2	hard-boiled eggs, sliced
2 tsp	high-oleic canola oil

Sauce

¼ cup	chopped onions
2 cups	diced red peppers
½ cup	canned no-salt-added diced tomatoes, drained
¼ cup	each: white wine and reduced-sodium chicken broth
3 tbsp	no-salt-added tomato paste
½ tsp	Italian herb seasoning

➤ Trim the fat off each chicken breast. Starting at the thickest section of each breast, butterfly cut each one without cutting through it and open up breast to form a thinner, larger working piece. Place plastic wrap or waxed paper on chicken and flatten by pounding with a mallet. Season with salt and pepper.

➤ To prepare the stuffing, coat a very large non-stick skillet with cooking spray and heat over medium-high heat. Add sausage meat, garlic and onions and cook, breaking up sausage into small pieces, until meat is no longer pink, about 3 minutes. Toss in spinach, peas and parsley and cook until peas are tender and ingredients are well incorporated, about 2 to 3 minutes.

➤ To assemble rolls, place chicken breast on a clean working surface. Top with one slice each of prosciutto cotto, provolone and a couple slices of egg. Place an equal amount of stuffing in the center of the chicken. Starting at the shortest end of the breast, roll up tightly, tucking in mixture and ends. Secure with two or three toothpicks. (Don't worry if they're not perfect.) Repeat with other breasts.

➤ Preheat oven to 350°F. Using the same non-stick skillet, heat oil on medium-high heat. Sear chicken breasts seam side down first, then turn with tongs onto remaining sides to cook until lightly browned, about 2 to 3 minutes per side. Transfer rolls to a small baking pan and keep warm while preparing sauce.

➤ To make the sauce, add onions and peppers to the same skillet and stir continuously, scraping up any bits at the bottom for 2 to 3 minutes. Add remaining ingredients and simmer for 2 to 3 more minutes until mixture is bubbling and heated through. Spoon sauce over rolls in pan and bake in oven for 10 to 15 minutes. Serve hot.

MAKE AHEAD Prepare the filling, including your hard-boiled eggs, the night before and refrigerate until the next day when you're ready to cook these bundles.

6 SERVINGS · GLUTEN-FREE* · MAKE AHEAD

PER SERVING 219 CALORIES | 8 G TOTAL FAT (2 G SATURATED FAT) | 127 MG CHOLESTEROL | 330 MG SODIUM | 6 G CARBOHYDRATE | 1 G FIBER | 29 G PROTEIN

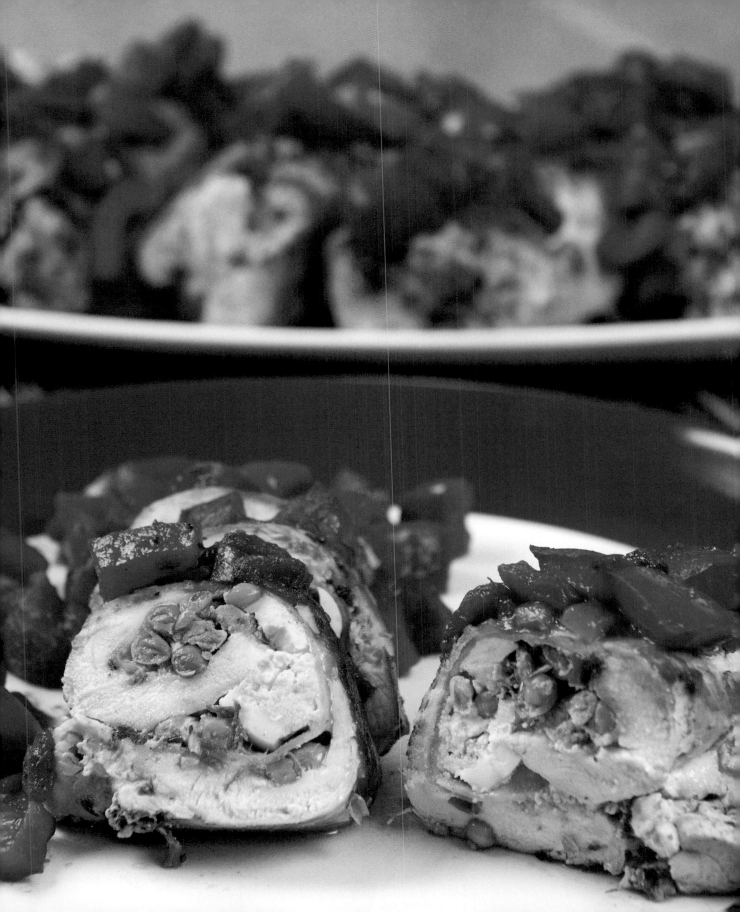

Baked Breaded Chicken Cutlets with Mushroom – Wine Sauce

Cotolette di pollo ai funghi e vino

IT'S HARD TO COMPETE WITH THE BEST RECIPES from the best cooks, so when I make my chicken cutlets, I'm always in "competition" with my mom. Her cutlets have long garnered the title "best cutlets in the whole wide world" voted by the finest tasters, her grandkids. Suffice to say, I've had the best teacher and she has taught me well (I'm going by what's left on everyone's plate after a meal).

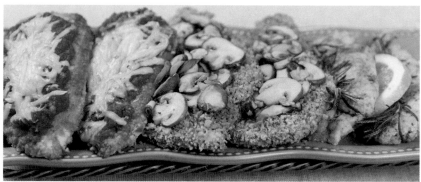

8	thinly sliced or butterfly-cut boneless skinless chicken breasts (about 1½ lbs/680 g)
¼ tsp	sea salt
Freshly ground black pepper to taste	
¼ cup	egg whites
1 cup	spelt dry breadcrumbs (*see tip, page 220*)
1 tbsp	freshly grated Parmigiano-Reggiano cheese
2 tsp	Italian herb seasoning
1 tsp	extra-virgin olive oil
1	clove garlic, minced
1½ cups	thinly sliced cremini or white button mushrooms
¼ cup	white wine
1 cup	no-salt-added chicken broth
Sea salt and freshly ground black pepper to taste	
¼ cup	minced fresh parsley

➤ Preheat oven to 375°F. Trim the fat off each chicken breast. Season breasts with salt and pepper. Pour egg whites in a shallow bowl or pie plate. In another dish, combine breadcrumbs, grated cheese and Italian herb seasoning until well blended. Line a baking sheet with foil paper and lightly coat with cooking spray.

➤ Dip one chicken breast into egg whites, then in breadcrumb mixture to coat well. Repeat with remaining pieces and place side by side on greased baking sheet. Lightly coat chicken tops with cooking spray. Cook chicken pieces in preheated oven for 8 minutes.

➤ In the meantime, heat olive oil in a large non-stick skillet over medium-high heat. Add garlic and mushrooms, tossing well to coat. Cook until slightly softened, about 2 to 3 minutes. Pour in wine and chicken broth. Stir and season with salt and pepper; simmer for 3 to 4 more minutes.

➤ Remove baking sheet with chicken from the oven. Spoon mushroom and wine sauce over cutlets; sprinkle with parsley and cook another 5 minutes or until chicken is no longer pink in the center and juices run clear when pierced with a fork. Serve hot.

 4 SERVINGS 40 MIN OR LESS

PER SERVING 189 CALORIES I 3 G TOTAL FAT (1 G SATURATED FAT) I 57 MG CHOLESTEROL I 237 MG SODIUM I 11 G CARBOHYDRATE I 1 G FIBER I 26 G PROTEIN

Gluten-Free Cutlets
Cotolette di pollo senza glutine

8	thinly sliced or butterfly cut boneless skinless chicken breasts (about 1½ lbs/680 g)
¼ tsp	sea salt
Freshly ground black pepper to taste	
¼ cup	egg whites
⅔ cup	chickpea flour (see tip, page 34)
1 tbsp	Italian herb seasoning
¼ tsp	ground nutmeg
4 tsp	coconut oil, divided
4	cloves garlic (whole), divided
4	sprigs fresh rosemary, divided
Juice and zest of ½ lemon	
2 tbsp	reduced-sodium chicken broth
2 tbsp	chopped fresh parsley for garnish

➤ Preheat oven to 350°F. Trim the fat off each chicken breast. Season breasts with salt and pepper. Pour egg whites in a shallow bowl or pie plate. In another dish, combine chickpea flour, Italian herb seasoning and nutmeg until well combined. Dip one breast into egg whites, then into flour mixture to coat well. Repeat with remaining pieces.

➤ In a large non-stick skillet, heat 2 tsp oil, 2 garlic cloves and 2 sprigs rosemary over high heat for 1 minute. Remove and discard garlic and rosemary — you just want to flavor the oil. Sear 4 pieces of chicken for about 1 to 2 minutes on each side. Transfer partially cooked chicken cutlets to a baking sheet. Add remaining 2 tsp coconut oil and repeat cooking with remaining chicken, garlic and rosemary. Add these cutlets to baking sheet.

➤ Combine lemon juice, zest and chicken broth in a small bowl. Pour lemon sauce on top of chicken cutlets. Finish cooking chicken in preheated oven for another 5 to 8 minutes or until chicken is no longer pink in the center and juices run clear when pierced with a fork. Serve with parsley.

 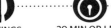

4 SERVINGS   30 MIN OR LESS   GLUTEN-FREE

PER SERVING 326 CALORIES | 8 G TOTAL FAT (5 G SATURATED FAT) | 117 MG CHOLESTEROL | 287 MG SODIUM | 9 G CARBOHYDRATE | 2 G FIBER | 50 G PROTEIN

Chicken Sorrentina
Cotolette di pollo alla Sorrentina

½ cup	no-salt-added chicken broth
1½ cups	prepared tomato or pasta sauce, divided (see recipe, page 10)
2	cloves garlic, minced
3 tbsp	chopped fresh basil
1 tsp	Italian herb seasoning
¼ cup	egg whites
⅔ cup	whole wheat dry breadcrumbs
4	skinless boneless chicken breasts (about 1½ lbs/680 g)
¼ tsp	sea salt
Freshly ground black pepper to taste	
1 cup	packed shredded part-skim mozzarella or light provolone cheese (4 oz/113 g)
1 tbsp	chopped fresh basil for garnish

➤ Preheat oven to 375°F. Combine broth, 1 cup tomato sauce, garlic, basil and Italian herb seasoning in a medium pot and simmer on medium-high heat for about 5 minutes. Set aside and keep hot.

➤ In the meantime, pour egg whites into a shallow bowl or pie plate. In another dish, add breadcrumbs. Trim the fat off each chicken breast. Season breasts with salt and pepper. Dip one chicken breast into egg whites, then coat well in breadcrumb mixture. Repeat with remaining chicken.

➤ Coat a 9 x 13-inch baking dish with cooking spray. Pour hot sauce into pan and add breaded chicken breasts, leaving a little bit of space around each. Spoon remaining tomato sauce evenly on top of chicken breasts. Cook in preheated oven for 25 minutes or until chicken is no longer pink in the center and juices run clear when pierced with a fork. Halfway through cooking, spoon sauce at the bottom of pan onto chicken and top evenly with shredded mozzarella. Serve hot garnished with chopped basil.

4 SERVINGS   40 MIN OR LESS

PER SERVING 409 CALORIES | 9 G TOTAL FAT (4 G SATURATED FAT) | 139 MG CHOLESTEROL | 447 MG SODIUM | 17 G CARBOHYDRATE | 1 G FIBER | 61 G PROTEIN

Veal Cutlet Roll-Ups in Tomato-Wine Sauce

Involtini di vitello al sugo

WE OFTEN ATE VEAL GROWING UP — either as a cutlet or as a fast-fry with a squeeze of lemon juice. Even though Mom always tried to find perfect cuts at our local butcher, veal's unpredictable texture didn't always deliver tender results; that is, until this recipe made it into the rotation. Stuffed with a surprise filling and braised in a tangy sauce, it's guaranteed to melt in your mouth.

Veal Roll-Ups

6	large veal cutlets, scallopini or inside round cut (about 1¼ lbs/565 g)
1	egg white
⅓ cup	spelt or whole wheat dry breadcrumbs*
⅓ cup	chopped reduced-sodium extra-lean deli-style prosciutto cotto/ham (2 oz/56 g)
¼ cup	chopped fresh parsley
3 tbsp	freshly grated Parmigiano-Reggiano cheese
1 tbsp	dried currants
2 tsp	pine nuts
1	clove garlic, minced
Sea salt and freshly ground black pepper to taste	
1 tbsp	high-oleic canola or sunflower oil

Sauce

¼ cup	chopped onions
2½ cups	no-salt-added tomato purée (passata)
½ cup	white wine
2 tbsp	chopped fresh basil
Sea salt and freshly ground black pepper to taste	

➤ Place heavy plastic wrap or waxed paper on veal slices and lightly pound each piece with a mallet, being careful not to puncture them. Place egg white and breadcrumbs in two separate shallow bowls or pie plates; dip one side of each piece of veal into egg white and then press wet side into crumbs until well coated. Set aside.

➤ In a medium bowl, combine prosciutto cotto, parsley, cheese, currants, pine nuts and garlic. Divide mixture equally among veal pieces (about 2 tbsp each) and spread over the uncoated side, leaving some room around the perimeter. Starting from one end, roll the veal piece tightly, tucking in mixture and securing rolled veal with a toothpick at the top and bottom. Repeat with other veal pieces. Season with salt and pepper.

➤ In a large non-stick skillet, heat oil over medium-high heat. Sear rolls, turning frequently until all sides are lightly browned, about 2 minutes. Remove veal from skillet and keep warm.

➤ Coat a medium-sized deep skillet or dutch oven with cooking spray and heat over medium-high heat. Add onions and stir until softened. Add tomato purée, wine, basil, salt and pepper and simmer for 2 to 3 minutes. Reduce heat to medium-low. Add veal rolls in a single layer and cover. Cook for about 35 to 40 minutes, turning occasionally or until veal is tender.

MAKE AHEAD Prepare the roll-ups and sear them the night before. Refrigerate them in the tomato-wine sauce and bake them just before serving.

6 SERVINGS

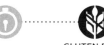

GLUTEN-FREE*
REPLACE WITH GF BREADCRUMBS

MAKE AHEAD

PER SERVING 287 CALORIES | 7 G TOTAL FAT (2 G SATURATED FAT) | 87 MG CHOLESTEROL | 185 MG SODIUM | 19 G CARBOHYDRATE | 3 G FIBER | 34 G PROTEIN

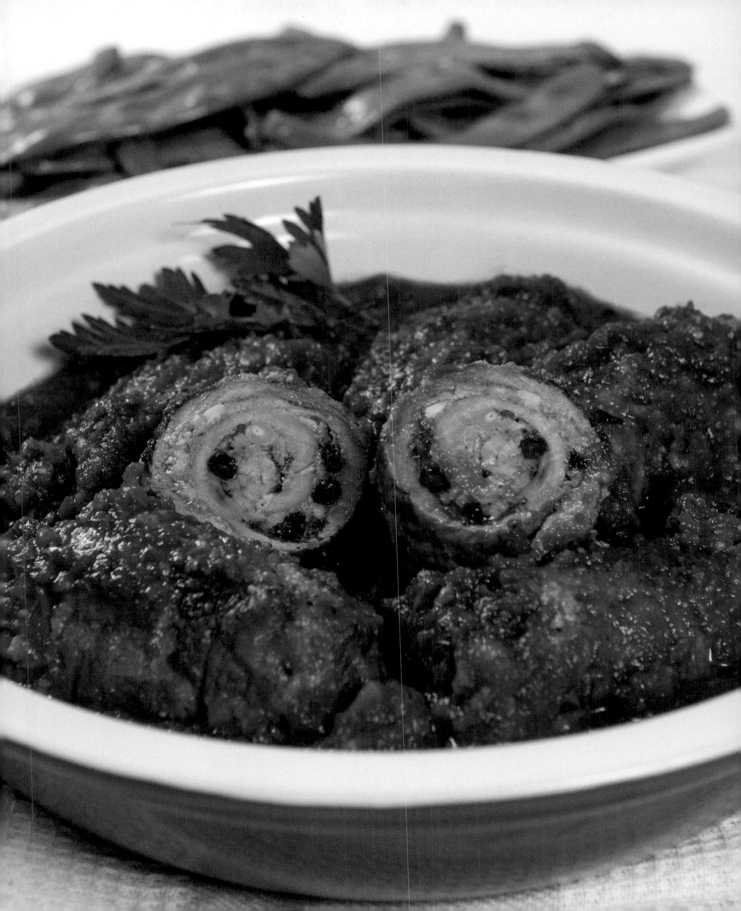

Florentine Tomato-Based Beef Stew

Stracotto alla fiorentina

IF YOU WERE INVITED FOR *STRACOTTO* at any of my Italian friends' homes, you'd typically be indulging in a large, mouth-watering chunk of succulent beef tenderized in an aromatic tomato sauce for about three hours. So what if I told you that you can enjoy the same comfort dish but get it to the table in less time and with more nutrients? Stew-pendous, right?

1 tbsp	extra-virgin olive oil
1½ lbs	(680 g) extra-lean beef stewing meat, cut into 1-inch/2.5-cm cubes
1	onion, diced
½ cup	chopped green onions
3	cloves garlic, minced
½ cup	red wine
1 cup	canned no-salt-added whole peeled tomatoes, chopped
1 can	(5.5 oz/156 mL) no-salt-added tomato paste
4 cups	reduced-sodium beef broth
¾ cup	water
1½ cups	diced celery
2 tbsp	chopped fresh sage leaves, or 1 tsp dried sage
2 to 3	bay leaves
1 tsp	Italian herb seasoning
Freshly ground black pepper to taste	
1 cup	cubed sweet potato
1 cup	diced carrots
½ cup	chopped fresh parsley
1 tbsp	cornstarch

➤ In a large stock pot, heat olive oil over high heat. Pat meat dry and add it to pot; stir continuously until browned, about 2 to 3 minutes.

➤ Add onions and garlic. Stir continuously, scraping up the bottom brown bits, about 2 minutes. Stir in wine, tomatoes and tomato paste until well combined. Add beef broth, water, celery (it's your choice how small or big you dice it), sage, bay leaves, Italian herb seasoning and black pepper. Reduce heat to medium-low. Cover and simmer, stirring occasionally, for 1½ hours. Add sweet potatoes, carrots and parsley during the last 30 minutes of cooking time.

➤ Combine cornstarch with 2 tbsp water, stir and add into the stew. Simmer for 5 minutes to thicken stew, remove and discard bay leaves and serve. I like this smothered over brown rice or whole wheat couscous but it's also great over whole-grain or rice pasta or a slice of Sweet Potato Polenta (*for recipe, see page 22*).

MAKE AHEAD Because extra-lean cuts of beef can vary in tenderness and texture, the longer they simmer the more fall-apart delicious they become. Make this stew the day before and heat it up just before serving.

↻LOW IN...CHOLESTEROL

Extra-lean beef offers an excellent source of protein similar to white meat, but lean beef has less cholesterol than many poultry pieces and similar amounts of fat. This stew uses chunks of extra-lean beef instead of whole beef rump or chuck roast, which is typically wrapped in pancetta and herbs, seared, then slowly braised. Here, we've left out the fatty pancetta, but you won't miss it — the bounty of herbs and spices makes up for it, while the sweet potato adds a welcome sweetness.

6 SERVINGS

GLUTEN-FREE

MAKE AHEAD

PER SERVING 310 CALORIES | 7 G TOTAL FAT (2 G SATURATED FAT) | 79 MG CHOLESTEROL | 182 MG SODIUM | 17 G CARBOHYDRATE | 3 G FIBER | 42 G PROTEIN

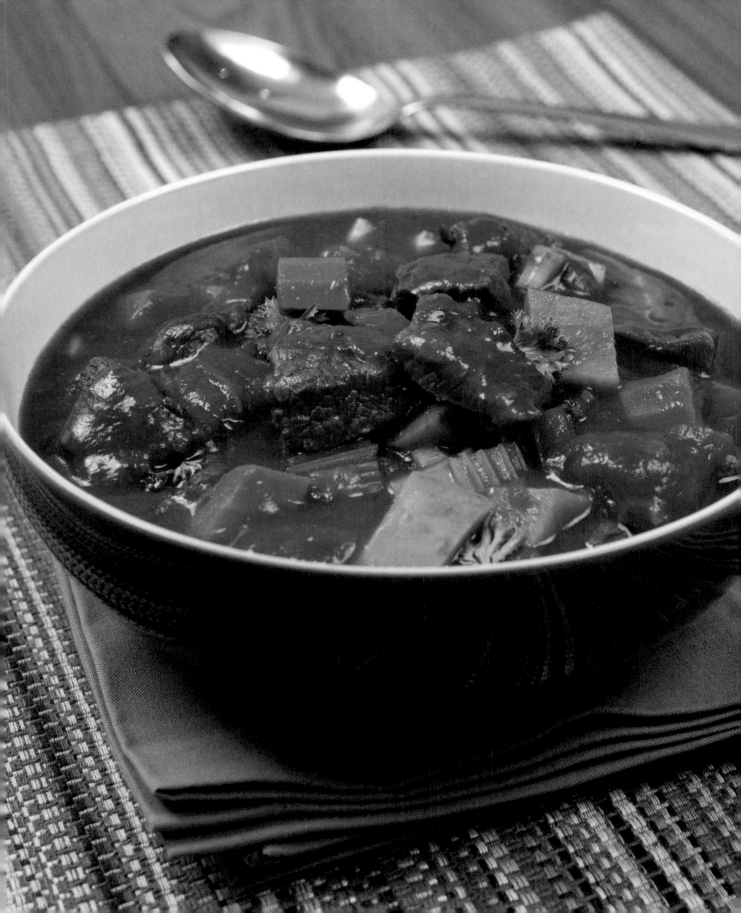

Herb & Prosciutto-Stuffed Pork Tenderloin
Filetto di maiale ripieno alle erbe e prosciutto

GROWING UP, PORK ROASTS AT OUR HOUSE were reserved for special occasions. Because the fattier cuts chosen required a slow, long roast, my parents would wrap them with bacon or prosciutto, celery leaves, herbs and orange peel. I use similar ingredients but I chose a leaner cut of pork and adapted it to accommodate a weekday dinner so you don't have to wait for special celebrations to enjoy it.

Pork

1½ lbs	(680 g) pork tenderloin
2	very thin slices prosciutto (0.5 oz/17 g)
3 to 4	leaves fresh sage
2 tbsp	each: chopped fresh basil and fresh parsley
¼ tsp	fennel seeds
1	clove garlic, pressed or minced

Rub

1 tbsp	extra-virgin olive oil + extra for basting
2 tsp	chopped fresh rosemary
1 tsp	grated orange zest
½ tsp	each: sea salt and garlic powder
¼ tsp	crushed red pepper flakes

Freshly ground cracked black pepper to taste

Balsamic Reduction Sauce (*see recipe, page 20. Prepare this before preparing loins*)

➤ Preheat oven to 400°F.

➤ Make a deep cut lengthwise in the center of tenderloin, making sure not to cut through it, so it opens like a book. Layer the prosciutto on the center cut, overlapping and folding where necessary. Scatter fresh herbs, fennel seeds and garlic over entire length of bottom half. Secure by tying the roast with butcher's twine at 2-inch (5-cm) intervals.

➤ In a small bowl, combine all rub ingredients, from olive oil to black pepper. Work in the rub all over the roast.

➤ Spray a large non-stick skillet with cooking spray and set on high heat. Add pork tenderloin and sear for 2 to 3 minutes each side, turning to ensure all sides are browned. Transfer to a greased baking pan. Pour ¼ cup water in hot skillet to lift pan drippings and pour them at the bottom of baking pan. Roast loin for 20 to 25 minutes or until internal temperature reaches 145°F. Add more water if liquid is drying up.

➤ Remove roast from oven, tent with foil and let rest for 5 minutes before removing string. Slice into ¾-inch (2-cm) round pieces. Serve with Balsamic Reduction Sauce — just a little drizzle packs a whole lot of flavor.

MAKE AHEAD Stuff the roast a day ahead, cover tightly with plastic wrap and refrigerate. Add the rub to the tenderloin just before roasting the next day. Prepare the balsamic reduction days ahead — it keeps for at least two to three weeks in the refrigerator.

⌂ HIGH IN...THIAMIN (VITAMIN B1)

A lean, inexpensive protein, pork loin is also high in thiamin, or vitamin B-1. Just one serving of this dish offers more than 75 percent of the daily recommended intake. Thiamin is crucial in helping your body convert carbohydrates to energy and aiding in digestion — because the body stores very little thiamin it needs to continually replenish its supplies.

6 SERVINGS   40 MIN OR LESS   GLUTEN-FREE   MAKE AHEAD

PER SERVING 189 CALORIES I 9 G TOTAL FAT (3 G SATURATED FAT) I 77 MG CHOLESTEROL I 303 MG SODIUM I 1 G CARBOHYDRATE I 0 G FIBER I 26 G PROTEIN

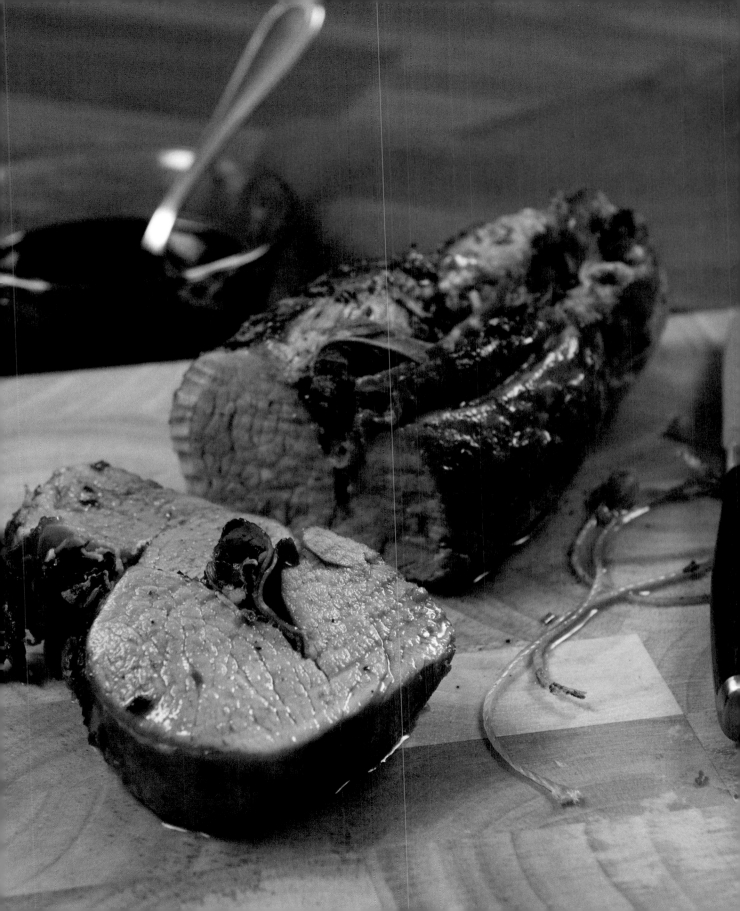

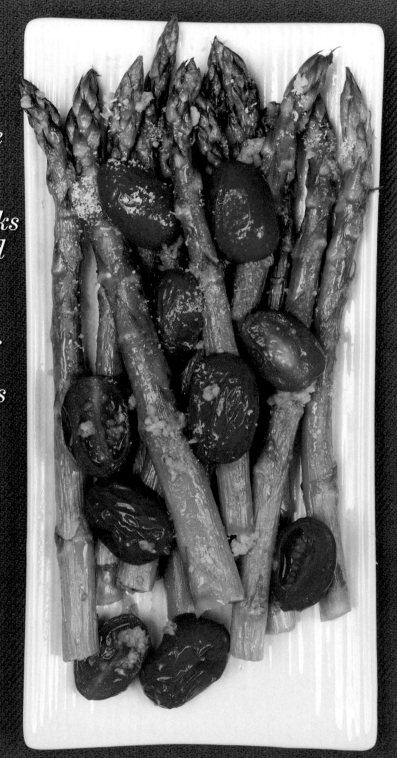

I can count on the kids eating their veggies when I serve asparagus, especially when the stalks are prepared al forno to serve up tender-crisp. Paired with the tanginess of roasted tomatoes and garlic, asparagus steals the show

Sides

Contorni

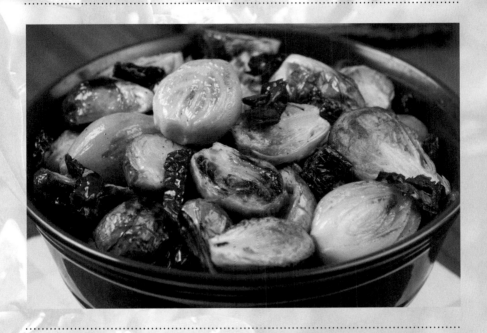

When Brussels sprouts mingle with typically Italian ingredients, they become the most passed around dish at the table

Roasted Fennel with Caramelized Onions

Finocchi arrostiti con cipolle caramellate

YOU KNOW HOW THEY SAY "IF YOU DON'T SUCCEED, try, try, try again" by reintroducing foods to picky eaters, well, this applies to all of you who've shun fennel over the years. That subtle licorice taste in the raw becomes slightly sweetened when roasted, even more so here when matched up with caramelized onions. Perhaps, then, once you've tried fennel again, you'll have the same fascination with it as do the fabulous cooks of Italy.

2 tbsp + 2 tsp extra-virgin olive oil

1 tsp   light butter

2   yellow onions, thinly sliced into rings

2   fennel bulbs (see tip)

¼ tsp   Italian herb seasoning

Sea salt and freshly ground black pepper to taste

Balsamic Reduction Sauce for serving (*see recipe, page 20*) or a good-quality balsamic vinegar (optional)

▶ In a large non-stick skillet, heat 2 tsp olive oil and butter on medium heat. When butter melts, toss in onion rings and stir to coat well. Simmer on low heat, stirring periodically, for 40 minutes.

▶ In the meantime, prepare fennel. Preheat oven to 375°F.

▶ Remove stalks and cut bulb in half. Cut out most of the inner core at the top of fennel bulb (don't cut the whole core or your wedges will fall apart) and slice each half lengthwise into 1-inch (2.5-cm) pieces to make 4 wedges for every half or 8 wedges per bulb. Place wedges on their sides on a large baking sheet lined with foil.

▶ Combine remaining 2 tbsp olive oil, Italian herb seasoning, salt and pepper in a small bowl. Brush fennel with dressing on both sides. Roast in oven for 30 to 35 minutes until lightly golden and softened, turning once halfway between cooking. Serve with a generous helping of caramelized onions and balsamic reduction.

TIP Although fennel is sometimes incorrectly labelled as anise (it's similar looking and tasting but a different plant), a fennel bulb has a round body with stalks and fronds at its tips.

⌂ HIGH IN...VITAMIN C

You might think that vegetables with little color offer very little nutrients but you'd be wrong to assume that of onions and fennel, both of which offer a quarter of the recommended daily dose of vitamin C in just one serving. Onions also contain a powerful compound called quercetin, which protects the heart by lowering cholesterol and high blood pressure. That's not the only thing onions lower — when onions are eaten raw or cooked, studies show they also bring down high blood sugar, so you're less likely to reach for sweets to quash a craving.

 4-6 SERVINGS

 GLUTEN-FREE

 MEATLESS

PER SERVING(6) 175 CALORIES | 9 G TOTAL FAT (1 G SATURATED FAT) | 1 MG CHOLESTEROL | 59 MG SODIUM | 21 G CARBOHYDRATE | 3 G FIBER | 2 G PROTEIN

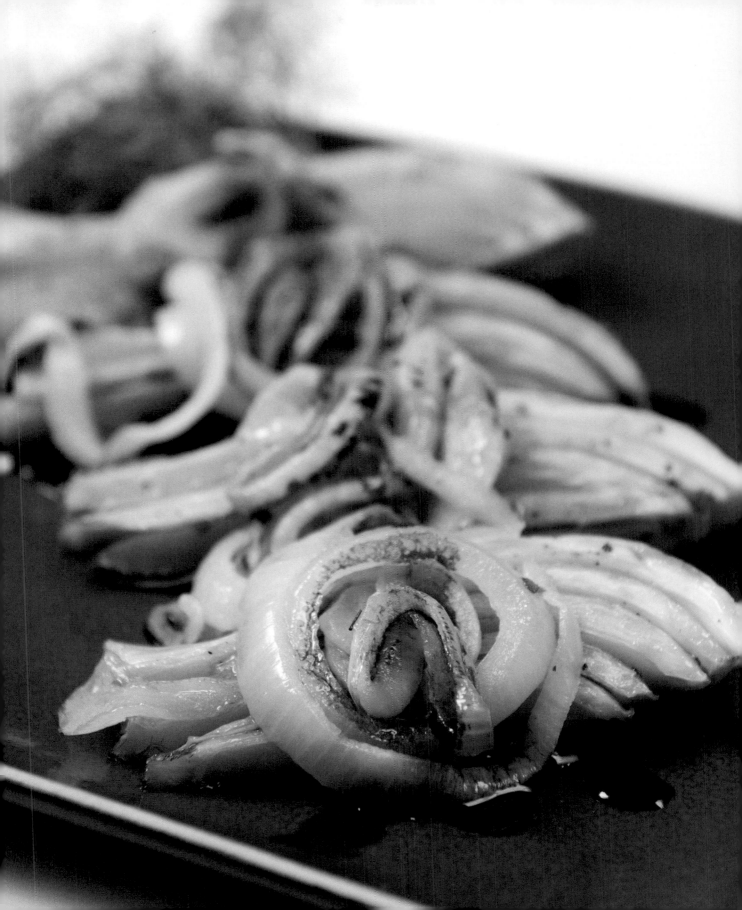

Dandelion Greens in Garlic

Cicoria con aglio e peperoncino

YOU MIGHT BE SURPRISED TO KNOW THAT THESE GREENS, which are the same leafy greens lawn companies spend millions of dollars a year to eradicate from our yards, are revered among Italian home cooks. Today, grocery stores stock cultivated varieties (without the dandelion flower) but I remember the early days when my neighbors would forage for them in public green spaces to cook up at home. However they make their way into the kitchen, they're a delight. My friend Angelo who grew up in Italy's hilly region of Molise adores them stewed with potatoes. At my house, we enjoy them simply prepared like this.

2	small bunches or 1 large bunch dandelion greens
2 tbsp	extra-virgin olive oil
4	cloves garlic, thinly sliced
¼ tsp	crushed red pepper flakes
Sea salt to taste	
Lemon wedges for serving	

➤ Trim tough ends of dandelion greens and leave about an inch or two of stem; you should have about 5 to 6 cups. Bring a large pot of salted water to a boil. Add the dandelion greens and cook until the stems are tender, about 3 minutes. Drain in a colander.

➤ Heat olive oil in a large non-stick skillet over medium heat. Stir in garlic and cook until lightly browned, about 2 minutes. Remove garlic slices with a slotted spoon and transfer to another dish until they're ready to serve. Add dandelion and crushed red pepper flakes to skillet; stir until leaves are a glossy green and well coated, about 3 to 4 minutes. Remove from the skillet, add salt to taste and top with crisp garlic. Serve with lemon wedges. Even though this green is somewhat bitter, avoid the temptation to drench it with salt — the zing of the red pepper flakes and tang of freshly squeezed lemon balance out the flavors.

⌒ HIGH IN...BETA-CAROTENE

This is no regular weed — dandelion greens are one of the most nutritious greens available. They're one of the richest sources of beta-carotene — the pigment found in colorful plants and vegetables that is transformed into vitamin A in the body. Vitamin A is important for boosting the immune system, maintaining healthy skin and protecting eye health. Dandelions are also loaded with vitamin C, iron and calcium.

4 SERVINGS   30 MIN OR LESS   GLUTEN-FREE   MEATLESS

PER SERVING 84 CALORIES | 7 G TOTAL FAT (1 G SATURATED FAT) | 0 MG CHOLESTEROL | 42 MG SODIUM | 5 G CARBOHYDRATE | 2 G FIBER | 1 G PROTEIN

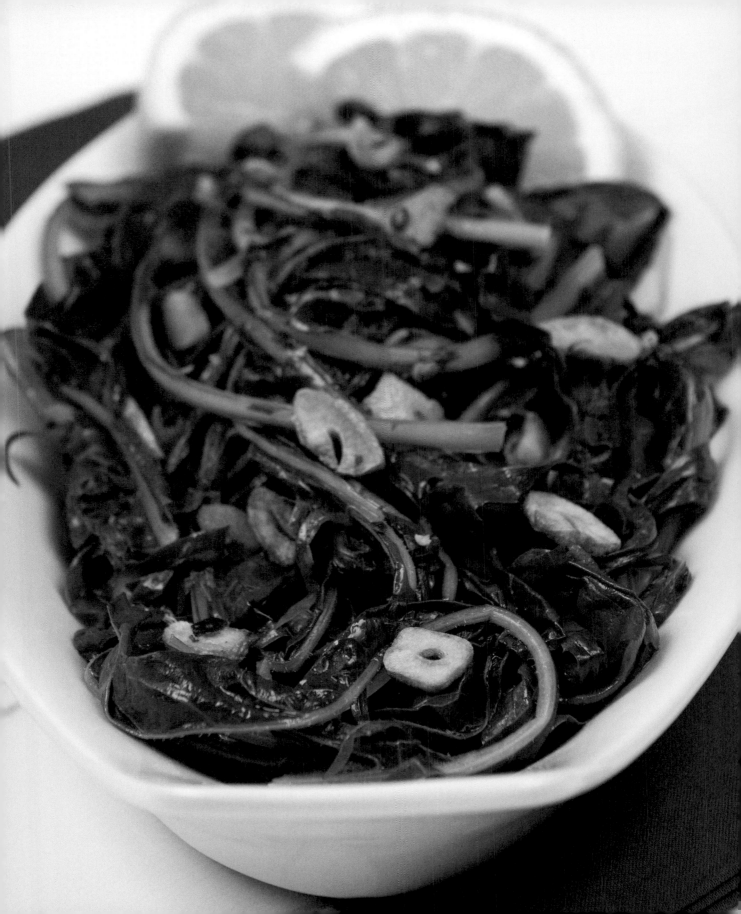

Baked Cardoons Au Gratin
Cardoni gratinati

FEW PEOPLE I KNOW — even among my fellow *Italo-Canadesi* — have heard of cardoons (see tip) let alone cooked with them. But Christmas Eve dinner just isn't the same without this Sicilian specialty that I've enjoyed since I was a little girl. Beyond just the nostalgic connection I have to this obscure vegetable, it's the taste that has me seeking them out in late fall. I'm building quite a following, too — every single person who's tasted them prepared like this has asked me for the recipe.

1	bunch cardoons (see tip)
1 tbsp	sea salt
¼ tsp	baking soda
3 tbsp	whole wheat dry breadcrumbs, divided
2 tbsp	extra-virgin olive oil
5 to 6	anchovy fillets in olive oil, rinsed, patted dry and minced
2 tbsp	freshly grated Parmigiano-Reggiano cheese
2 tbsp	ripe dry-cured (infornate) black olives, pitted and halved (*see tip, page 242*)
3 tbsp	chopped fresh parsley
1	clove garlic, minced
3 tbsp	white wine
Freshly ground black pepper to taste	

TIPS Although anchovy fillets are found in cans or jars, look for them in the refrigerated section and not the tuna section at your grocery store.
➤ Cardoons, also known as cardone or artichoke thistles, are close cousins of the artichoke plant. Though widely consumed in Italy, cardoons have been traced as far back as ancient Egypt and even referenced in Greek mythology. These gems have a long growing season so you'll typically find them in grocery stores only between October and January, although producers are starting to make them available in early spring, too.

➤ Clean cardoon stalk by removing ends, leaves and thorny buds. Cut each stalk horizontally into 3 equal pieces, pulling threads if hanging.

➤ Bring a large pot of water to a boil. Add salt, baking soda and cardoon stalks. Immerse stalks fully in water. Reduce heat to medium-high and cook stalks for 10 minutes. Drain and set aside.

➤ Preheat oven to 375°F. Coat a 9 x 13-inch baking pan with cooking spray. Sprinkle pan with 1 tbsp breadcrumbs. Add half the parboiled cardoons in a single layer, pressing them gently to flatten out. Sprinkle 1 tbsp olive oil, another 1 tbsp breadcrumbs and half of anchovy fillets, cheese, olives, parsley and garlic on top of cardoons. You'll be making a second layer like you would when making lasagna. Add the remaining cardoons over the first layer, sprinkle with white wine, then repeat toppings: remaining olive oil, breadcrumbs, anchovy fillets, cheese, olives, parsley and garlic. Season with black pepper.

➤ Bake for 25 to 30 minutes until cardoons are tender. Cut into pieces like a lasagna and serve.

⇄ VARIATION The salty bits of anchovies are a welcome addition to this naturally bitter stalk. But if you "don't do" anchovies, replace them with about 6 pieces (3 tbsp) of chopped sun-dried tomatoes.

🎧 HIGH IN...FIBER

Cardoons are low in calories while providing a good source of fiber, about 3 grams per serving here — that's about the same as a cup of strawberries or ¾ cup of cooked brown rice. Cardoons are also high in potassium, calcium and magnesium.

6 SERVINGS   MEATLESS

PER SERVING 72 CALORIES | 5 G TOTAL FAT (1 G SATURATED FAT) | 1 MG CHOLESTEROL | 479 MG SODIUM | 4 G CARBOHYDRATE | 1 G FIBER | 1 G PROTEIN

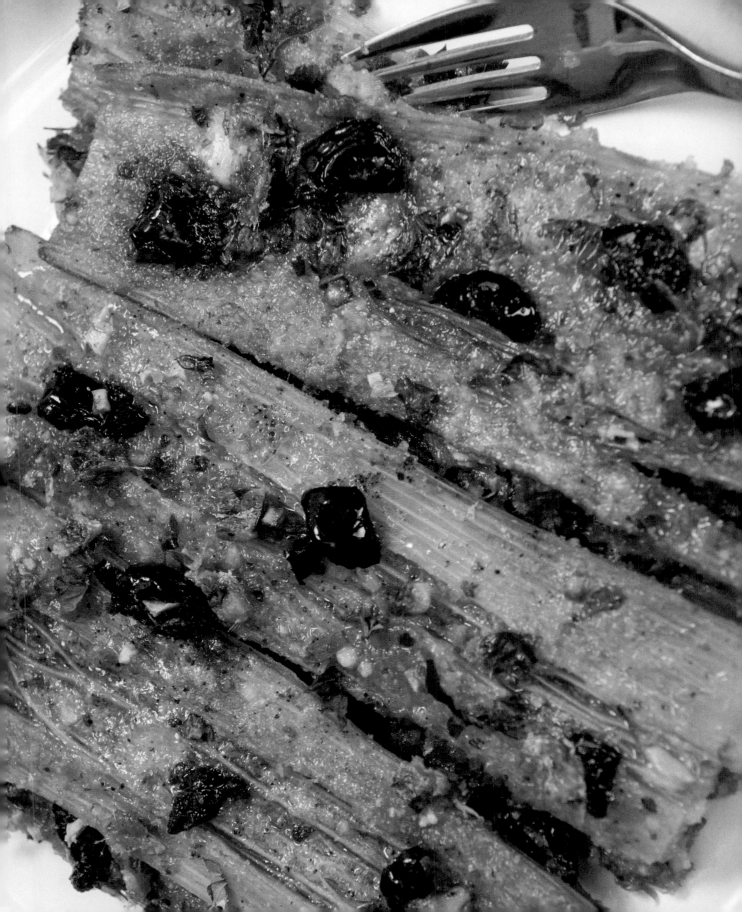

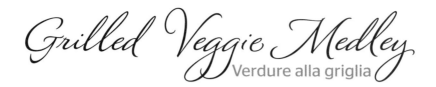

Grilled Veggie Medley
Verdure alla griglia

THE PERFECT LINES OF SYMMETRY AND THE PROFUSION OF COLOR in the produce section is enough to inspire the artist in all of us. Perhaps all those years of working in grocery stores is what shaped my dad's stylish penmanship that he used to craft in-store signage long before computers took over the work. Whatever the motivation, I was always enamored of the shadowed lettering and curved numbers he'd etch with thick felt markers. The signs were as decorative as the stocked tables of fruits and vegetables, many of which I use here in this grilled medley. It, too, is a tableau of color, waiting to be explored.

3	medium portobello mushrooms, stems detached
2	medium zucchini
3	medium shallots, peeled
2	red peppers, preferably Sheppard or red bell
1	small bunch asparagus (about 15 medium-sized spears)
2 tbsp	extra-virgin olive oil, divided
1 tbsp	balsamic vinegar
3 tbsp	chopped fresh basil
2 tbsp	chopped fresh thyme
¼ tsp	sea salt
	Freshly ground black pepper to taste
2 tbsp	crumbled light goat's cheese (1 oz/28 g)

➤ Preheat grill to medium setting.

➤ Place mushrooms caps and stems on a large baking sheet. Trim ends of zucchini and slice vertically into thin slices, about ¼ inch (0.5 cm) thick; add in a single layer to baking sheet. Coat vegetables on both sides with cooking spray.

➤ Cut shallots in half or quarters and place in a large bowl. Trim tops of red peppers, seed and cut into about 6 wedges per pepper; add to bowl. Trim or snap tough ends of asparagus; add to bowl. Pour 1 tbsp olive oil over vegetables and toss gently with your hands to coat well. Take 2 large sheets of foil paper and double them up. Add asparagus and shallots in the center of one piece of foil, flattening them so they form no more than two layers. Fold in the sides of foil paper and pinch seams together to create a closed packet. Add red peppers in the center of the second piece of foil and fold to create a closed packet.

➤ Place foil packages on preheated grill rack that has been lightly brushed with oil; cook for 7 to 8 minutes each side. Grill mushrooms and zucchini directly on the grill for 4 to 5 minutes each side. Combine all grilled vegetables in a large bowl or serving platter. Slice mushrooms in 3 to 4 long strips; cut asparagus in half. Season with remaining olive oil, balsamic vinegar, basil, thyme, salt and pepper. Top with crumbled goat's cheese and serve.

⌂ HIGH IN…VITAMINS ABC

With plenty of vegetables in this dish, there's no shortage of health-boosting vitamins. In fact, these veggies are perfectly paired to bring you vitamins A (asparagus), B (mushrooms) and C (red peppers, zucchini, onions), in addition to a laundry list of other nutrients like potassium and folate. Eating your ABCs has never been easier!

 6 SERVINGS   30 MIN OR LESS   GLUTEN-FREE   MEATLESS

PER SERVING 74 CALORIES | 5 G TOTAL FAT (1 G SATURATED FAT) | 2 MG CHOLESTEROL | 31 MG SODIUM | 5 G CARBOHYDRATE | 1 G FIBER | 2 G PROTEIN

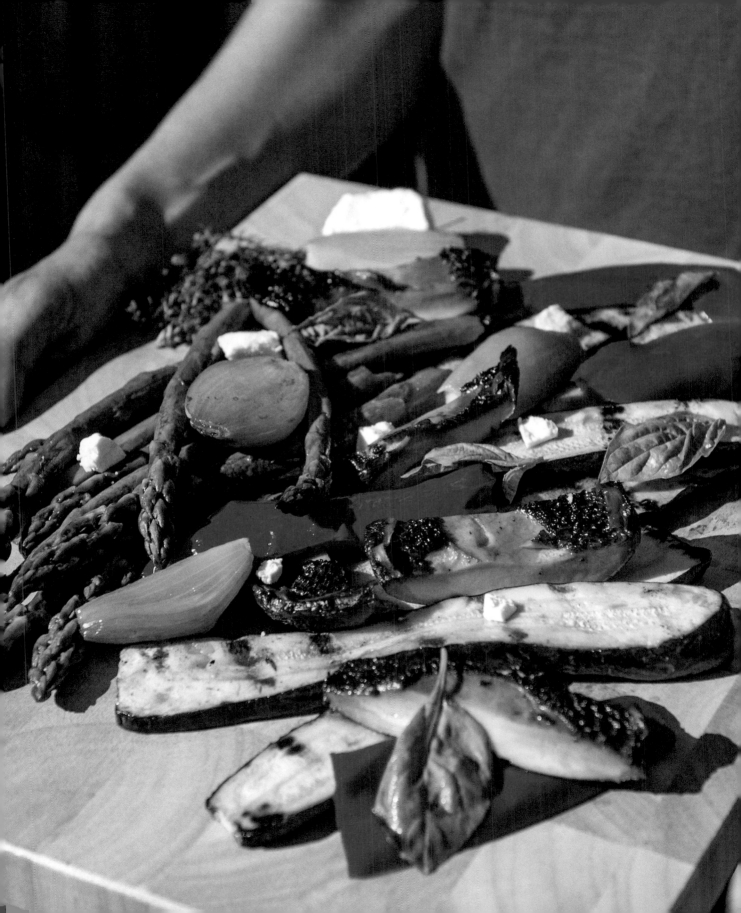

Broiled Eggplant Bake with Tomatoes & Parsley

Melanzane ripiene con pomodori e prezzemolo

I WAS SURPRISED WHEN A COLLEAGUE OF MINE ONCE TOLD ME she had no idea what to do with eggplants except to grill them. Italians have been cooking with this versatile vegetable since it made its way to the country from India more than seven centuries ago. In my own kitchen, it's second nature to dish it up in so many ways — whether grilled, marinated, sautéed and stuffed like in both of these recipes. If you're like my colleague, serve these up to your family, your girlfriends, your neighbours and they'll be saying, "What?! Eggplant!? I never knew it could taste like this!"

4	mini eggplants or 2 large eggplants (see tip)
½ tsp	sea salt
5	cloves garlic, minced
½ cup	minced fresh parsley
1½ cups	no-salt-added diced tomatoes, drained
2 tbsp	extra-virgin olive oil, divided
Freshly ground black pepper to taste	
2 tbsp	whole wheat dry breadcrumbs
2 tbsp	freshly grated Parmigiano-Reggiano cheese
1 tsp	Italian herb seasoning
½ cup	water

➤ Preheat oven to 375°F.

➤ Trim tops of eggplants and cut in half lengthwise; don't remove skin. (If you're using large eggplants, cut them into half horizontally and then vertically). Score deeply twice lengthwise, then across three times, being careful not to cut outer skin. Lightly salt eggplant halves.

➤ Combine garlic and parsley in a small bowl. Distribute mixture evenly among eggplant halves and stuff as much of it as possible inside cuts.

➤ Place tomatoes in a medium bowl and, using your hands, press tomatoes slightly to break them up into smaller pieces. Stir in 1 tbsp olive oil and pepper. Spoon tomato mixture evenly on top of seasoned eggplant and press down slightly. Combine breadcrumbs, cheese and Italian herb seasoning in a small bowl. Spoon evenly over halves and press down slightly.

➤ Coat an extra-large baking pan with remaining 1 tbsp olive oil and water. Fit in eggplants so they're snug but not too tight. Cover with foil and cook for 40 minutes. Remove foil, reset oven to broil setting and bring pan to *middle* oven rack. Broil on high for 10 minutes, until tops turn slightly brown.

TIPS You can use regular-sized aubergine eggplants and cut them into quarters for this recipe, but I prefer the smaller globe variety because they have less seeds and, therefore, aren't as bitter. While Rosa Bianca eggplants are sweeter, they're typically too robust for this recipe. (*For more information about eggplant varieties, see Eggplant Parmigiana with Quinoa, page 172.*)
➤ If you love Eggplant Parmigiana but want to skip the steps to make it, this is a close cousin. It tastes even better the next day when flavors are soaked in.

6-8 SERVINGS

GLUTEN-FREE

MEATLESS

PER SERVING(8) 84 CALORIES | 4 G TOTAL FAT (1 G SATURATED FAT) | 1 MG CHOLESTEROL | 179 MG SODIUM | 11 G CARBOHYDRATE | 5 G FIBER | 2 G PROTEIN

Ground Turkey-Stuffed Eggplant

Melanzane ripiene con carne di tacchino

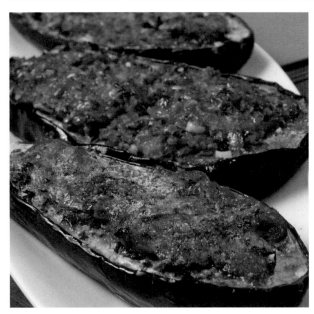

3	aubergine eggplants (about 1 lb/454 g each)
1 tsp	extra-virgin olive oil
7 oz	(200 g) lean ground turkey
½ cup	chopped onions
2	cloves garlic, minced
1 cup	chopped ripe tomatoes
¼ cup	white wine
⅓ cup	quick-cooking oats*
1	egg white
¼ cup	packed shredded part-skim mozzarella cheese (1 oz/28 g)
2 tbsp	chopped fresh basil
½ tsp	sea salt
¼ tsp	dried oregano
Freshly ground black pepper to taste	
2 tbsp	freshly grated Parmigiano-Reggiano cheese

➤ Preheat oven to 350°F.

➤ Trim tops of eggplants and cut each vertically into two equal halves. Coat cut halves lightly with cooking spray and place on a baking sheet lined with foil and lightly greased. Bake in oven for 30 minutes.

➤ Carefully use a sharp knife to cut a ½-inch (1 cm) perimeter around the sides and bottom of eggplant. Use a spoon to scoop out the flesh, being careful not to puncture the bottom. Place flesh in a large bowl, break it up into large pieces and mash until you get a creamy-chunky mixture. Set skins aside on baking sheet.

➤ In a large non-stick skillet, heat olive oil on medium-high heat. Add ground turkey, onions and garlic and stir frequently to break up turkey pieces; cook until onions begin to soften, about 4 to 5 minutes. Stir in tomatoes and white wine and cook for 4 to 5 minutes, until turkey is no longer pink. Cool mixture for 5 minutes and place in the bowl with eggplant flesh.

➤ Add oats, egg white, mozzarella cheese, basil, salt, oregano and black pepper; mix until well combined. Divide mixture into 6 equal portions and fill each eggplant skin, handling carefully so skin doesn't tear. Sprinkle each lightly with 1 tsp grated cheese.

➤ Bake in preheated oven on the *middle* rack for 25 minutes, then reset oven to broil setting and cook for another 5 minutes, until tops are lightly browned. Serve hot.

> **MAKE AHEAD** Bake eggplants the night before, scoop out their flesh and keep skins separate until you're ready to use them the next day.

6 SERVINGS   GLUTEN-FREE* CHECK LABEL   MAKE AHEAD

PER SERVING 91 CALORIES | 4 G TOTAL FAT (1 G SATURATED FAT) | 21 MG CHOLESTEROL | 242 MG SODIUM | 6 G CARBOHYDRATE | 3 G FIBER | 8 G PROTEIN

Farro with Tomatoes, Spinach & Bacon

Farro al pomodoro con spinaci e pancetta

DESPITE ITS MOST RECENT CLAIM TO FAME in North American kitchens, farro has had a long history. In fact, it was a main staple in the Roman Empire diet after it was brought over from Egypt. Although I don't remember eating it as a kid — the fact that it wasn't imported might have something to do with it — I've now made it a pantry staple. It's great for soups, salads and sides — my little emperors agree.

1 tsp	extra-virgin olive oil
½ cup	chopped onions
2	slices turkey or chicken bacon-style, chopped (1.8 oz/52 g)
2	cloves garlic, minced
¾ cup	chopped no-salt-added whole peeled tomatoes, drained and chopped
1 cup	semi-pearled farro (see tip)
¼ cup	white wine
1¼ cup	reduced-sodium chicken or vegetable broth
1 cup	packed fresh baby spinach leaves, torn
2 tbsp	chopped fresh basil
Pinch	dried oregano
Sea salt and freshly ground black pepper to taste	
Chopped fresh parsley for serving	
Freshly grated Parmigiano-Reggiano cheese for serving	

➤ In a medium pot, heat olive oil over medium-high heat. Add onions, bacon and garlic and stir continuously until onions are softened, about 2 minutes. Stir in tomatoes and farro and stir until well coated.

➤ Add remaining ingredients, except parsley and cheese, and combine well. Reduce heat to medium-low, cover and let simmer for about 25 minutes, stirring occasionally. Serve hot with fresh parsley and a sprinkle of freshly grated cheese.

TIP Don't confuse farro with spelt. While they have a similar aesthetics, farro — which is Italian for emmer wheat — has a nutty flavor like spelt but doesn't require the prerequisite soaking and it holds its chewy texture while cooking quickly.

⌂ HIGH IN...FIBER

Farro contains more fiber than other healthy grains, including brown rice, barley and quinoa. It's also considered a complex carbohydrate that not only breaks down slowly but also stimulates the immune system. Even though this dish gets a boost of protein from the bacon, farro on its own is also an excellent source of protein.

6 SERVINGS   40 MIN OR LESS

PER SERVING 142 CALORIES | 2 G TOTAL FAT (0 G SATURATED FAT) | 5 MG CHOLESTEROL | 77 MG SODIUM | 24 G CARBOHYDRATE | 4 G FIBER | 7 G PROTEIN

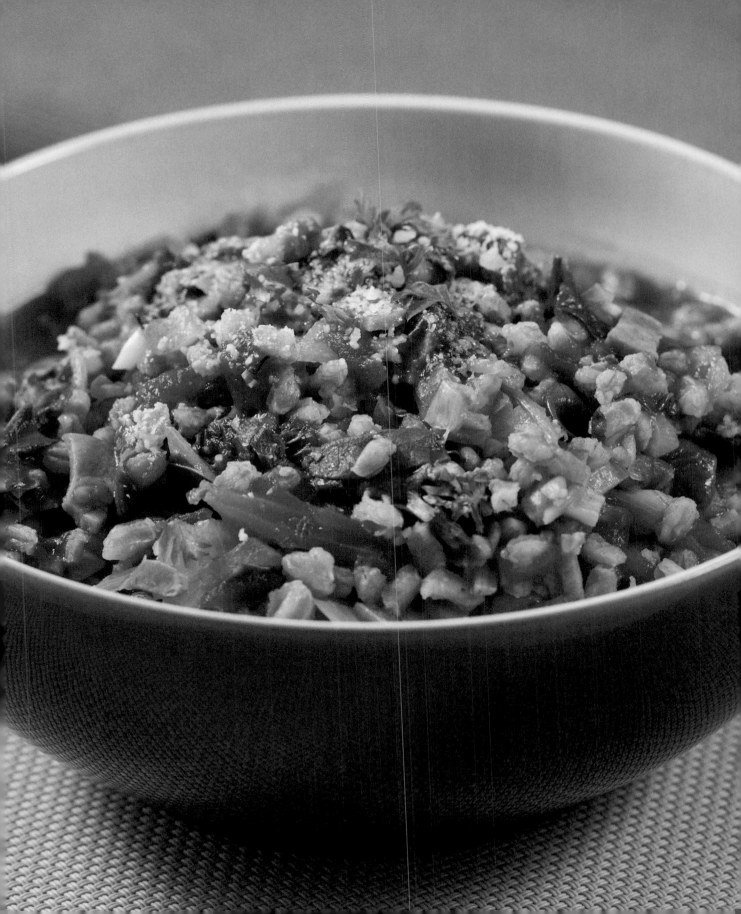

"Fried" Battered Cauliflower
Cavolfiori in pastella

LONG BEFORE I DISCOVERED TEMPURA on Japanese menus, I had been exposed to *la pastella*, a paste made with white flour, water and salt to coat a host of vegetables before landing in a fry pan to become crisp sensations. I always pulled up a stool and volunteered to help Ma dip the vegetables, from cauliflower and broccoli to zucchini and eggplant — not only for the ultimate reward of being the first to eat them but also for the therapeutic pleasure of working with food. Perfect for big and little hands alike, this pastella uses corn flour to give the dish more fiber, no gluten and a little more sunshine.

1	medium head cauliflower
1 cup	yellow or white corn flour
2 tbsp	minced fresh parsley
1 tsp	sea salt
¼ tsp	baking soda
1	clove garlic, minced
⅔ cup	water
2 tbsp	freshly grated Parmigiano-Reggiano cheese
¼ tsp	freshly ground black pepper
1 tbsp	extra-virgin olive oil
¼ cup	thinly sliced red onions

▶ Remove and discard leaves and large stalk from cauliflower. Pull apart florets to make several fist-sized pieces. Cut large pieces in half so they have a flat side (this will work best later when you need to cook them in the skillet). Bring a large pot of water to a boil. Add cauliflower and cook for about 6 to 7 minutes, until tender-crisp. Drain, rinse with cold water and thoroughly drain again.

▶ In a large bowl, combine flour, parsley, salt, baking soda and garlic. Whisk in water until well combined. Using tongs (or your hands), fully immerse each cauliflower floret into batter. Shake off excess batter and place onto a plate. Repeat with other florets. Sprinkle battered cauliflower with grated cheese and black pepper.

▶ In a large non-stick skillet, heat olive oil over medium-high heat. Add cauliflower and cook for 8 to 10, turning a few times to brown all sides and tops of cauliflower. Transfer to a serving dish and keep warm. Coat the same skillet with cooking spray and cook red onions for 2 minutes. Sprinkle onions on top of cauliflower and serve.

MAKE AHEAD You can parboil the cauliflower and refrigerate one to two days before dipping them in the batter and cooking them in the skillet.

◡ LOW IN...FAT

Eliminating the deep-fryer makes this cauliflower in pastella leaner by at least 25 percent. Corn flour also adds more fiber and flavor.

6 SERVINGS   30 MIN OR LESS   GLUTEN-FREE   MEATLESS   MAKE AHEAD

PER SERVING 122 CALORIES | 4 G TOTAL FAT (1 G SATURATED FAT) | 2 MG CHOLESTEROL | 487 MG SODIUM | 20 G CARBOHYDRATE | 3 G FIBER | 4 G PROTEIN

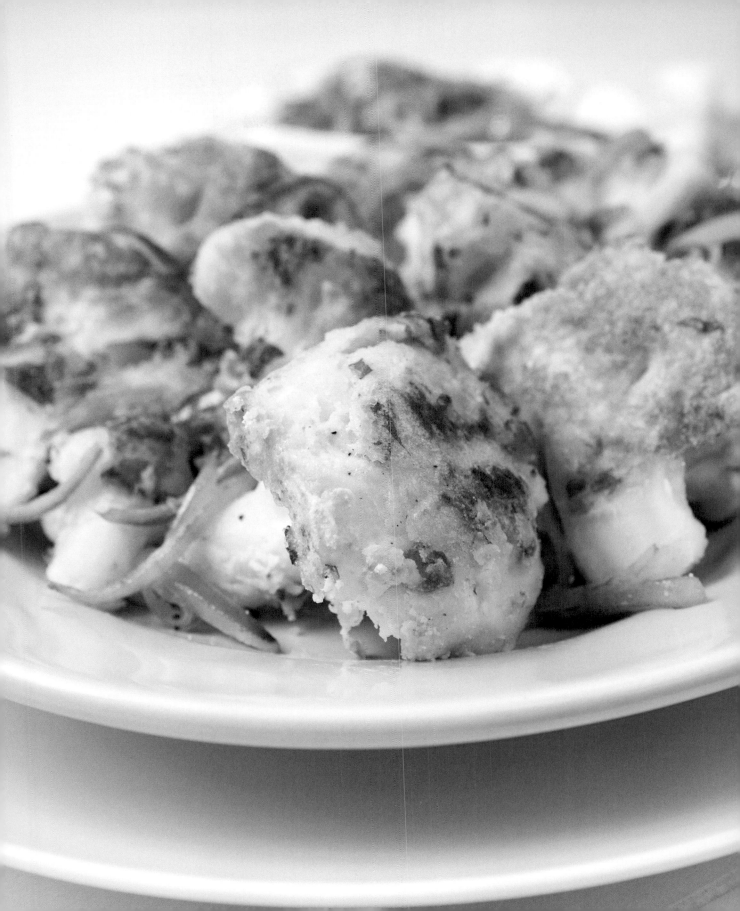

Peperonata—Braised Peppers
Peperonata

COME LATE SUMMER, my dad and I get busy sourcing the perfect peppers — typically it's the Sheppard variety that we buy by the bushels to preserve for later consumption. Dad is passionate about produce. When he emigrated from Italy to Canada in 1957, he landed his first job at the Ontario Food Terminal, getting to know firsthand what buyers were looking for when they came to select the finest fruits and vegetables to sell later in stores. He worked in produce until retirement. I still rely on him today to pick out the best — whether it's the perfect melon, tomatoes or the Sheppards and Cubanelles used here. At most Italian homes, you'll find peperonata alongside grilled chicken, or as a topper in a veal cutlet sandwich.

1 tbsp	extra-virgin olive oil
2	onions, thinly sliced
2	cloves garlic, minced
¼ cup	red wine
4	Cubanelle peppers, seeded and sliced into large wedges
4	Sheppard peppers, seeded and sliced into large wedges
12	ripe cherry or grape tomatoes, halved
2 tbsp	chopped fresh basil
½ tsp	dried oregano
¼ tsp	sea salt
1 tsp	chopped fresh thyme or ½ tsp dried thyme

➤ In a large non-stick skillet, heat olive oil over medium-high heat. Add onions and garlic and cook until onions are softened. Add wine and simmer for 2 minutes. Add peppers; reduce heat to medium and cook, covered, for about 15 minutes, stirring often.

➤ Stir in remaining ingredients and cook for 5 more minutes. Serve peppers on their own as a side or top on grilled meats, cutlet sandwiches or over cooked quinoa.

⌒ HIGH IN...CAROTENOIDS

Red peppers have an enormous amount of potent antioxidants called carotenoids. In fact, red peppers are one of only a few vegetables that are packed with so many of these types of phytochemicals, including beta-carotene and lycopene. Research shows that when women consume a high amount of vegetables rich in carotenoids, they can lower their risk of breast cancer by up to 20 percent.

 4 SERVINGS   30 MIN OR LESS   GLUTEN-FREE   MEATLESS

PER SERVING 114 CALORIES | 4 G TOTAL FAT (1 G SATURATED FAT) | 0 MG CHOLESTEROL | 163 MG SODIUM | 18 G CARBOHYDRATE | 6 G FIBER | 3 G PROTEIN

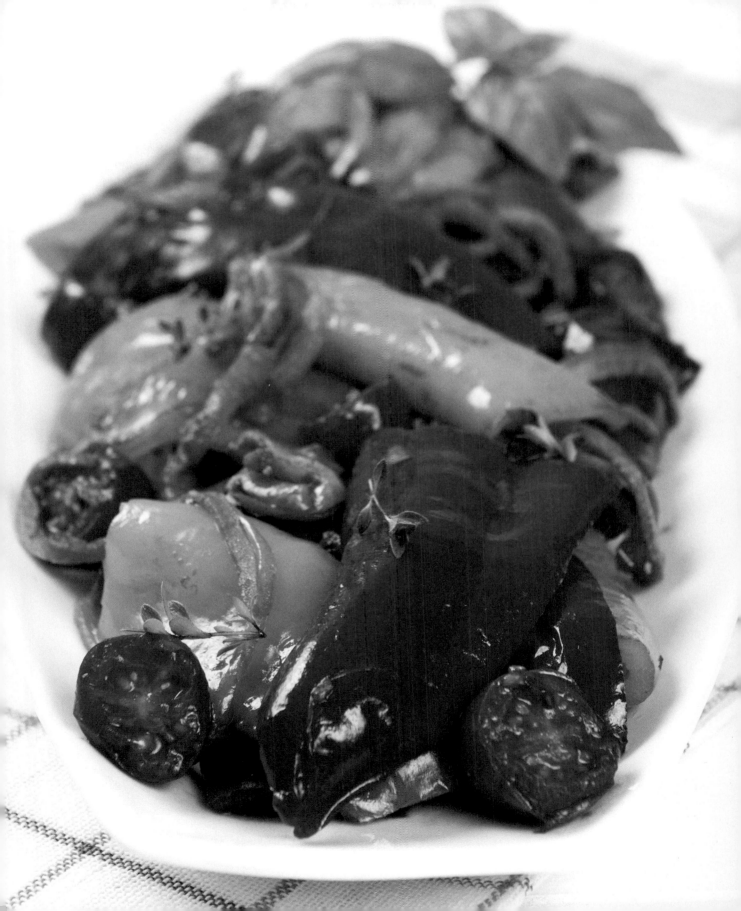

Garlic-Parsley Stuffed Artichokes
Carciofi ripieni

THE FRESH ARTICHOKE TAKES A PRIZED PLACE IN MY KITCHEN. It did in my parents' kitchen and in their parents' kitchen, too, because of its native Mediterranean origins. Naturally, we've never been intimidated by this vegetable's sometimes thorny demeanor, prying it open to add a garlicky blend that simmers to perfection and is enjoyed along with the choke's meaty leaves. In Italian cooking, the practice of stuffing vegetables is far-reaching — from the fleshy tomato to the tender pepper to the spongy eggplant — enhancing the flavors of the vessel itself. In the next recipe, plump tomatoes house a savory meatless mix that brings out their juicy goodness.

6	cloves garlic, minced
½ cup	minced fresh parsley
¼ cup	minced celery hearts
3 tbsp	whole wheat dry breadcrumbs
3 tbsp	egg white
2 tbsp	freshly grated Parmigiano-Reggiano cheese
2 tbsp + 1 tsp	extra-virgin olive oil, divided
3 tbsp	freshly squeezed lemon juice, divided
Freshly ground black pepper to taste	
6	medium artichokes
Sea salt to taste	

➤ In a medium bowl, combine garlic, parsley, celery hearts, breadcrumbs, egg white, cheese, 2 tbsp olive oil, 1 tbsp lemon juice and black pepper. Set aside.

➤ Trim the stems of each artichoke and about one-quarter of each top with a serrated knife. Remove tough brown outer leaves and discard. Cut any remaining thorny tips with scissors. Quickly immerse artichokes into a bath of cold water and remaining 2 tbsp lemon juice to prevent them from turning brown. Once all the artichokes have been cut and rinsed, pat dry with a paper towel and pry open the leaves (without pulling them off) with your thumbs to open up spaces for stuffing. Season with salt.

➤ Spoon about 1 tbsp of stuffing on top of each artichoke; use your thumbs to push stuffing down into the cavities between leaves. Add a bit more stuffing on the top.

➤ In a medium pot, arrange artichokes so they're sitting upright and snugly side by side. Pour water slowly into the pot until it reaches about two-thirds of the way up artichokes. Sprinkle with salt and drizzle with remaining 1 tsp olive oil.

➤ Bring water to a boil. Reduce heat to medium-low and simmer, covered, until artichoke leaves are tender and easy to pull, about 40 minutes. You may need to add a little bit more water if liquid is low. Use tongs to remove artichokes and serve.

TIP Use 1 or 2 medium whole potatoes to fill in the gaps when placing artichokes side by side in the pot to keep them sitting upright while cooking. The potatoes also absorb the artichokes' bitterness.

6 SERVINGS   MEATLESS

PER SERVING 128 CALORIES | 6 G TOTAL FAT (1 G SATURATED FAT) | 2 MG CHOLESTEROL | 170 MG SODIUM | 16 G CARBOHYDRATE | 7 G FIBER | 6 G PROTEIN

Baked Stuffed Tomatoes
Pomodori ripieni al forno

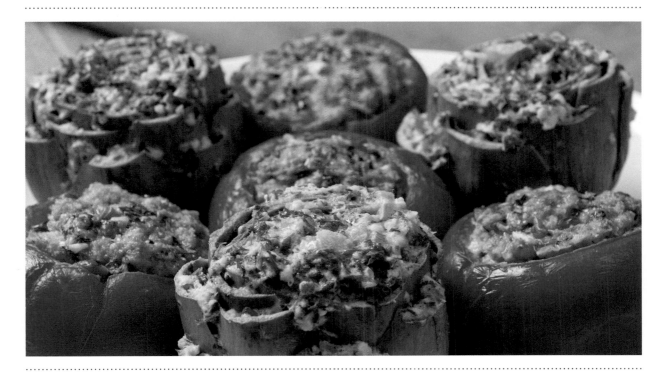

6	large vine-ripened tomatoes (ripe but firm)
3 cups	cubed whole-grain bread (crust removed)
½ cup	canned no-salt-added brown lentils, drained and rinsed
¼ cup	chopped fresh basil
2	cloves garlic, minced
⅓ cup	no-salt-added vegetable or chicken broth
1	egg, beaten
4 tbsp	freshly grated Asiago or Pecorino Romano cheese

Freshly ground black pepper to taste

Sea salt to taste

➤ Gently cut out tops of tomatoes with a paring knife. Spoon out seeds and membranes until hollow. Save tops, seeds and membranes for another dish. Set aside hollowed tomatoes. Preheat oven to 350°F.

➤ In a large bowl, combine bread cubes, lentils, basil and garlic. Wet mixture well with broth. Add egg, cheese and black pepper and mix until well combined (using your hands to work in).

➤ Lightly salt inside of tomatoes and fill evenly with stuffing until just slightly above opening. Spray a small baking pan or deep-dish pie plate. Place stuffed tomatoes close together but not touching. Bake in preheated oven for 30 minutes. Handle gently when serving so you don't puncture tomatoes.

⇆ VARIATION Make this a gluten-free recipe by replacing bread cubes with 2 cups cooked quinoa.

6 SERVINGS

GLUTEN-FREE
SEE VARIATION

MEATLESS

PER SERVING 124 CALORIES | 3 G TOTAL FAT (1 G SATURATED FAT) | 33 MG CHOLESTEROL | 194 MG SODIUM | 19 G CARBOHYDRATE | 4 G FIBER | 7 G PROTEIN

Stuffed Mushroom Caps
Funghi ripieni

IN NORTH AMERICA, THE UNSUNG HERO in the produce section is the underrated mushroom. Yet this dark and mysterious fungus is revered among Italian cooks — so much so that in Italy the hunt for the perfect fungus (the white truffle is highly prized) has resulted in the overharvesting of many fungi, and strict guidelines are now in place to enforce quotas. The sport has even gone to the dogs, which are trained to sniff out the pungent prize from damp forest floors. My family doesn't dig for them in the wild (neither does my dog) but my dad has made cooking them an art, stuffing them to perfection with pointed peaks using a fragrant blend of herbs and spices. At family gatherings, we all hunt for them once we sit at the table and enjoy popping them in our mouths.

1 pkg	(8 oz/ 227 g) cremini or white button mushrooms
1 tsp	extra-virgin olive oil
1 tsp	light butter
2	cloves garlic, minced
1	slice (1.6 oz/45 g) whole-grain bread (crust removed), crumbled
1	egg white
¼ cup	minced fresh parsley
1½ tbsp	freshly grated Parmigiano-Reggiano cheese
Freshly ground black pepper to taste	
Sea salt to taste	
4 tbsp	reduced-sodium vegetable broth
3 tbsp	white wine

➤ Preheat oven to 375°F.

➤ Remove stems of mushrooms and finely chop them up and set aside. Keep mushroom caps separate.

➤ In a small non-stick skillet, heat olive oil and butter over medium-high heat. Add garlic and mushroom stems and sauté until softened, about 3 to 4 minutes. Cool slightly.

➤ In a small bowl, add mushroom-garlic mixture along with bread pieces, egg white, parsley, cheese and black pepper. Use your fingertips to combine and work in all the ingredients.

➤ Sprinkle mushroom caps with a little salt and fill each one with about 1 tsp of filling, pressing it in slightly with the back of the teaspoon and rounding the filling on the top.

➤ Combine broth and white wine and pour into a small baking pan. Add stuffed mushrooms in a single layer. Bake until mushrooms are tender, about 15 to 20 minutes

⌂ HIGH IN...PHYTOCHEMICALS

Button and cremini mushrooms have been linked to protection against breast cancer. For example, in one study, when researchers evaluated five commonly consumed or specialty mushrooms, it found that they significantly suppressed the growth of cancerous cells.

4 SERVINGS   40 MIN OR LESS   MEATLESS

PER SERVING 103 CALORIES | 5 G TOTAL FAT (1 G SATURATED FAT) | 3 MG CHOLESTEROL | 148 MG SODIUM | 8 G CARBOHYDRATE | 1 G FIBER | 5 G PROTEIN

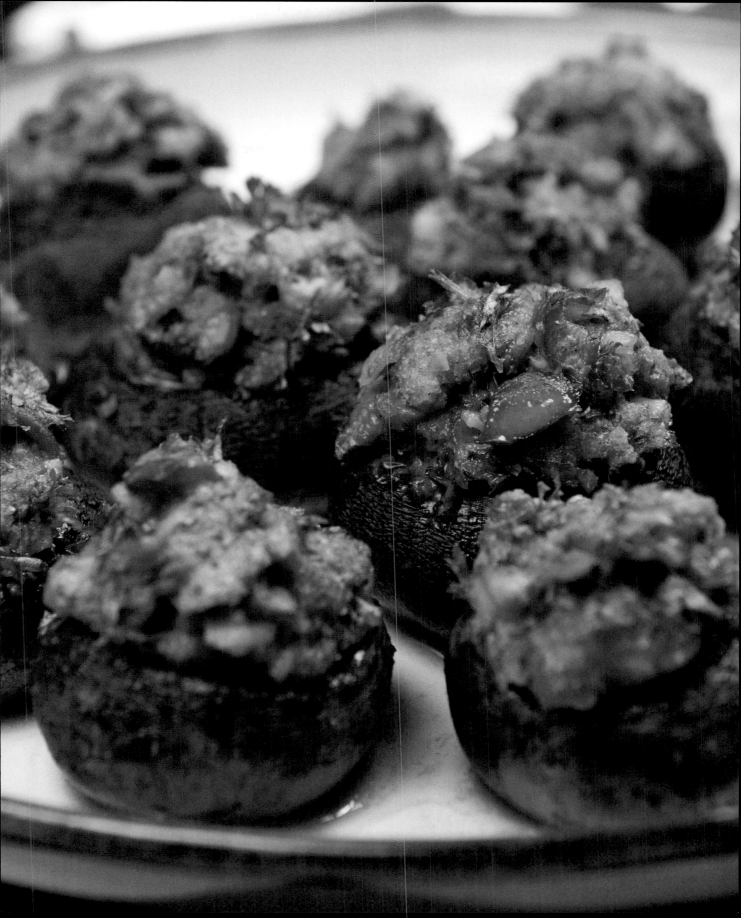

Sweet Potato & Fresh Herb Croquettes
Crocchette di patate dolci alle erbe aromatiche

MY IDEA OF HOMEMADE FRIED POTATOES has no resemblance to the variety you get from the drive-through window. Instead, I think of my mom's croquettes, which are patties made with mashed potatoes and an aromatic bouquet of garden-fresh herbs, bound together with eggs and a dollop of grated cheese. I can still remember their intoxicating scent wafting out of the basement window (where Mom had an "extra" kitchen) as she deep-fried them in a sizzling bath of oil. These croquettes don't require a basement kitchen, nor do they get showered with oil to achieve their crispy exterior and velvety smooth center.

3	large baking potatoes
1	large sweet potato
2 tbsp	1% milk
1 tbsp	light butter, melted
1	egg, beaten
¼ cup	packed shredded light provolone or part-skim mozzarella cheese (1 oz/28 g)
4 tbsp	freshly grated Parmigiano-Reggiano cheese
1	clove garlic, minced
¼ cup	minced fresh parsley
2 tbsp	minced fresh basil
½ tsp	sea salt
Freshly ground black pepper to taste	
2 cups	spelt dry breadcrumbs (see tip)
½ cup	egg white

TIP Spelt breadcrumbs are light and airy to give baked dishes like this one a crispy exterior. Find them in the grocery aisle where other breadcrumbs are sold.

➤ Cut potatoes in half and cover completely in a pot of water. Bring to a boil and cook for 30 minutes, until tender when centers are poked with a fork. Drain and let cool slightly until easier to handle.

➤ Remove skins and hand mash potatoes in a large bowl until completely mashed. Add milk and butter and toss to cool a little more before handling. Add egg, cheeses, garlic, parsley, basil, salt and pepper; toss well to combine. Refrigerate mixture for 30 minutes.

➤ Preheat oven to 425°F.

➤ Pour breadcrumbs into a shallow dish or pie plate, half at a time to avoid clumps. In another shallow dish, pour egg white. Measure out 2 heaping tbsp of potato mixture and shape into 1 x 3-inch-long (2.5 x 7.5-cm) rolls. Coat with breadcrumbs, dip one side into egg white and roll it in the palm of your hand to coat all sides, then dip again into breadcrumbs. Place on a baking sheet lined with foil paper. Spray tops and sides (about 5 seconds) with cooking spray and cook until lightly golden, about 20 to 25 minutes on *middle* oven rack.

➤ Serve with Quick Marinara Sauce (*see recipe, page 13*).

MAKE AHEAD You can boil the potatoes and refrigerate for up to three days before you reheat and mash them to make the mixture.

↻ LOW IN...FAT

Low-fat cheeses and a no-fry dunk give these croquettes irresistible crunch without the fat — at least 50 percent less. Minus all the added fat, white potatoes can make a nutritious contribution, especially since they bring a wallop of essential minerals, but just the same we've added in some sweet potato for its fiber — more than double the amount in white spuds.

25-28 CROQUETTES   MEATLESS   MAKE AHEAD

PER SERVING (28) 293 CALORIES | 4 G TOTAL FAT (1 G SATURATED FAT) | 31 MG CHOLESTEROL | 294 MG SODIUM | 52 G CARBOHYDRATE | 6 G FIBER | 13 G PROTEIN

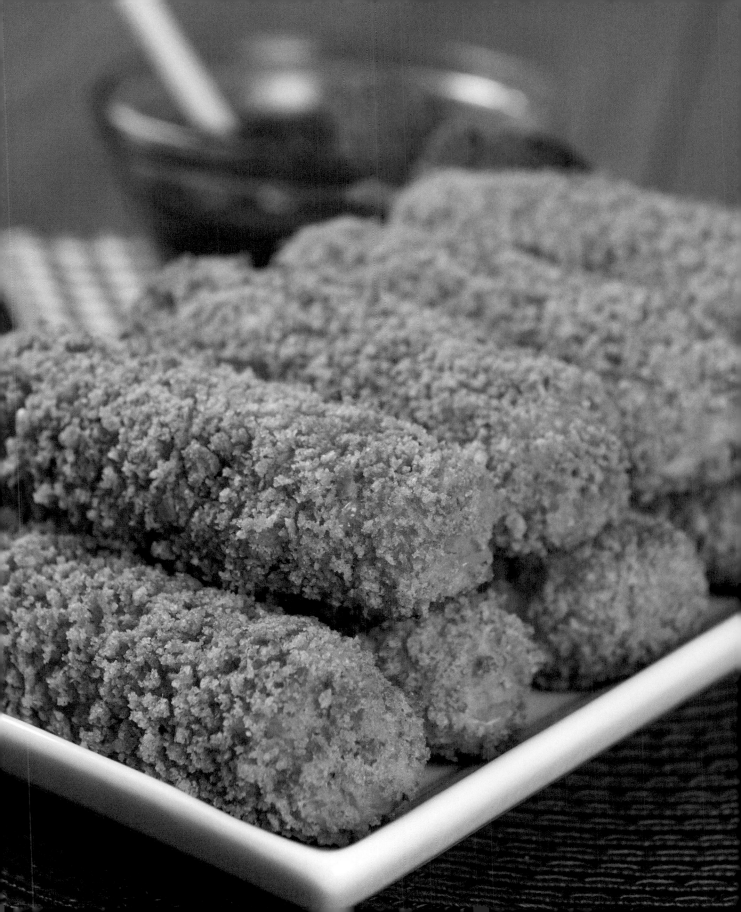

Stuffed Zucchini Boats
Zucchine in barchetta

MY DAD IS AMONG THE MANY ITALIANS who love pairing the versatile zucchini with other delicious foods. He combines them with potatoes as toppers on pizza, fills them with a savory stuffing like in this recipe and mixes them with eggs in a stir-fry to make a *pasticcio*, or "a mess" in English (see opposite page). Stuffed or sliced, you might also adopt it as your new favorite vegetable.

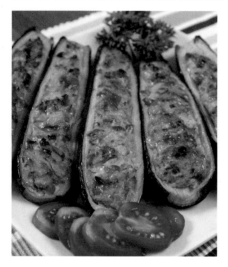

4	medium zucchini
2 cups	cubed eggplant (skin removed)
1	egg, beaten
⅓ cup	whole wheat dry breadcrumbs*
1	thin slice lean mortadella (about 0.5 oz/15 g), minced
2 tbsp	finely diced red peppers
1 tbsp	freshly grated Parmigiano-Reggiano cheese
1	clove garlic, minced
1 tsp	extra-virgin olive oil
Sea salt and freshly ground black pepper to taste	

➤ Trim ends of zucchini and carefully slice them vertically in half to create 8 boats.

➤ Fill a large pot with a couple inches of water and bring to a boil. Choose a pot that's wide enough to lay down zucchini without bending them. When water comes to a boil, add eggplant cubes and place zucchini halves on top. Reduce heat to medium high; cover and cook until zucchini are tender-crisp, about 5 minutes.

➤ Preheat oven to 375°F.

➤ Remove zucchini and set aside to cool. Drain eggplant, making sure to squeeze out all the water. Add eggplant to a large bowl. Take zucchini halves and carefully scoop out their middle flesh with a serrated spoon, being careful not to tear them or dig too deeply. Chop zucchini flesh. You'll want to create a cavity with enough flesh around it to hold the stuffing. Set boats aside.

➤ Use your hands or a potato masher to mash zucchini and eggplant. Stir in egg, breadcrumbs, mortadella, red peppers, cheese and garlic; mix until well combined.

➤ Coat a large baking pan with olive oil. Lightly sprinkle boats with salt and pepper and fill each with about 3 tsp of filling. Arrange boats side by side in baking pan. Bake in preheated oven for 30 minutes. Reset oven to broil setting and cook on top oven rack about 6 inches from broiler element until tops are lightly browned, about 3 to 4 minutes. Let stand for 5 minutes before serving.

MAKE AHEAD Prepare the stuffing the night before.

 4 SERVINGS

  GLUTEN-FREE*
REPLACE WITH GF BREADCRUMBS

 MAKE AHEAD

PER SERVING 93 CALORIES | 4 G TOTAL FAT (1 G SATURATED FAT) | 49 MG CHOLESTEROL | 122 MG SODIUM | 10 G CARBOHYDRATE | 3 G FIBER | 5 G PROTEIN

Zucchini, Potato & Egg Stir-Fry

Pasticcio di zucchine, patate e uova

4	medium zucchini
3	eggs
1 tbsp	freshly grated Parmigiano-Reggiano cheese
2 tsp	extra-virgin olive oil
1 cup	thinly sliced mini red potatoes (skin on)
½ cup	chopped onions
3 tbsp	chopped fresh parsley
¼ tsp	sea salt

Freshly ground black pepper to taste

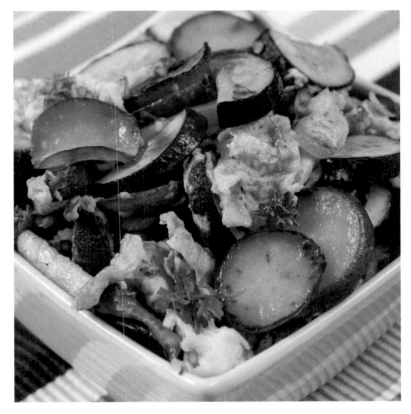

➤ Slice zucchini in ¼-inch (0.5-cm) circles and cut circles in half (you should have about 4 cups).

➤ In a medium bowl, whisk together eggs and cheese. Set aside.

➤ In a large non-stick skillet, heat olive oil over medium-high heat. Pat potatoes dry and add to skillet; stir occasionally until slightly softened and lightly browned, about 4 to 5 minutes. Toss in zucchini and onions; cook until zucchini are softened, about 6 to 7 minutes. Add parsley, salt and pepper. Pour egg mixture evenly over vegetables. Let eggs set slightly, then toss mixture, scraping the sides and bottom of skillet until eggs are fully cooked. Serve hot with freshly cut cherry tomatoes.

6 SERVINGS 4 AS A MAIN DISH   **30 MIN OR LESS**   **GLUTEN-FREE**   **MEATLESS**

PER SERVING(6) 78 CALORIES | 4 G TOTAL FAT (1 G SATURATED FAT) | 92 MG CHOLESTEROL | 38 MG SODIUM | 6 G CARBOHYDRATE | 1 G FIBER | 4 G PROTEIN

Fava Beans & Peas with Mint

Fave e piselli alla menta

FAVA BEANS HAVE BEEN AS FAMILIAR to me as any other beans, albeit it wasn't always the fresh variety that we ate growing up. We regularly enjoyed them as dried salted finger foods — served by the bowlfuls when company visited or at the cottage during a card game of *briscola*. But, with a regular bounty now appearing in grocers, the best way to savor their undeniably creamy texture is by eating them fresh, tossed with tender sweet peas and a jolt of thyme and mint. So simple yet so delicious.

2 cups	fresh or frozen fava beans, pods removed (see tip)
1 cup	fresh or frozen green peas (thawed)
1 tbsp	extra-virgin olive oil
½ cup	chopped onions
3	sprigs fresh thyme
2 tbsp	chopped fresh mint
2 tsp	light butter
3 tbsp	reduced-sodium vegetable broth

Sea salt and freshly ground black pepper to taste

➤ Bring a pot of water to a boil. Add fava beans and peas and cook for 5 minutes. Drain, rinse and drain again.

➤ In a medium bowl, pop out the fava beans from their outer shell — use your hands, but you may need a knife to pierce the skin first.

➤ In the same pot, heat olive oil over medium-high heat and add onions; cook until softened. Add cooked fava beans and peas, along with fresh herbs, and mix for 1 minute. Add butter and broth. Season with salt and pepper. Remove thyme stems and serve.

TIP Fava beans, also known as broad beans, grow in thick, long pods and require double peeling — first, to remove them from a thick, sturdy pod and then to discard their waxy, outer shells by blanching them. Despite their similar appearance, fava and lima beans are not the same. Lima pods are smaller and brighter than favas and don't require peeling, but they're less "meaty" than favas.

⇆ VARIATION Serve with a shaving of Parmigiano-Reggiano cheese or ricotta insalata.

⌒ HIGH IN...VITAMIN C

There's a reason why mom said "Eat your peas, please!" They're loaded with a host of vitamins, most notably vitamin C. Just ½ cup (or two servings here) offers half of a day's worth or as much vitamin C as a clementine. Vitamin C keeps your immune system healthy so you're protected from infections. Both green peas and fava beans also make this dish a rich source of fiber and protein.

4 SERVINGS

30 MIN OR LESS

GLUTEN-FREE

MEATLESS

PER SERVING 150 CALORIES | 8 G TOTAL FAT (3 G SATURATED FAT) | 8 MG CHOLESTEROL | 61 MG SODIUM | 16 G CARBOHYDRATE | 2 G FIBER | 7 G PROTEIN

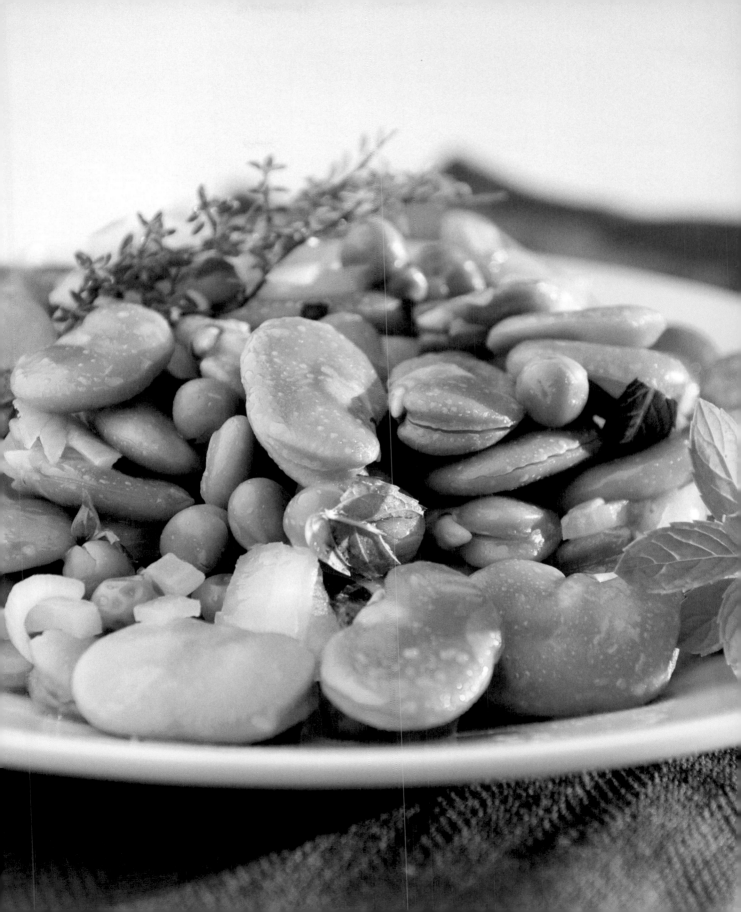

Broiled Asparagus with Cherry Tomatoes

Asparagi con pomodorini

ASPARAGUS IS ONE VEGGIE THAT I CAN COUNT ON THE KIDS TO EAT, especially when the vegetable is prepared *al forno* to serve up tender-crisp. Anytime my mom surprises me with a take-home meal, whether it's her baked sausages or chicken in the oven, she'll always toss in a handful of stalks. Paired with the tanginess of roasted tomatoes and garlic, asparagus steals the show.

1	bunch asparagus, about 20 medium-sized spears
1 tbsp	extra-virgin olive oil, divided
1 cup	halved cherry tomatoes
2	cloves garlic, pressed or minced
Pinch	sea salt
Freshly ground black pepper to taste	
1 tbsp	freshly grated Parmigiano-Reggiano cheese

➤ Preheat oven to broil setting. Position top oven rack about 6 inches from broiler element.

➤ Snap off tough sections from each asparagus stalk. You're guaranteed to remove the tough ends if you snap them off instead of guessing where to cut them. Coat a baking sheet with about half of the olive oil. Place asparagus in a single layer and scatter cherry tomatoes in between or at the end of stalks; top with garlic, salt and pepper. Drizzle remaining olive oil over vegetables, turning stalks and tomatoes a little with your hands to make sure they're well coated.

➤ Place on top rack and cook for 4 to 5 minutes on each side until asparagus is glossy green but not browned. Remove from oven and sprinkle with cheese while hot before serving.

∩ HIGH IN...FOLATE (FOLIC ACID)

In the vegetable kingdom, asparagus is one of the highest ranked foods for its amount of folate, which is a B-complex vitamin found naturally in fruits and vegetables (incidentally, folic acid is its synthetic form). Folate is known not only to decrease the risk of birth defects, but also to prevent anemia, Alzheimer's disease and several types of cancers, including breast, colon and lung. You can get one-quarter of your daily requirement of folate from just six spears of tender asparagus so load up on this side dish.

4 SERVINGS   **30 MIN OR LESS**   **GLUTEN-FREE**   **MEATLESS**

PER SERVING 60 CALORIES | 4 G TOTAL FAT (1 G SATURATED FAT) | 1 MG CHOLESTEROL | 79 MG SODIUM | 5 G CARBOHYDRATE | 2 G FIBER | 3 G PROTEIN

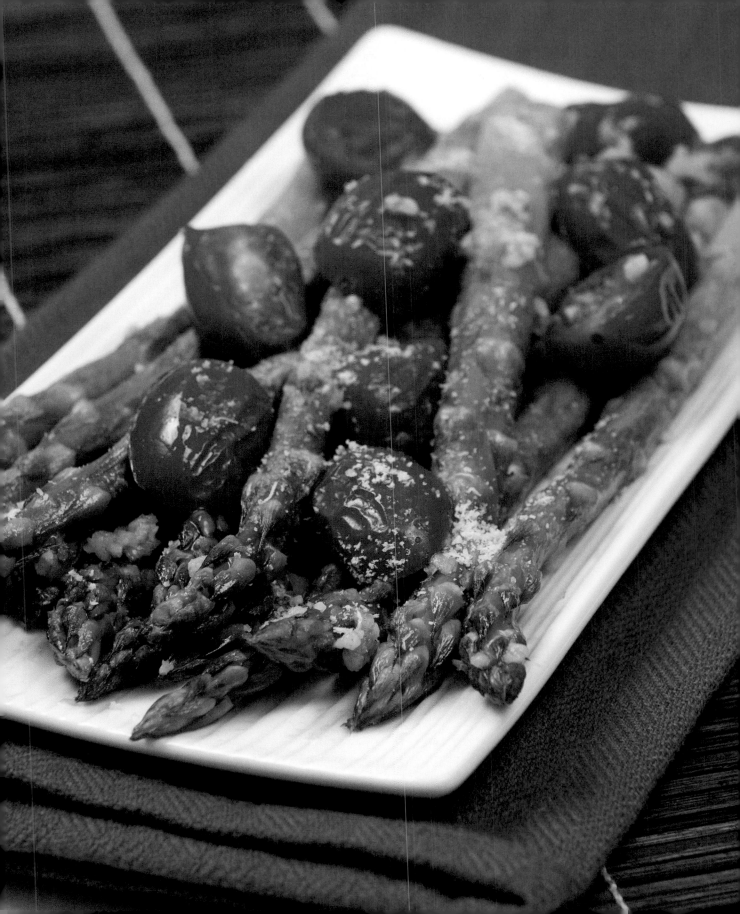

Roasted Brussels Sprouts with Shallots & Sun-Dried Tomatoes

Cavoletti di bruxelles con scalogni e pomodori secchi

BRUSSELS SPROUTS HAVE A BAD REPUTATION among some of my friends who grew up with tasteless versions of them alongside the mashed potatoes for a holiday dinner. But when they mingle with typically Italian ingredients, they become the most passed around dish at the table. A traditional dish usually calls for crisp pancetta to coat and flavor these green nuggets — and that does a fine job — but my recipe takes a vegetarian approach with a variety of different textures from the shallots and sun-dried tomatoes.

4 cups	Brussels sprouts, trimmed and halved (about 1 lb/454 g)
8	medium shallots, peeled and halved
¼ cup	thinly sliced sun-dried tomatoes, reconstituted in warm water (see tip)
¼ cup	white wine
2 tbsp	extra-virgin olive oil
½ tsp	sea salt
Freshly ground black pepper to taste	

➤ Preheat oven to 375°F.

➤ In a large bowl, toss Brussels sprouts and shallots with remaining ingredients. Pour into a shallow baking pan lined with foil and cook for 30 minutes or until sprouts are tender and golden brown, stirring once during cooking time.

TIP Once the sun-dried tomatoes have softened, use kitchen shears to cut them into thin strips.

⌂ HIGH IN...VITAMIN C

Green can be as powerful as orange — at least when it comes to vitamin C. And Brussels sprouts, loaded with more than the daily requirement of vitamin C in just one serving here, is no exception. This cruciferous vegetable, which belongs to the same family as broccoli, cauliflower, cabbage, kale and rapini, also has the most plant omega-3s out of any in the group and is tied for first with broccoli in its ranking of folate (folic acid) per serving.

 4 SERVINGS   40 MIN OR LESS   GLUTEN-FREE   MEATLESS

PER SERVING 133 CALORIES | 7 G TOTAL FAT (1 G SATURATED FAT) | 0 MG CHOLESTEROL | 328 MG SODIUM | 14 G CARBOHYDRATE | 4 G FIBER | 4 G PROTEIN

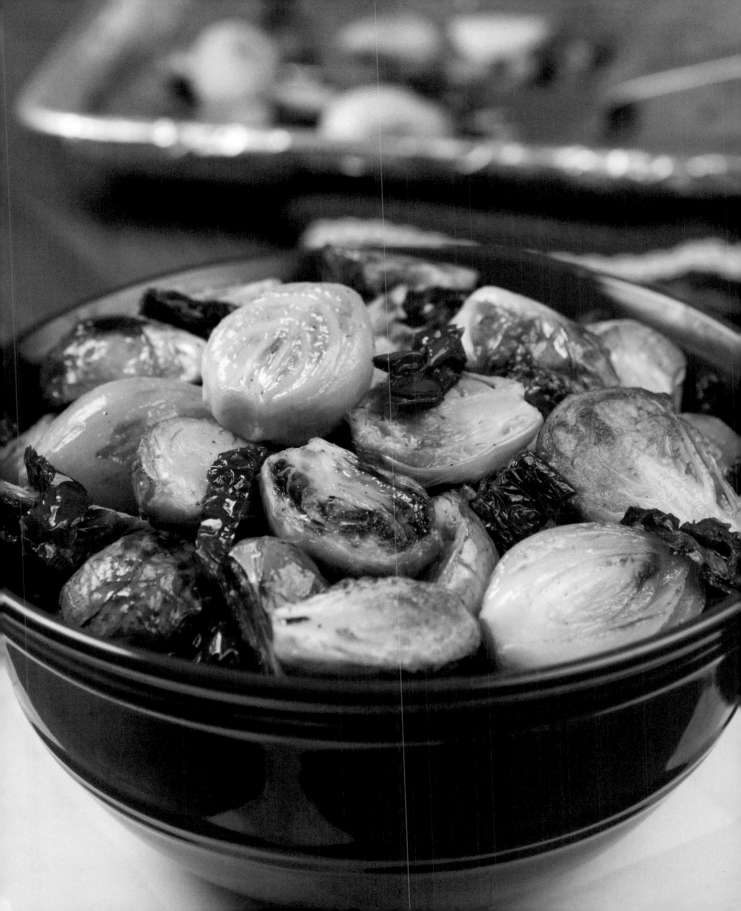

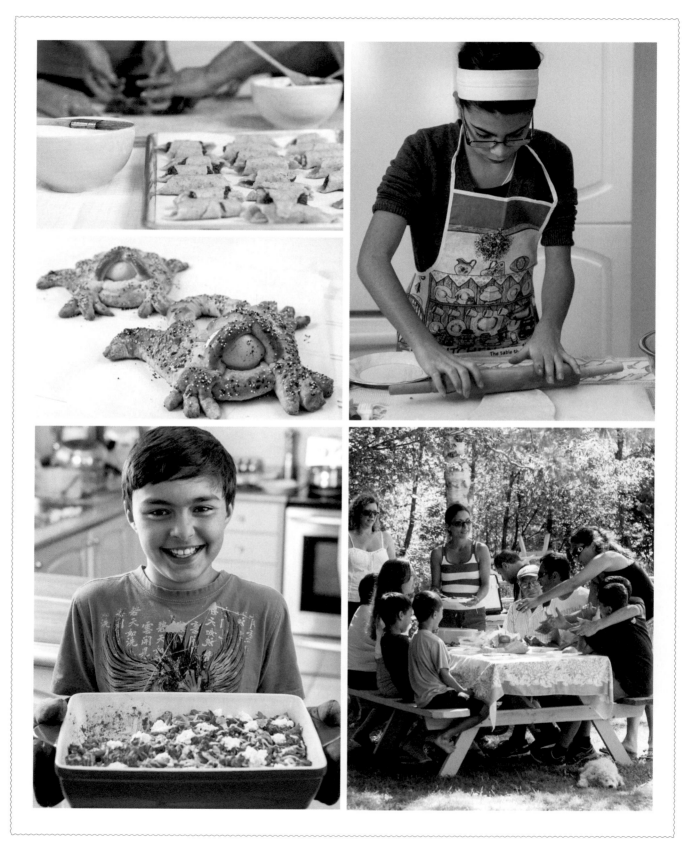

Traditions
Passing Along Family Treasures

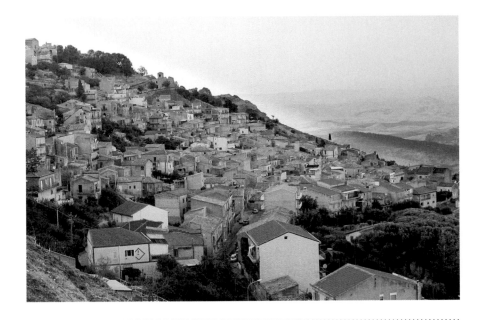

There are no greater teachers than those from generations past. So I consider myself fortunate that my cooking credentials came from the lessons dished out by my mother, father, grandmother, aunts and uncles. Our low-tech kitchen was the classroom, whether the lesson was learning to knead fresh pasta dough, make Sunday tomato sauce or bake traditional Christmas cookies. When my parents left their native home in small-town Sicily, they brought with them a font of knowledge — from customary cooking methods to a familiarity with Mediterranean ingredients to time-tested recipes that are as precious as family heirlooms. Today, it's my sister, brother, in-laws and me passing along those culinary traditions to our children. One of my nieces has taken my place at the pasta machine to roll out her own concoctions with my mom, her beloved nonna; my boys take pride in serving up a pasta dish they help me cook; my nephews have taken up the flipper to make their own breakfasts; and another niece loves to stir the cookie mix with her extraordinarily talented baker mom. When the kids aren't hands on, they're the designated taste-testers to help create even better recipes, learning that it's not just wholesome ingredients that make an exceptional dish but the teamwork involved, too. In the end, that's what it's all about. It's about cherishing lifetimes of recipes that have been nurtured by so many passionate home cooks before them. It's about cooking for the love of food *and* family.

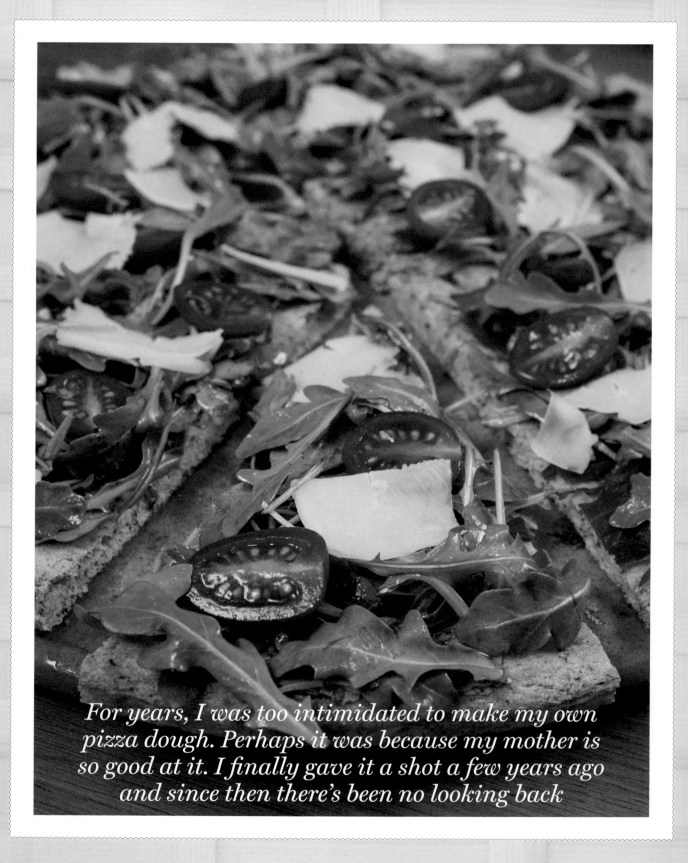

For years, I was too intimidated to make my own pizza dough. Perhaps it was because my mother is so good at it. I finally gave it a shot a few years ago and since then there's been no looking back

Pizzas & Frittatas

Pizze e frittate

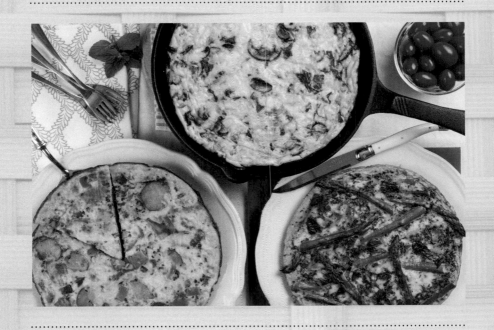

When I unfolded my unconventional lunch in class — this one was a mushroom frittata — it piqued the curiosity of my classmates, including my professor, who helped themselves to a tasting

Sicilian Pizza

Pizza alla Siciliana

WHENEVER I'VE VISITED ITALY (oh, how I miss you!), I've always been struck by the changes in the country's topography as you travel from north to south. What's even more fascinating to me is the incredible abundance of agriculture that flourishes on the dry arid land in its southern regions. Succulent tomatoes, zesty olives, wild fennel, fragrant herbs — there just isn't a meal that can't benefit from these Mediterranean treasures. They're the same culinary delights my ancestors used in their everyday cooking from living off the land and I celebrate that by bringing them together in this pizza.

1	lean Italian sausage link (about 3.5 oz/100 g)
1 tsp	fennel seeds
¼ tsp	crushed red pepper flakes
1	14-inch multigrain pizza dough (*see recipe, page 236*) or store-bought pizza dough
2	vine-ripened tomatoes, sliced
1 cup	packed shredded part-skim mozzarella cheese (4 oz/113 g)
10	ripe dry-cured (infornate) black olives, pitted and halved
¼ tsp	dried oregano
6	pieces sun-dried tomatoes, reconstituted and cut into strips (see tip)
6	fresh basil leaves, torn

TIP Reconstituting sun-dried tomatoes (a soak in warm water for 10 minutes) is necessary here since they'll burn if they're not softened.

➤ Preheat oven to 550°F or as hot as your oven can go.

➤ Remove casing from sausage. In a small non-stick skillet over medium-high heat, cook sausage meat, fennel seeds and crushed red pepper flakes for 10 minutes or until sausage is lightly browned, breaking meat up into smaller chunks while stirring occasionally. Set aside.

➤ Spread out pizza dough on a greased round 14-inch pizza pan. Layer evenly with tomato slices. Sprinkle mozzarella over entire crust on top of tomatoes. Top evenly with cooked sausage and fennel seeds, black olives and oregano.

➤ Bake in preheated oven for about 10 minutes; top evenly with sun-dried tomatoes (they'll burn if you add them in earlier). Cook pizza for another 2 to 3 more minutes, until crust is golden brown. Let stand for 2 to 3 minutes before cutting into 10 equal slices. Serve with fresh basil scattered over top.

⇆ VARIATION Give this pizza even more Sicilian flair with anchovies. Cut back the sun-dried tomatoes to at least half the quantity and add three anchovy fillets, rinsed and chopped.

⌢ HIGH IN...ANTIOXIDANTS

You might be surprised to learn that the tiny fennel seed is chock-full of powerful phytonutrients. Not only is it very high in calcium and fiber (every teaspoon offers an additional gram of fiber), but it also houses a host of antioxidants like flavonoids, carotenoids and fenchone, which combat free radicals in the body and fight inflammation. Its carminative properties also help aid digestion and bloating and help prevent intestinal cancers.

MAKES 1 14-INCH PIZZA 10 SLICES   30 MIN OR LESS

PER SLICE 168 CALORIES | 5 G TOTAL FAT (2 G SATURATED FAT) | 14 MG CHOLESTEROL | 288 MG SODIUM | 23 G CARBOHYDRATE | 2 G FIBER | 8 G PROTEIN

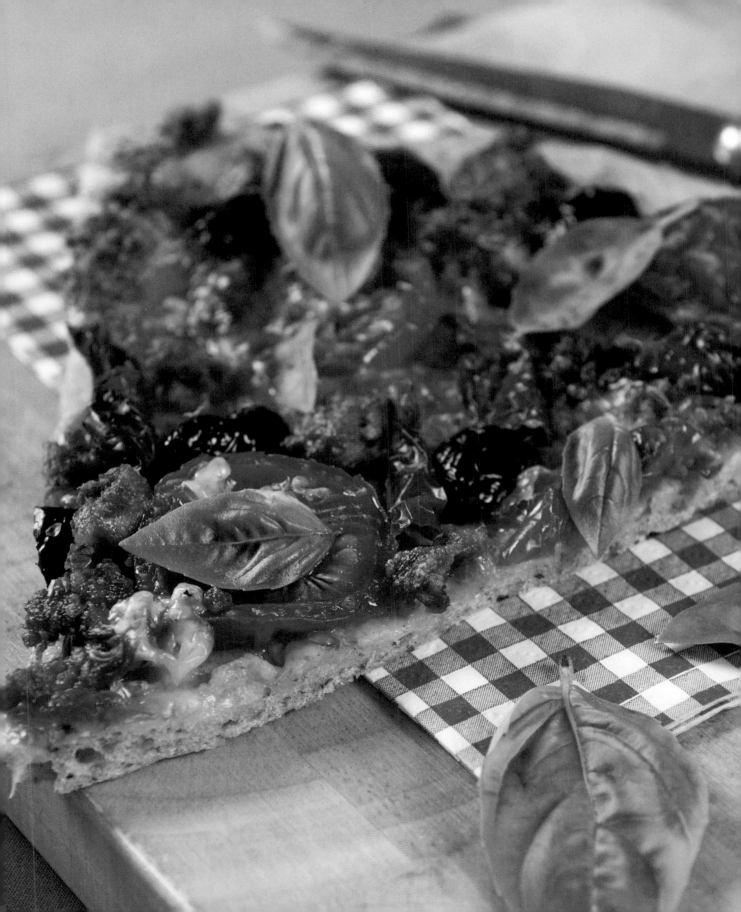

Multigrain Thin-Crust Pizza Dough

Impasto per pizza integrale

FOR YEARS, I WAS TOO INTIMIDATED TO MAKE MY OWN PIZZA DOUGH. Perhaps it was because my mother is so good at it. Or that my dear friend Liza has been a pro at it since our university days, and I knew it would be tough to top her homemade crust. (We often joke that someone mixed up the I's when she was born into an Irish family and not into an Italian *famiglia*). With her inspiration and a few family secrets from my cousin's bustling pizzeria in Italy, I finally gave it a shot a few years ago and since then there's been no looking back. Topped with a zesty tomato sauce or crafted into a traditional monochromatic pie like the one featured on the next page, making pizza dough is now a "pizza cake."

1½ cups	100% whole durum wheat semolina flour (see tip)
1¼ cups	unbleached all-purpose flour
1¼ cup	whole wheat flour
2 tbsp	ground flaxseed
4 tsp	pizza or quick-rising yeast
1 tsp	sea salt
1¾ cups	warm water
½ tsp	honey
1½ tbsp	extra-virgin olive oil

TIP Durum and semolina flours are usually combined together and sold in the same package — semolina is the coarse grains from milling the flour; durum is the fine powder left from the milling process. Look for them wherever other regular baking flours are sold at your grocery store.

MAKE AHEAD Prepare the pizza dough and once it has had time to rise, refrigerate for one to two days. Bring to room temperature before baking.

➤ In a large bowl, combine flours, flaxseed, yeast and salt. Mix well and set aside.

➤ Run the tap until the water is as hot as it can get. Fill a measuring cup with water; dissolve honey and add olive oil. Make a well in the middle of flour mixture and pour in water mixture. Mix thoroughly. When a ball forms, transfer to a flat, floured surface. Knead, dusting with flour if sticky, until dough is silky.

➤ Lightly oil a large ceramic or glass bowl and place dough ball into it. Cover with plastic wrap and a tea towel and let rise in a warm spot for 1 hour or until doubled in size. Divide ball into two doughs.

➤ When working with dough, use a spatula to scrape out of bowl and grease hands if dough is sticky to the touch.

➤ Coat two 14-inch pizza pans with cooking spray, sprinkle some durum flour and spread out pizza doughs evenly. This crust spreads very easily! Add your favorite toppings. Bake in a preheated 550°F oven for about 10 to 12 minutes or until preferred doneness. If you like it extra crispy, remove pizza from pan and place it directly on *middle* oven rack for 5 more minutes.

⌂ HIGH IN...FIBER

The addition of whole wheat flour and flaxseed offers more fiber and assorted phytochemicals that you don't usually see in pizza dough. Both durum and semolina flours come from milling only the endosperm of the durum wheat (*Triticum turgidum*) kernel, which has a high-protein content. With up to 25 percent more protein than all-purpose or whole wheat flours, durum/semolina makes pizza dough more elastic or pliable.

MAKES 2 14-INCH PIZZA CRUSTS
10 SLICES EACH

MEATLESS MAKE AHEAD

PER SLICE 117 CALORIES | 2 G TOTAL FAT (0 G SATURATED FAT) | 0 MG CHOLESTEROL | 119 MG SODIUM | 21 G CARBOHYDRATE | 2 G FIBER | 4 G PROTEIN

Potato-Zucchini Pizza

Pizza di patate e zucchine

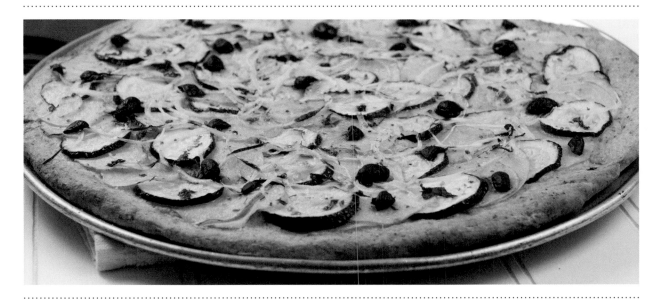

1 to 2	medium Yukon Gold potatoes (see tip)
1	zucchini, thinly sliced
2 tbsp	extra-virgin olive oil
2 tbsp	chopped fresh basil
2 tsp	dried oregano
Sea salt and freshly ground black pepper to taste	
1	14-inch multigrain pizza dough (*see opposite page*) or store-bought pizza dough
1 cup	thinly sliced sweet or cooking onions
1 tbsp	freshly grated Parmigiano-Reggiano cheese
2 tbsp	chopped pitted black olives

➤ Preheat oven to 550°F or as hot as your oven can go.

➤ Remove eyes of potatoes but don't peel skin. Thinly slice potatoes; you want them paper thin and almost see through (you'll have about 1½ cups).

➤ In a large bowl, combine potatoes and zucchini. Drizzle with olive oil; add basil, oregano, salt and pepper. Toss well until potatoes and zucchini are evenly coated.

➤ Spread out pizza dough on a greased round 14-inch pizza pan. Starting from the outside edge and working your way in to the center of pizza, layer crust evenly with zucchini and potato slices, alternating and slightly overlapping them. Scatter onion slices and sprinkle cheese evenly over vegetables. Top with olives.

➤ Bake in preheated oven for about 12 to 14 minutes, or until crust is golden brown. Cut into 10 equal slices and serve hot or at room temperature.

TIPS Choose potatoes that are more narrow than round in shape so their cuts are similar to the size of the sliced zucchini.

➤ Use a mandoline to slice the potatoes and zucchini for an even thickness.

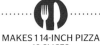

MAKES 1 14-INCH PIZZA
10 SLICES

30 MIN OR LESS

MEATLESS

PER SLICE 155 CALORIES | 3 G TOTAL FAT (1 G SATURATED FAT) | 3 MG CHOLESTEROL | 206 MG SODIUM | 26 G CARBOHYDRATE | 3 G FIBER | 5 G PROTEIN

Arugula & Asiago Pizza
Pizza con rucola e Asiago

ARUGULA AND ASIAGO are not only great alliterative companions but also impressive gusto matches. My family typically enjoys them together as a salad — my boys love to create their own masterpieces by shaving slivers of cheese on the arugula and topping it with slivers of sweet pear to balance the peppery body. With this pizza, it's all hands on deck again; this time it's a fun exercise in keeping the zesty salad balanced on top of the oh-so-crunchy thin crust.

1	14-inch multigrain pizza dough (*see recipe, page 236*) or store-bought dough
4 to 5	very thinly slices prosciutto (about 1.2 oz/33 g)
1 tbsp	extra-virgin olive oil
1 tsp	freshly squeezed lemon juice
¼ tsp	sea salt
Freshly ground black pepper to taste	
2 cups	packed baby arugula leaves
½ cup	halved ripe cherry tomatoes
2 oz	(56 g) Asiago cheese shavings

➤ Prepare pizza crust as per recipe.

➤ Preheat oven to 550°F or as hot as your oven can go.

➤ Spread out pizza dough on a greased round 14-inch pizza pan. Tear prosciutto into large slices and scatter evenly over dough. Press prosciutto gently into dough. Bake until crust is golden brown, about 10 to 12 minutes.

➤ In the meantime, whisk together olive oil, lemon juice, salt and pepper in a small bowl. Add dressing to arugula and tomatoes in a large bowl and toss well.

➤ Remove hot pizza from oven. Cut immediately on a cutting board into 10 slices. Scatter dressed arugula and tomatoes evenly over cut crust and top with Asiago shavings. Serve immediately.

ᯤ HIGH IN...IRON

If you're comparing the amount of iron in greens, spinach ranks close to the top, but it also contains substances such as oxalate that limits the absorption of iron. On the other hand, arugula's modest dose of iron is readily absorbed, even more so because of the abundance of vitamin C from the cherry tomatoes in this recipe.

MAKES 1 14-INCH PIZZA
10 SLICES

30 MIN OR LESS

PER SLICE 160 CALORIES | 5 G TOTAL FAT (2 G SATURATED FAT) | 9 MG CHOLESTEROL | 400 MG SODIUM | 22 G CARBOHYDRATE | 2 G FIBER | 6 G PROTEIN

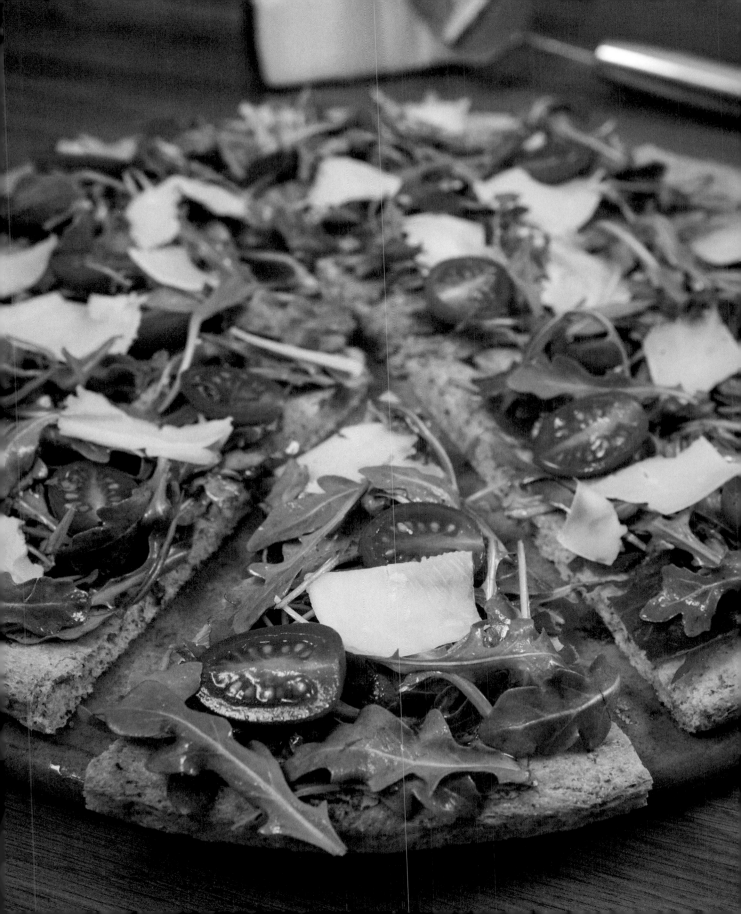

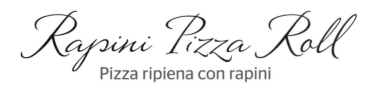

Rapini Pizza Roll

Pizza ripiena con rapini

MY GIRLFRIEND GRACE IS QUEEN OF THE RAPINI ROLL. When our families come together for an afternoon or a night of gab and laughter, I can count on her roll to be on the appetizer table along with a glass of wine as we both put our feet up. Like most Italians, my family has always had a love affair with rapini — before it was widely available throughout the seasons in stores, it wasn't uncommon for my parents to buy the freshly picked green from a local farm in early fall, blanch it and bag it for the freezer so we had a full winter's supply. We love it simply sautéed in garlic, tossed in pasta or stuffed in a pizza crust like this.

1	large bunch rapini (broccoli rabe)
1½ tbsp	extra-virgin olive oil
3	cloves garlic, minced
Pinch	crushed red pepper flakes
Pinch	sea salt
1	14-inch multigrain pizza dough (*see recipe, page 236*) or store-bought pizza dough
1 tbsp	basil pesto (*see recipe, page 18*) or store-bought pesto
2 tbsp	crumbled light goat's cheese (1 oz/28 g)
1 tbsp	egg white
½ tsp	dried oregano

MAKE AHEAD Prepare the rapini mixture a day or two before. Refrigerate until ready to use.

➤ Preheat oven to 450°F.

➤ Trim tough ends of rapini. Bring a large pot of water to a boil. Add rapini (you'll have about 7 cups) and cook until stems are tender, about 3 minutes. Drain well and squeeze out any excess water in a colander. Cut cooked rapini into large pieces.

➤ In a large non-stick skillet, heat olive oil on medium-high heat. Add garlic and cook until lightly browned, about 2 to 3 minutes. Toss in drained rapini, crushed red pepper flakes and salt. Cook for 1 minute until well combined and heated through.

➤ Spread out pizza dough on a greased, rectangular pizza pan to make a 9 x 16-inch (23 x 40-cm) rectangle. Spread basil pesto over entire crust. Place rapini mixture down the center of the rectangle, leaving about 1-inch (2.5-cm) perimeter. Sprinkle cheese evenly over rapini mixture. Roll pizza dough like a jelly roll, starting on the shorter end and loosely tucking in rapini as you roll. Fold ends and pinch dough to close up seams. Transfer pizza roll, seam side down, to a baking sheet lined with parchment paper.

➤ Brush top and sides of dough with egg white and sprinkle with oregano. Bake in preheated oven until golden brown, about 20 minutes. Let stand 5 minutes; cut into 1½-inch (4 cm) slices.

⌂ HIGH IN... VITAMINS K AND C

Rapini is one of those rare nutritional powerhouses that contains vitamins K, C, E, B, folate, fiber and calcium. One of the most significant is vitamin K — every serving here exceeds the daily requirement (and contains about 40 percent of a day's worth of vitamin C). The vitamin can lower the risk of osteoporosis, non-Hodgkin lymphoma and heart disease. And since vitamin K needs a little fat to be readily absorbed, you won't need to skimp on the goat's cheese sprinkled in between.

8-10 AS AN APPETIZER   40 MIN OR LESS   MEATLESS   MAKE AHEAD

PER SERVING(10) 54 CALORIES | 3 G TOTAL FAT (1 G SATURATED FAT) | 1 MG CHOLESTEROL | 93 MG SODIUM | 3 G CARBOHYDRATE | 2 G FIBER | 4 G PROTEIN

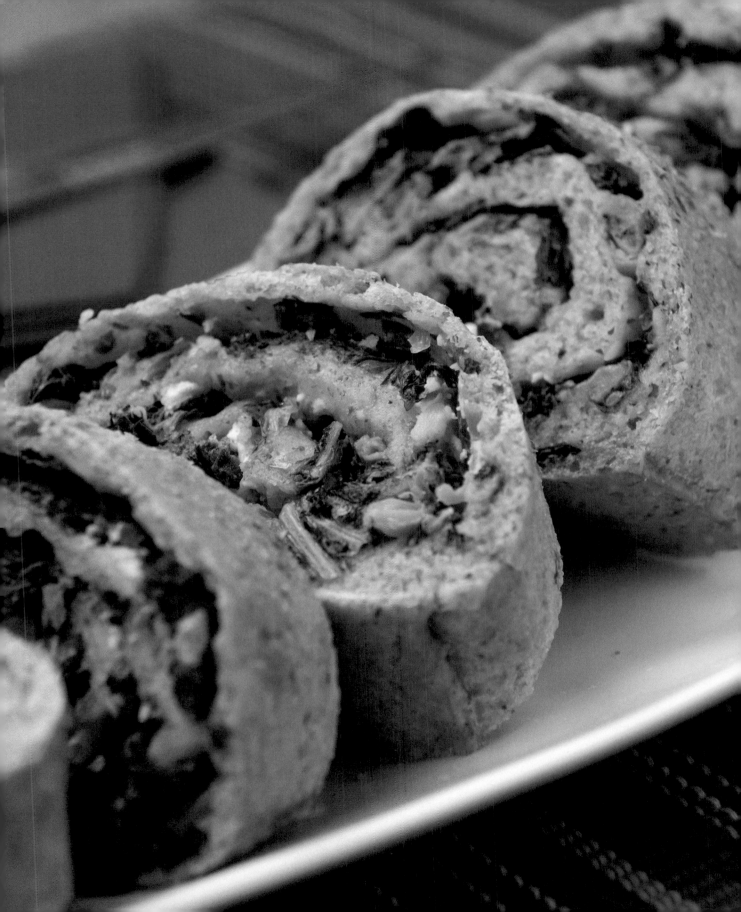

Dad's Swiss Chard-Stuffed Pizza
Impanata di bietole

ALTHOUGH NOT PROPER ITALIAN, we called Dad's delicious creation "banata," derived from the term "impanata" or stuffed bread or pastry. Besides a crispy crust, bundles of Swiss chard are essential — hence the reason we coax Mother Nature to help Dad yield an enormous crop of tender greens from his small vegetable patch each summer. The more chard, the more banata. With three kids and six grandkids all living nearby, when word spreads that Dad is making his specialty, he has to makes sure there's enough to pass around.

3	large bunches Swiss chard
2 tbsp	extra-virgin olive oil
4	cloves garlic, minced
3 tbsp	chopped fresh basil
Freshly ground black pepper to taste	
2	14-inch multigrain pizza dough (*see recipe, page 236*) or store-bought dough
4 tbsp	chopped sun-dried tomatoes, reconstituted (*see tip, page 234*)
4 tbsp	ripe dry-cured (infornate) black olives, pitted and chopped (*see tip*)
3 tbsp	freshly grated Parmigiano-Reggiano cheese
2	anchovy fillets in olive oil, rinsed, patted dry and minced (optional)
1	egg white
1 tsp	garlic powder

TIP Look for infornate or dry-cured olives at your grocer's salad bar or in jars in the aisle where other olives are sold. Just a few provide lots of flavor.

➤ Preheat oven to 475°F.

➤ Bring a large pot of water to a boil. Trim most of stems from Swiss chard — the center ribs will tenderize when cooked so don't discard them. Cut chard into bite-sized pieces. Add Swiss chard and parboil for about 2 to 3 minutes. You'll likely need to cook them in at least two batches. Drain well and squeeze out any excess water by using your hands to press them in a colander.

➤ In a large non-stick skillet, heat olive oil on medium-high heat. Add garlic and cook for 1 to 2 minutes, until lightly browned. Add drained chard and toss with basil and black pepper. Transfer chard to a bowl; set aside.

➤ You'll need two rectangular pizza pans, about 11 x 17 inches (28 x 43 cm). Line one pan with foil and lightly coat with cooking spray. Spread out one pizza dough. Lightly coat the other pan with cooking spray and spread out the second pizza dough.

➤ Top the second pizza dough (not in the lined pan) evenly with Swiss chard mixture. Sprinkle sun-dried tomatoes, olives, cheese and anchovies, if using, evenly over chard. Carefully flip and place reserved pizza dough on top of toppings. Gently peel away the foil paper as you position it directly over the bottom pizza. Pinch dough all around perimeter to close up seams.

➤ Brush top of dough with egg white and sprinkle evenly with garlic powder. Bake in preheated oven for 20 to 25 minutes or until golden brown, placing pan on upper rack to brown crust during the last 5 minutes of cooking. Let stand for 5 minutes before cutting into squares.

MAKE AHEAD Prepare the Swiss chard mixture a day or two before. Refrigerate until ready to use.

12 PIECES   MEATLESS   MAKE AHEAD

PER PIECE 155 CALORIES | 6 G TOTAL FAT (1 G SATURATED FAT) | 2 MG CHOLESTEROL | 475 MG SODIUM | 21 G CARBOHYDRATE | 3 G FIBER | 5 G PROTEIN

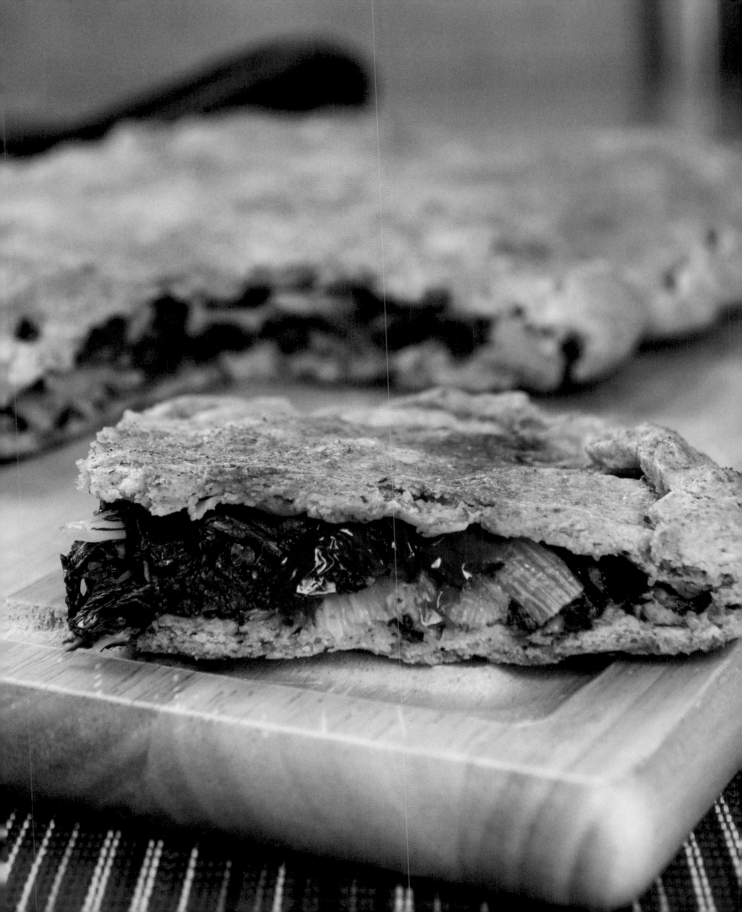

Mushroom–Kale Frittata
Frittata con funghi e cavolo nero

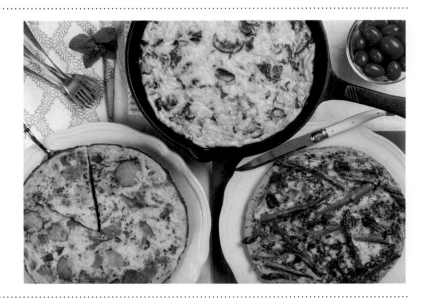

IT WASN'T UNTIL I WAS IN UNIVERSITY that I realized just how special my mother's frittatas were. I found any way to eat them, whether fashioned with mushrooms, asparagus or potatoes. One day, when I unfolded my unconventional lunch in class — a mushroom frittata in between a bun — it piqued the curiosity of my classmates and professor, who helped themselves to a bite, while the sandwich circled the group until only crumbs remained. It obviously made the honor role! So do these yummy frittatas.

7	eggs, beaten
2	egg whites
¾ cup	1% reduced-sodium cottage cheese
1 tbsp	freshly grated Parmigiano-Reggiano cheese
2 tbsp	chopped fresh basil
1 tbsp	chopped fresh parsley
½ tsp	sea salt
Freshly ground black pepper to taste	
2 tsp	extra-virgin olive oil
1	onion, chopped
1	clove garlic, minced
2 cups	thinly sliced cremini or porcini mushrooms
1½ cups	packed baby kale leaves or shredded kale (see tip)
½ cup	shredded light provolone cheese, (2 oz/56 g)

➤ Preheat oven to 350°F.

➤ In a large bowl, combine eggs and egg whites, cottage cheese, grated cheese, basil, parsley, salt and pepper.

➤ In a 10-inch cast-iron or non-stick skillet with a heatproof handle, heat olive oil over medium heat. I recommend a cast-iron skillet, which gives the sides a slightly crunchy texture once cooked. Add onion and garlic and cook until onions are softened, about 1 to 2 minutes. Add sliced mushrooms and baby kale; cook until mushrooms are slightly softened, about 2 to 3 minutes.

➤ Pour egg mixture over vegetables, making sure they're evenly distributed. Top with provolone.

➤ Transfer skillet to preheated oven (if the skillet handle is not ovenproof, wrap it in foil). Bake on *middle* oven rack until center is set and edges are golden, about 20 minutes. Let cool for 5 minutes before slicing and serving.

TIP You can find baby kale in boxed salad containers in the refrigerated lettuce section of your grocery store. If you can't find it, use regular kale — remove the middle stalk and shred leaves; cook for a few minutes longer.

6 SERVINGS   40 MIN OR LESS   GLUTEN-FREE   MEATLESS

PER SERVING 123 CALORIES | 6 G TOTAL FAT (2 G SATURATED FAT) | 70 MG CHOLESTEROL | 381 MG SODIUM | 9 G CARBOHYDRATE | 2 G FIBER | 9 G PROTEIN

Asparagus & Herb Frittata
Frittata con asparagi ed erbe

1	small bunch asparagus, about 15 spears
5	eggs, beaten
1	egg white
¼ cup	minced fresh mint
2 tbsp	minced fresh basil
½ tsp	Italian herb seasoning

Sea salt and freshly ground black pepper to taste

2 tsp	extra-virgin olive oil
¼ cup	chopped onions
2	cloves garlic, chopped
¼ cup	reduced-sodium vegetable broth
2 tbsp	freshly grated Parmigiano-Reggiano cheese

➤ Trim ends of asparagus and cut into halves or thirds.

➤ In a large bowl, combine eggs and egg white, mint, basil, Italian herb seasoning, salt and pepper.

➤ In a 9- or 10-inch non-stick skillet, heat olive oil over medium-high heat. Add onions and garlic and cook until onions are softened, about 1 to 2 minutes. Stir in broth, followed by asparagus pieces, cooking until slightly softened, about 5 minutes.

➤ Pour egg mixture over asparagus, making sure asparagus is evenly distributed in skillet. Turn down heat to medium-low and cover skillet with a tight-fitting lid for about 8 to 10 minutes. When eggs are set, sprinkle grated cheese over top, cover to cook for 1 more minute. Slice into 4 equal pieces and serve hot with a salad and/or whole-grain bread.

⇄VARIATION Want a meatier option, add a handful of crumbled cooked lean sausage (casing removed) or ½ cup of peameal bacon (cured pork loin) or turkey bacon-style.

4 SERVINGS   30 MIN OR LESS   GLUTEN-FREE   MEATLESS

PER SERVING 137 CALORIES | 9 G TOTAL FAT (3 G SATURATED FAT) | 231 MG CHOLESTEROL | 118 MG SODIUM | 3 G CARBOHYDRATE | 1 G FIBER | 10 G PROTEIN

Red Potato & Ham Frittata
Frittata con patate rosse e prosciutto

7	eggs
1	egg white
¼ cup	1% milk
¼ tsp	dried oregano

Sea salt and freshly ground black pepper to taste

1½ tbsp	extra-virgin olive oil
1½ cups	mini red potatoes, thinly sliced
½ cup	chopped onions
½ cup	chopped green bell peppers
1½ tbsp	minced fresh rosemary
⅓ cup	chopped reduced-sodium extra-lean deli-style prosciutto cotto or ham (about 2 oz/56 g)
¼ cup	packed shredded part-skim mozzarella cheese (1 oz/28 g)

➤ In a large bowl, combine eggs, egg white, milk, oregano, salt and pepper.

➤ In an extra-large non-stick skillet, heat olive oil over medium-high heat. Add potato slices in a single layer and cook for about 4 to 5 minutes, flipping them halfway between cooking. Reduce heat to medium-low and stir in onions, green peppers and rosemary. Cook for 3 to 4 more minutes, until vegetables soften. Distribute prosciutto cotto pieces, along with vegetables, evenly in skillet.

➤ Pour egg mixture evenly over potatoes and other vegetables. Wiggle pan a little to make sure eggs are evenly distributed. Cover skillet with a tight-fitting lid for about 10 to 12 minutes. (Be careful that the lid isn't touching the eggs or it'll be stuck for good!) When eggs are set, sprinkle shredded cheese over top, cover to cook for 1 more minute. Loosen sides and slice frittata into 6 equal pieces. Serve hot or at room temperature.

6 SERVINGS   30 MIN OR LESS   GLUTEN-FREE

PER SERVING 175 CALORIES | 10 G TOTAL FAT (3 G SATURATED FAT) | 221 MG CHOLESTEROL | 156 MG SODIUM | 9 G CARBOHYDRATE | 1 G FIBER | 11 G PROTEIN

Ricotta-Mint Mini Frittatas

Frittata con ricotta e menta

MY CHILDHOOD FRIEND Anna Rita has been demonstrating her cooking prowess since we were wee, whipping up sweet and strange concoctions in our toy ovens. Forward a decade or two or three, and it's been her signature regional dishes from her Molise ancestry in south-central Italy that make my mouth water and my heart sing. Yours would too if you tasted her casciatelli (half-moon cheese-filled pasta), egg noodle pasta, walnut-crusted cod fish (see page 180) and pepper cookies. This super-easy frittata recipe, in particular, is a favorite, always awaiting us as we arrive for Anna's annual summer brunch at her Georgian Bay cottage.

2 tsp	extra-virgin olive oil
½ cup	chopped onions
6	eggs
2	egg whites
⅓ cup	packed coarsely chopped fresh mint
¼ tsp	sea salt
Freshly ground black pepper to taste	
3 tbsp	part-skim ricotta cheese

➤ Preheat oven to 350°F.

➤ In a small non-stick skillet, heat olive oil over medium heat. Add onions and cook until softened and slightly yellow, about 2 to 3 minutes. Set aside to cool.

➤ In a large bowl, combine eggs, egg whites, mint, salt and pepper. Stir in the cooked onions.

➤ Coat six 3-inch (125 mL) ramekins with cooking spray and arrange on a baking sheet. Pour equal amounts of the egg mixture into each ramekin. Take 2 tsp of ricotta at a time and drop in two or three places into each egg mixture (the idea here is to drop in blobs of ricotta but not stir it into the egg).

➤ Bake in preheated oven for 15 to 17 minutes or until eggs are set in the center. They'll puff out like little soufflés but will shrink up a little as they cool. Serve frittatas in ramekins or flip them out onto a serving plate with sliced strawberries or tomatoes drizzled with olive oil, salt and pepper.

☟ LOW IN...FAT

Frittatas are a great meal any time of the day and are a perfect dish to pack in the savory qualities of herbs and veggies. But you could counteract those healthy benefits when you load a frittata with fats in cheeses, pancetta and butter. Combine high-protein eggs with a dab of low-fat ricotta and a handful of aromatic mint and you have a dish that not only adequately fuels you until your next meal but also stays off the hips.

 6 MINI FRITTATAS   30 MIN OR LESS   GLUTEN-FREE   MEATLESS

PER SERVING 106 CALORIES | 7 G TOTAL FAT (2 G SATURATED FAT) | 188 MG CHOLESTEROL | 187 MG SODIUM | 2 G CARBOHYDRATE | 0 G FIBER | 8 G PROTEIN

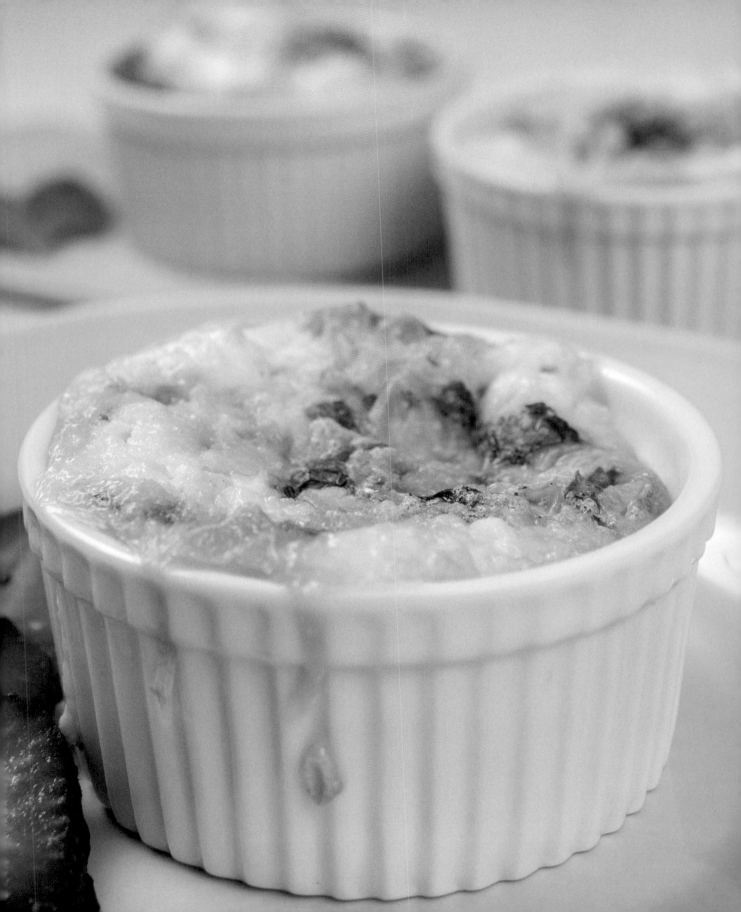

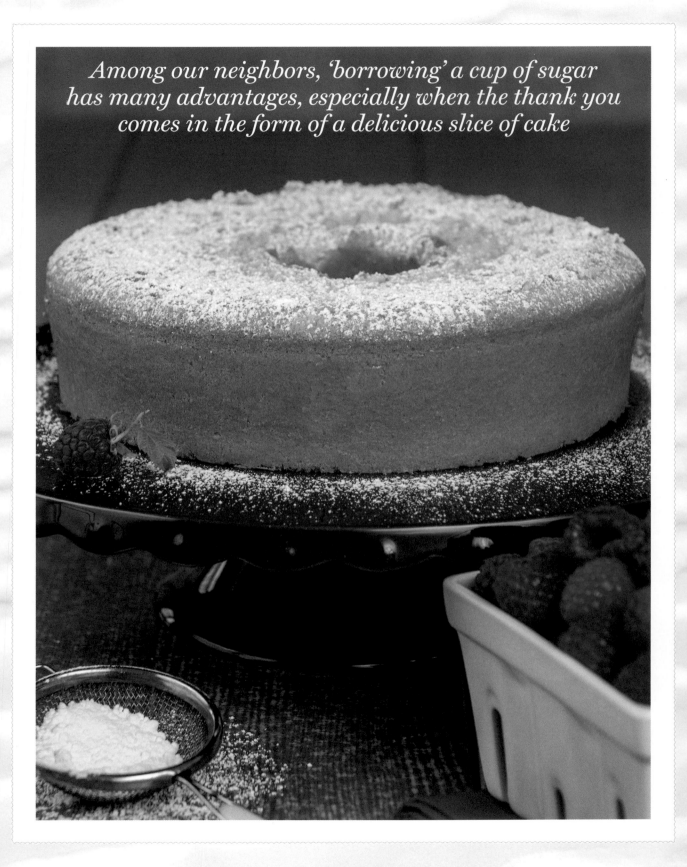

Among our neighbors, 'borrowing' a cup of sugar has many advantages, especially when the thank you comes in the form of a delicious slice of cake

Desserts

Dolci

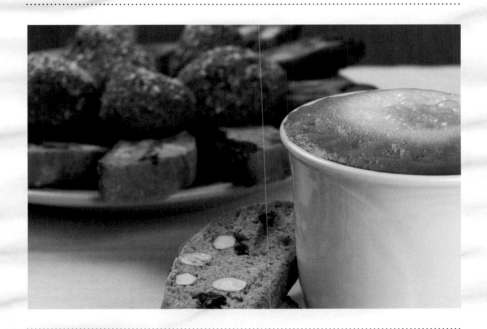

My dad's coffee mug became a dunking pot for biscotti like these ones. The kids would climb onto his lap, and once he set down the mug, the dunking frenzy began

Lemon Polenta Cake

Torta di polenta con limone

MY LOVE OF LEMONS HAS GROWN SINCE tasting them from my late grandfather's orchard in Sicily. There you'll find them in desserts like granita, gelato and almond cookies. Although you may not expect them paired with a savory ingredient like cornmeal, lemons give this slightly gritty, slightly sweetened cake the perfect touch of tanginess.

¾ cup	yellow cornmeal (see tip)
½ cup	unbleached all-purpose flour
½ cup	oat flour (see tip, page 254)
⅓ cup	raw cane sugar
1 tsp	baking powder
¼ tsp	baking soda
Pinch	salt
2	large eggs, beaten
¾ cup	low-fat 2% vanilla Greek yogurt
⅓ cup	1% buttermilk or milk
3 tbsp	light butter, melted
Zest of 1 lemon	
4 tbsp	freshly squeezed lemon juice

Lemon Syrup (optional)

½ cup	icing (confectioner's) sugar
2½ tbsp	freshly squeezed lemon juice
2 tbsp	limoncello liqueur
Zest of ½ lemon	

⇆ VARIATION For an added burst of color, add a handful of blueberries (blue and yellow are so Mediterranean!). Or add fresh or frozen cranberries during Thanksgiving or Christmastime for a dazzling festive match. Try cake accompanied with grilled peaches, too.

➤ Preheat oven to 350°F.

➤ In a large bowl, combine cornmeal, flours, sugar, baking powder, baking soda and salt and stir until fully incorporated.

➤ Whisk together eggs, yogurt, buttermilk, butter and lemon zest and juice in a medium bowl. Add wet ingredients to dry ingredients and combine well with a spatula until fully blended.

➤ Grease a 9-inch round non-stick cake pan. Pour cake batter into pan. Bake in preheated oven for 25 minutes, or until a pick inserted in the center of cake comes out clean. Let cool for 15 minutes.

➤ While the cake is cooling, prepare the lemon syrup. Whisk all ingredients in a small bowl until well combined.

➤ Serve cake slice with a drizzle of lemon syrup and a sprig of fresh mint. If you like a sweeter cake, take a toothpick and prick the cake every few inches to create little "funnels." Pour and spread syrup over entire cake.

TIPS If you like less texture, look for an extra-fine cornmeal or give it a whirl in the bowl of a food processor for 5 minutes before using.
➤ When zesting the lemon, don't over-grate it. Rotate your lemon evenly as you grate and be sure to stop grating once you've reached the white membrane (pith), which adds bitterness.

↻ LOW IN...FAT

To smooth out the sandy texture of the cornmeal, some traditional recipes add a wallop of fat, up to 1 cup of oil. This scrumptious cake leaves the oil in the bottle and serves up a moist treat that goes exceptionally well with a frothy cappuccino, steeped tea or a tall glass of milk. Bottoms up!

8-10 SERVINGS   40 MIN OR LESS

PER SERVING(10) 210 CALORIES | 6 G TOTAL FAT (3 G SATURATED FAT) | 56 MG CHOLESTEROL | 249 MG SODIUM | 34 G CARBOHYDRATE | 2 G FIBER | 8 G PROTEIN

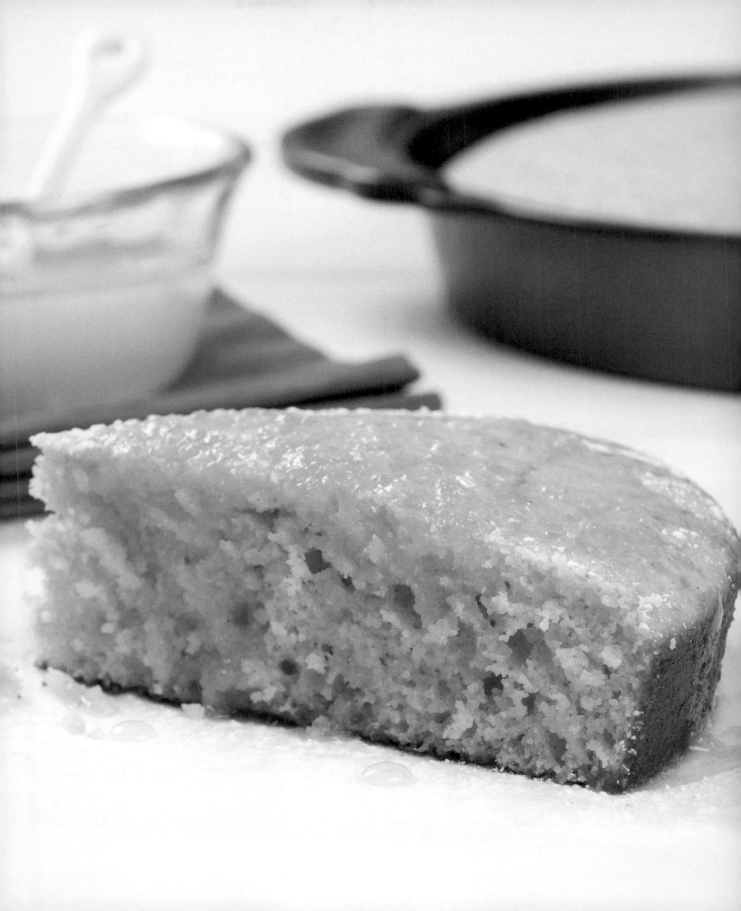

Poached Pears in Marsala

Pere cotte al marsala

WE MOVED INTO A BRAND NEW FAMILY HOME when I was 12 years old, and one of the first things Dad did was plant a pear tree in the backyard. It flourished so quickly that within two years we had more pears than we knew what to do with, so that encouraged us to reach into the family vault to unearth new ways to enjoy their plump, juicy flesh, including poaching them in a fortified wine like marsala. The effect is a light, bold-tasting dessert with fragrant spices that instantly tells guests they're in for a real treat.

4	ripe red, forelle or Bartlett pears
1½ cups	sweet marsala (*see tip, page 264*)
¾ cup	water
½ cup	packed brown sugar
1 tsp	ground cinnamon
1 tsp	pure vanilla extract
¼ tsp	ground cloves
Zest and juice of ½ orange	
1 cup	white seedless grapes
½ cup	strawberries, hulled and halved
8 tbsp	low-fat 2% vanilla Greek yogurt or vanilla frozen yogurt*
8 tsp	toasted sliced almonds

➤ Peel pears, being careful to leave their stem intact. Slice pears in half lengthwise and remove seeds with a melon baller.

➤ In a large pot, add all ingredients, except pears, grapes and strawberries; stir well. Bring mixture to a boil. Turn down heat to medium-low and gently place pear halves into liquid, covering them as much as possible. Sprinkle in grapes and strawberries. Cover and simmer for about 15 to 20 minutes, until pears are tender.

➤ To serve, spoon out pear half and a few grapes and strawberries with poached liquid on a dessert plate and top with 1 tbsp vanilla yogurt and 1 tsp sliced almonds.

MAKE AHEAD You can prepare this dessert (minus the yogurt and almonds) one to two days before, store in the refrigerator and warm up just before serving.

⌂HIGH IN...PHYTOCHEMICALS

Adding cinnamon to desserts adds instant sweetness without the sugar. Recent studies have shown that it can also lower blood sugar, in particular in people with pre-diabetes or type 2 diabetes.

    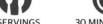

8 SERVINGS | 30 MIN OR LESS | GLUTEN-FREE | DAIRY-FREE* | MAKE AHEAD
TOP WITH DAIRY-FREE YOGURT

PER SERVING 214 CALORIES | 2 G TOTAL FAT (0 G SATURATED FAT) | 1 MG CHOLESTEROL | 13 MG SODIUM | 38 G CARBOHYDRATE | 4 G FIBER | 2 G PROTEIN

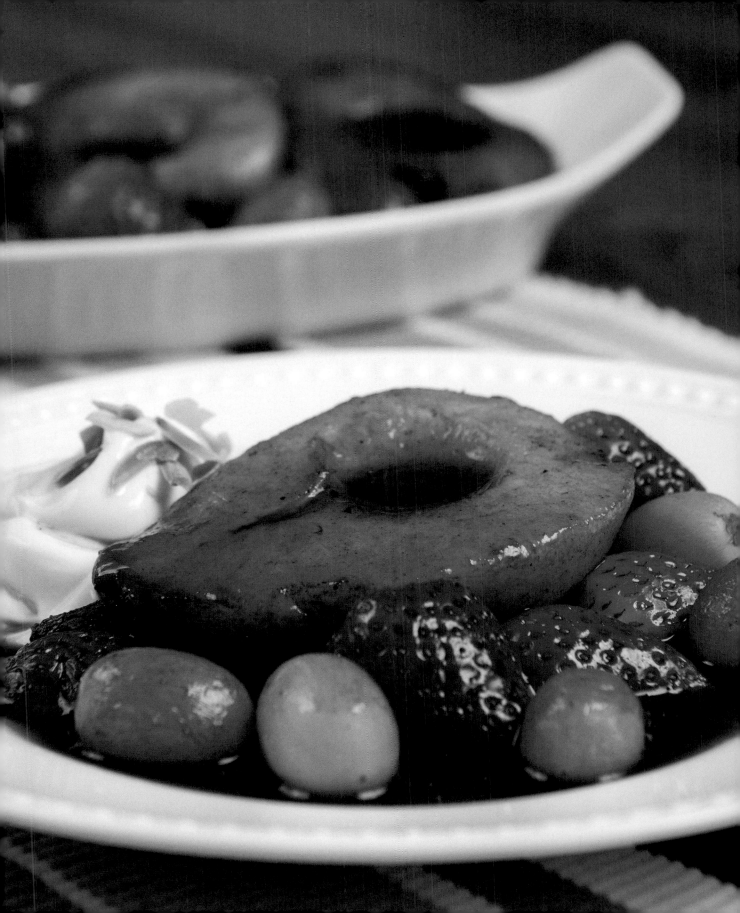

Chocolate-Pear Torte

Torta di cioccolato e pere

MOST WOULD SAY THAT CHOCOLATE PAIRED WITH ANY FRUIT is a match made in heaven, and I'd have to agree. But there's something about the celestial pairing of chocolate and pears — a traditional combination in the Italian dessert repertoire — that makes it special. Sweet, succulent pears are a favorite fruit in our house, so matching them up with our top dessert ingredient makes this torte even better.

Pear Topping

1	large ripe Bartlett pear, cored and peeled
1 tbsp	freshly squeezed orange juice
2 tsp	brown sugar
¼ tsp	each: ground cinnamon and ground ginger
2 tbsp	toasted almond slices

Cake

¾ cup	whole wheat flour
½ cup	oat flour (see tip)
½ cup	unsweetened cocoa powder
1 tsp	baking powder
1 tsp	ground cinnamon
¼ tsp	salt
2	large eggs
¾ cup	granulated sugar
½ cup	canned pure pumpkin (see tip)
2 tbsp	high-oleic safflower oil
1 tsp	pure vanilla extract
½ cup	1% buttermilk
¼ cup	dark (at least 60% cocoa) chocolate chips

TIPS If you don't have oat flour, take the same amount + 2 tbsp of quick-cooking oats (not instant oats) and whirl in a food processor until it becomes flour. For more fiber, pulse oat bran.
➤ Look for 100% pure pumpkin (not seasoned pumpkin) in the baking aisle of your grocery store.

➤ Slice pears thinly, about ½ inch (1 cm) thick, and toss with orange juice, brown sugar, cinnamon and ginger in a medium bowl.

➤ To make the cake batter, sift flours and cocoa powder into a large bowl. Add baking powder, cinnamon and salt and combine well. Set aside.

➤ Preheat oven to 350°F. In a stand mixer fitted with a paddle attachment, beat eggs and sugar together on medium-high speed until light and fluffy. While mixer is running, add pumpkin, oil and vanilla; beat just until well combined. Gradually add flour-cocoa mixture, alternating with buttermilk and ending with the flour mixture. Scrape down the sides of the bowl as needed. Fold chocolate chips into batter.

➤ Line the bottom of a 9-inch springform pan with parchment paper. Coat the sides with cooking spray and dust them with flour. Pour cake batter into pan, coaxing it to the sides. Layer the seasoned pears carefully on top of the batter, arranging wedges in a circular pattern. Sprinkle toasted almond slices evenly over pears. Bake in preheated oven for 45 minutes, or until a pick inserted in the center of cake comes out clean. Let cool for 5 minutes.

➤ Gently loosen the edges of the cake with the tip of a knife while removing side pan. Place on a serving plate and serve warm or at room temperature.

♡ LOW IN...CHOLESTEROL

A diet high in oats is effective in lowering LDL (bad) cholesterol levels. Oat bran, the outer hull of the oat grain, is particularly high in soluble fiber, which is said to reduce the absorption of cholesterol in the bloodstream. Flavonols in dark chocolate have also shown to reduce cholesterol and lower blood pressure.

8 SERVINGS

PER SERVING 323 CALORIES | 12 G TOTAL FAT (4 G SATURATED FAT) | 49 MG CHOLESTEROL | 37 MG SODIUM | 55 G CARBOHYDRATE | 8 G FIBER | 10 G PROTEIN

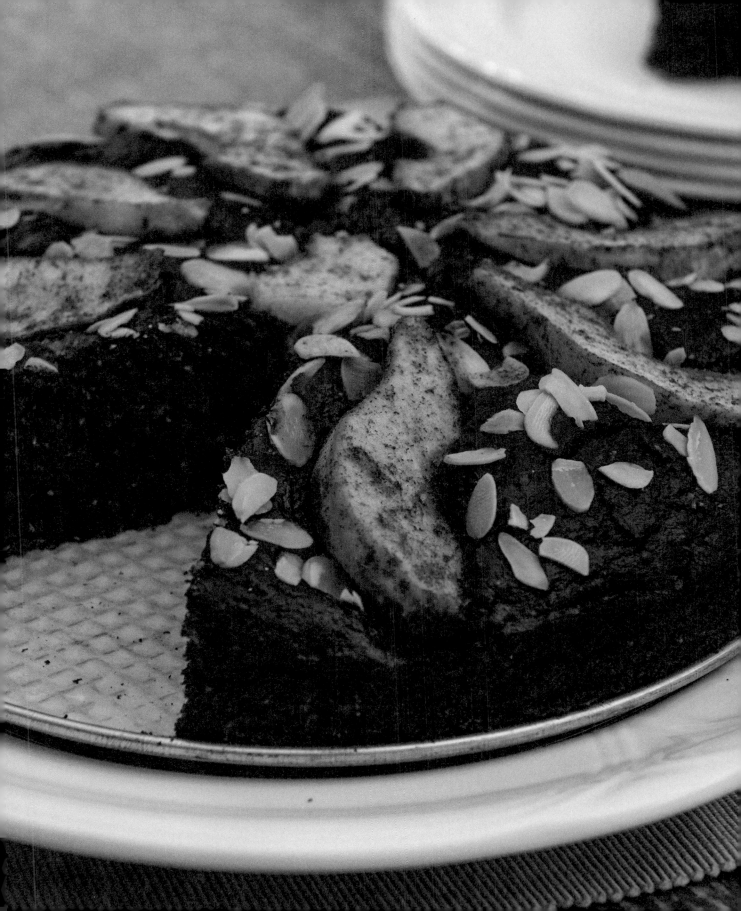

Quinoa Crepes with Berry Compote
Crepes con composta di bacche

WE HAVE A LONG HISTORY OF CREPE-MAKING in our family. No, the recipe didn't get passed down to us from a relative in Italy or France, where crepes have their origins; rather, my mom began experimenting with gluten-free versions decades ago to replace the pasta sheets she used to wrap her cannelloni fillings so my sister, who has Celiac disease, could eat them. Mom's recipe gave me a foundation to try other variations, in particular this one using protein-rich quinoa flour, for a crepe that is marvelous, *meravigliosa, merveilleux*...however you want to say it.

Crepes

2	large eggs
1 cup	warm water
½ cup	quinoa flour (see tip)
½ cup	whole wheat flour
1 pkg	(0.3 oz/8 g) vanillin sugar (see tip)
Pinch	each: ground cinnamon and salt

Fresh strawberries and blueberries for garnish

Vanilla frozen yogurt (optional)

Berry Compote

2 cups	frozen berries (raspberries, strawberries, blackberries, blueberries)
2 tbsp	freshly squeezed orange juice
1 tsp	maple syrup

⇆ VARIATION Use crepes for a healthy breakfast option — spread crepes with natural peanut butter, almond butter or sunflower butter and roll. Use fruit purée as a dip. Or use crepe as a sandwich wrap, stuffed with shaved meats, low-fat dressing and crisp lettuce or julienned carrots.

➤ In a large bowl, beat eggs. Whisk in warm water. Set aside.

➤ In medium bowl, combine flours, vanillin sugar, cinnamon and salt. Whisk dry ingredients into egg mixture until well combined.

➤ Lightly coat a medium non-stick skillet with cooking spray and heat over medium-low heat. Add a half ladleful of batter and rotate skillet in a circular motion as you pour batter from the center out to edges of skillet to fully cover the bottom. Cook for 30 seconds to 1 minute, flip with spatula and cook other side for another 30 seconds or just until no longer sticky to the touch. Repeat with remaining batter, coating skillet with cooking spray each time.

➤ Prepare compote by placing berry compote ingredients into the bowl of a food processor. Pulse a few times until chunky.

➤ Serve crepes with compote as a filling or a topping along with fresh berries. If you're filling crepe with frozen yogurt, let crepe cool down, add a couple of scoops down the center of crepe and roll as you shape. Place on a parchment-lined baking sheet and freeze for 1 hour. Serve with compote and fresh berries.

TIPS To make your own quinoa flour, use a coffee grinder or mill (a food processor won't work) to grind the quinoa. Add a small amount (only filling the grinder's basket halfway), grind for about 2 minutes, mixing with a spoon in between grinding. A cup yields ⅔ cup flour.
➤ Vanillin sugar is a powdered vanilla product added to baked goods. You'll find it in the baking section of your grocery store.

⌂ HIGH IN...FIBER

These crepes get a big jolt of added fiber with the addition of whole wheat and quinoa flours. Top with a wallop of berries and the fiber count is even more impressive.

6 CREPES   **30 MIN OR LESS**   **DAIRY-FREE**

PER CREPE 137 CALORIES | 3 G TOTAL FAT (1 G SATURATED FAT) | 79 MG CHOLESTEROL | 32 MG SODIUM | 23 G CARBOHYDRATE | 7 G FIBER | 5 G PROTEIN

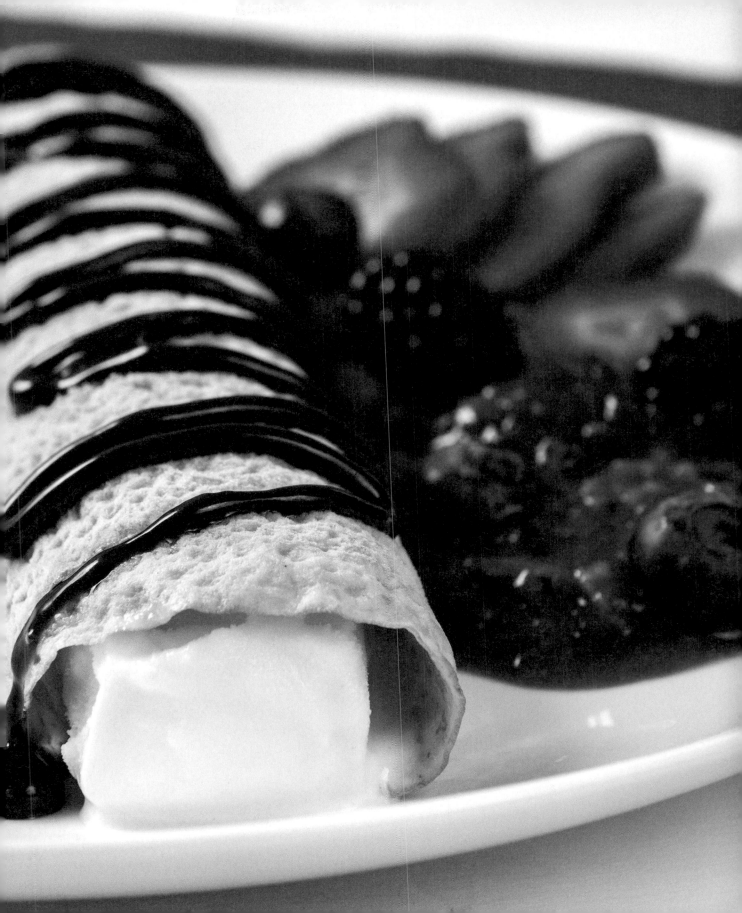

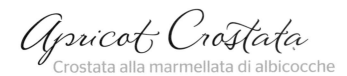

Apricot Crostata
Crostata alla marmellata di albicocche

CALL IT IRONIC (OR LUCK!) THAT NO MATTER WHERE MY FAMILY HAS LIVED, we've been surrounded by neighbors who are gifted bakers, in particular outstanding crostata makers. I've tasted enough of them to know that they are among the finest. Some have filled their sweet crusts with ricotta, others with apples or peaches from their own fruit trees, and still others with a homemade mincemeat filling or syrupy fruit jam. Among our neighbors, "borrowing" a cup of sugar has many advantages, especially when the thank you comes in the form of a delicious slice of crostata heaven.

Crust

1¼ cups	unbleached all-purpose flour
1¼ cups	whole-grain spelt flour
1 tbsp	ground flaxseed
1 pkg	(0.6 oz/16 g) Bertolini Lievito Vaniglinato (see tip)
¼ tsp	salt
3 tbsp	unsalted butter, softened
¼ cup	granulated sugar
3	large eggs
¼ cup	low-fat 2% vanilla Greek yogurt

Milk for brushing

Apricot Jam-Almond Topping

½ cup	toasted sliced almonds
1¼ cups	reduced-sugar apricot jam

Icing (confectioner's) sugar for dusting

TIP Bertolini Lievito Vaniglinato is a premixed product that combines baking powder and vanillin. A suitable substitute is 3 tsp baking powder + 1 tsp vanillin (or ½ tsp pure vanilla extract). Find it next to the yeast in the baking section of a well-stocked grocery store. It's also available online. The product is gluten-free.

➤ In a large bowl, combine flours, flaxseed, Lievito Vaniglinato and salt. Set aside.

➤ In a stand mixer fitted with a paddle attachment, cream the butter and sugar together on medium speed until light and fluffy. Add eggs, one at a time, beating well after each addition. Mix in yogurt.

➤ With the mixer running on medium-low speed, gradually add the flour mixture just until all the ingredients are combined. Turn the dough out onto a lightly floured surface and knead for 1 to 2 minutes. Reserve about 1 cup (or a handful) of dough to make lattice-patterned crust on top.

➤ Grease a deep, round 12-inch non-stick baking pan or 12.5-inch non-stick fluted tart pan with removable bottom. Using a rolling pin, roll out dough to about ½ inch (1 cm) thick, large enough to fit pan size. The dough will rise so don't be afraid to roll it out thinly. Transfer dough to greased pan and gently press dough up the sides of the pan. (If you don't have an extra-large deep pan, use a round pizza pan to flatten out dough and pinch up the edges).

➤ Preheat oven to 350°F.

➤ Scatter almonds evenly over the entire crust and gently press pieces into dough. Drop apricot jam by the teaspoonful over almonds, leaving ½ inch (1 cm) perimeter of dough bare.

➤ Take the reserved dough, sprinkle with extra flour and flatten with a rolling pin to form a rectangle about 6 x 10 inches (15 x 25 cm). Cut dough into six long strips, about ¾ inch (2 cm) wide. Place over filling, evenly spaced from end to end. Lay the remaining strips diagonally over the first strips. Cut off any remaining dough at ends and pinch dough at the perimeter.

12 SERVINGS

PER SERVING 268 CALORIES | 6 G TOTAL FAT (2 G SATURATED FAT) | 8 MG CHOLESTEROL | 81 MG SODIUM | 44 G CARBOHYDRATE | 5 G FIBER | 7 G PROTEIN

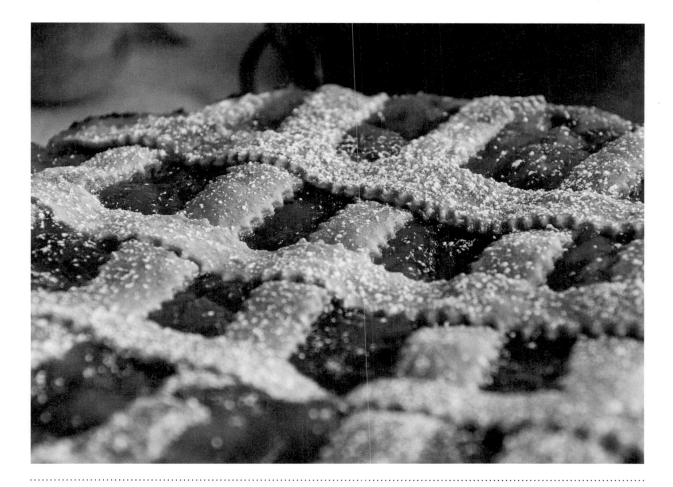

➤ Bake for about 40 minutes or until crostata is lightly browned. Remove crostata from oven and let cool for about 10 minutes before removing from pan. Once cooled, sprinkle with icing sugar and serve.

| ⇆ VARIATION | **Prune-Plum Topping** |

3 cups	prune plums, pitted and cut evenly into quarters (about 1½ lbs/680 g), (see tip)
2 tsp	honey
	Zest of ½ orange
1 tbsp	freshly squeezed orange juice
1 tbsp	light butter, melted
½ tsp	ground cinnamon

➤ In a large bowl, combine prune-plum quarters, honey, orange zest and juice, butter and cinnamon. Gently toss until prune plums are well coated.

➤ Arrange prune plums in a circular pattern in a single layer onto crust, starting from the outer edge until you get to the center. You'll want to overlap them only slightly as your arrange them. Drizzle any syrup left in bowl over the prune plums.

➤ Follow the directions on the opposite page to create the lattice-patterned top crust.

➤ Bake in 350°F preheated oven for about 45 minutes. Remove crostata from oven and let cool for about 10 minutes before dusting with icing sugar, cutting and serving.

TIP Prune plums are also known as blue plums, typically available in late summer.

⌂ HIGH IN...FIBER

Although we're talking about a dessert here, this recipe is actually high in fiber, thanks to the addition of an ancient grain, potent nut and versatile seed — spelt flour, almonds and flaxseed. While I wouldn't advocate eating dessert for breakfast, most cereals contain as much sugar, more fat and a lot less fiber than a slice of this crostata. Try the prune-plum topping variation for even greater fiber benefits.

Light Raspberry Tiramisu
Tiramisù light ai lamponi

I HAVE TIRAMISU MASTER BUILDERS SURROUNDING ME — my mother, sister and sister-in-law Christina all craft their own lusciously decadent tiramisus. So to outdo them was a real battle. Add the fact that I'm replacing mascarpone cheese, the key ingredient that gives tiramisu its velvety finish, and some aficionados would say winning the lottery is easier. I've never won the lottery, but this recipe has a winning combination.

1 tub	(1 lb/500 g) 1% reduced-sodium cottage cheese
¼ cup	light (5%) cream
2	large eggs
2 tbsp	granulated sugar
1 tub	(1 lb/500 g) low-fat 2% vanilla Greek yogurt
1½ cups	strongly brewed coffee
2 tbsp	coffee-flavored liqueur, such as Tia Maria or Kahlúa
33 to 36	lady finger cookies (savoiardi)*
2 cups	fresh or frozen raspberries
2 tsp	unsweetened cocoa powder
1	square (1 oz/28 g) dark chocolate for grating and shavings

➤ Combine cottage cheese and cream in the bowl of a food processor or blender and purée until smooth and fluffy (don't use a stand mixer or pieces won't cream). Set aside.

➤ In a stand mixer fitted with a paddle attachment, beat eggs and sugar on medium-high speed until light and fluffy. Stir in the creamed cottage cheese mixture and yogurt just until well blended.

➤ In a medium bowl, add warm coffee and liqueur.

➤ To assemble, use a glass trifle or round bowl. Begin the first layer by dipping lady finger cookies, one at a time, in coffee just until fully wet. Let coffee drip before placing cookies along the sides and at the bottom of trifle dish, cutting cookies to fit in between spaces. Scatter one-third of raspberries over cookies. Scoop out one-third of cream mixture and spread evenly over cookies/raspberries. Repeat layers two more times.

➤ On the final layer, sift cocoa powder and grate chocolate evenly over cream. Garnish with remaining raspberries. Refrigerate for 2 to 4 hours before serving.

ᴗ LOW IN...FAT

Ultra-decadent mascarpone cheese and 35% cream are the signature ingredients in most tiramisu recipes. They get swapped here with another ultra-rich blend of cheese and cream but with an extraordinarily less amount of fat — the mascarpone in the traditional recipe has more than four times the amount of fat and 10 times the amount of saturated fat than a light cottage cheese.

10-12 SERVINGS   GLUTEN-FREE* SEE PAGE 276 FOR GLUTEN-FREE CAKE IN PLACE OF COOKIES

PER SERVING(12) 216 CALORIES | 4 G TOTAL FAT (2 G SATURATED FAT) | 59 MG CHOLESTEROL | 127 MG SODIUM | 34 G CARBOHYDRATE | 2 G FIBER | 12 G PROTEIN

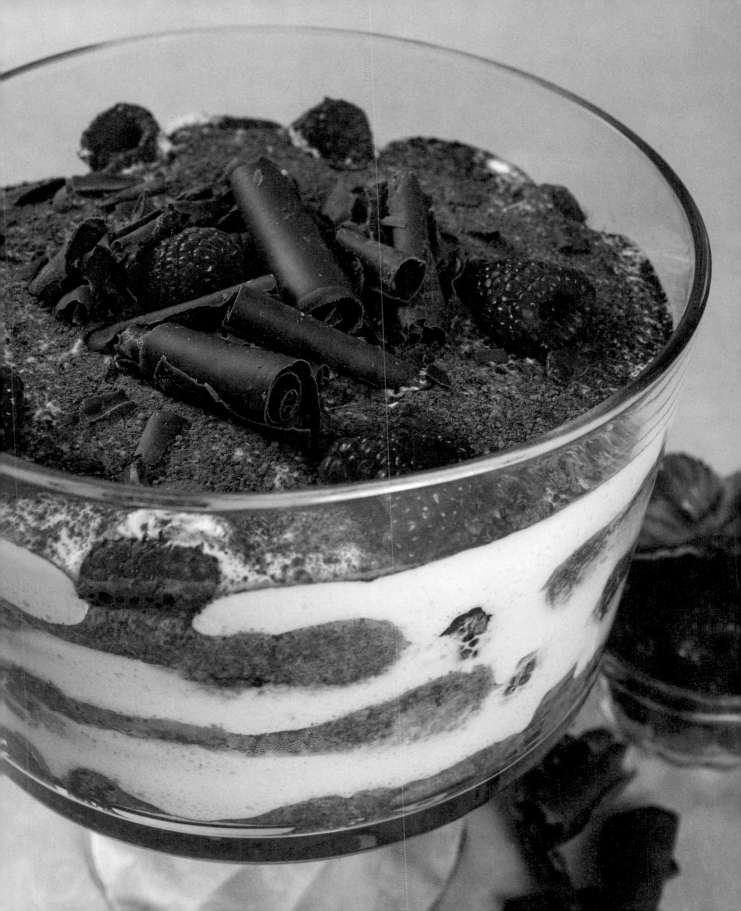

Sicilian Cassata Cake

Cassata Siciliana

LIKE THE CHRISTMAS HOLIDAYS, Easter has its fair share of traditional baked goods and decadent desserts. My mom crafts her chick-shaped Easter bread for each grandchild, my mother-in-law makes her mother's rice crostata and I like to add this citrusy ricotta cake — a homage to ancestral customs and a nod to newer, sweet beginnings.

Cake

1	prebaked 9 x 9-inch square sponge cake or 9-inch round sponge cake or 1 recipe Rosa's Gluten-Free Super Sponge Cake (*see page 276*)

Ricotta Filling

1 tub	(1 lb/475 g) part-skim ricotta cheese, well drained
¼ cup	low-fat 2% honey or vanilla Greek yogurt
3 tbsp	granulated sugar
Zest of 1 orange	
¼ tsp	pure vanilla extract
1 tbsp	rum

Glaze

2 tbsp	milk
1 tsp	cornstarch
¼ cup	icing (confectioner's) sugar
1 tsp	freshly grated orange zest
2 tbsp	chopped unsalted dry-roasted pistachios, shelled
2	kiwi fruit, peeled and thinly sliced, for garnish

➤ If preparing sponge cake using Rosa's Gluten-Free Super Sponge Cake, pour batter into a greased 9 x 13-inch oblong cake pan lined with parchment paper. Bake in a preheated oven at 350°F on oven rack slightly higher than bottom rack for 30 minutes. Once cooled, gently loosen cake with the tip of a knife around the sides of the pan and invert. Slice cake slab horizontally into two equal thick halves. Save one for another use (or use to double this recipe). Cut the other half vertically with a sharp knife to make two halves. Trim sides of cake to make the 2 layers even. Set them aside.

➤ In a stand mixer fitted with a paddle attachment on medium speed, beat ricotta cheese, yogurt and sugar until well combined, about 4 to 5 minutes. Scrape down sides and stir in orange zest and vanilla.

➤ To assemble cake, place bottom layer on a serving dish and brush rum evenly over cake. Spread ricotta mixture evenly over cake layer. Carefully transfer the other cake layer on top of ricotta. If ricotta mixture spills over sides, use a knife to tuck it in and smooth it along sides.

➤ In a small cup, combine milk and cornstarch. Whisk milk mixture with icing sugar in a small bowl. Stir in orange zest. Spread a thin layer over top cake layer. Top with pistachios and garnish with kiwi. Refrigerate cake for 2 to 4 hours or overnight to fully set. Cut into 9 pieces and serve.

MAKE AHEAD You can prepare the sponge cake the day before. Store in an air-tight container until ready to use.

VARIATION Stir 3 tbsp of dark chocolate chips into ricotta mixture.

TIP When cutting the layers, use sewing thread for a more even cut.

9 SERVINGS

PER SERVING 249 CALORIES | 8 G TOTAL FAT (3 G SATURATED FAT) | 9 MG CHOLESTEROL | 106 MG SODIUM | 34 G CARBOHYDRATE | 2 G FIBER | 10 G PROTEIN

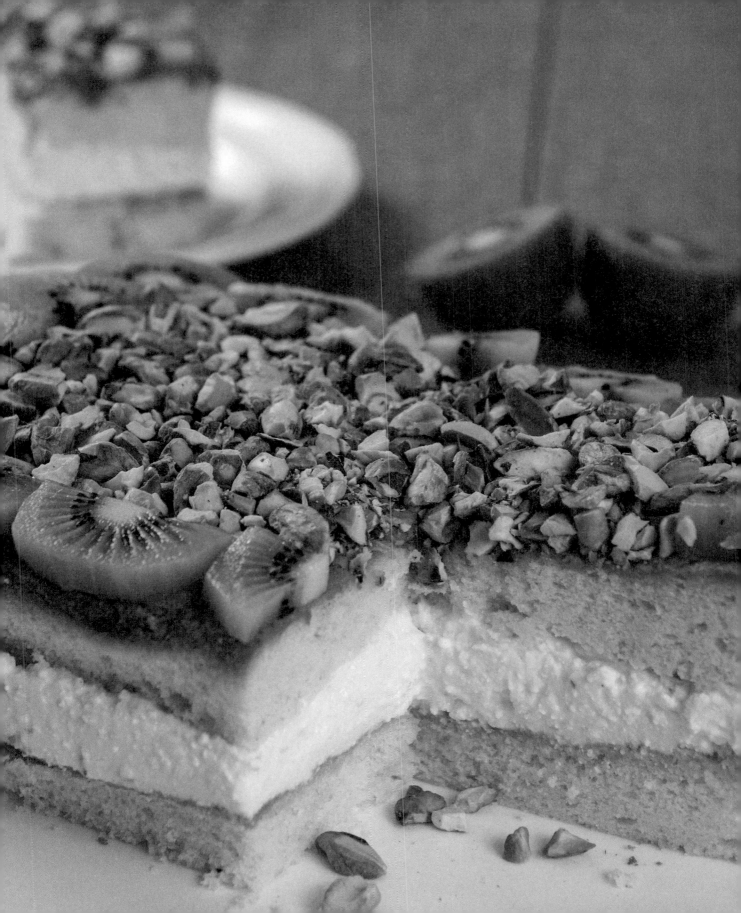

Nonna's Cookies in Cream
Biscotti con crema e marsala

WHEN NONNA CAME TO VISIT US FROM ITALY, she'd stay for six months at a time. We were showered with hugs and kisses — and food — because, of course, food is love for all Italian nonnas. This was her signature dessert, whipped up *just because*. Made from simple ingredients already in our pantry, Nonna never had to make a special trip to the grocery store to surprise us with it. But we already knew it was coming as soon as our noses caught a whiff of the simmering sweet marsala. You might say it was a call to action either to help dunk the layered cookies, drizzle the sweet cream or scatter our favorite sprinkles.

½ cup	sweet marsala (see tip)
½ tsp	agave syrup or honey
2 cups	almond milk, divided
2½ tbsp	cornstarch
1 tsp	granulated sugar
½ tsp	pure vanilla extract
Pinch	ground nutmeg
20	Maria tea biscuits* (round)
2 tsp	hemp seeds
Candy sprinkles (optional)	

⇆ VARIATION Make individual servings of this recipe in glass dessert bowls or cups and let the kids choose their favorite garnishes: nuts, mini chocolate chips or shaved chocolate or candy sprinkles (just a little!).
➤ If you're looking for more fiber, substitute whole-grain cookies or unsalted whole-grain crackers for tea biscuits.

➤ In a small pot, combine marsala with agave and bring to a gentle simmer over medium-high heat. Cook for 3 to 4 minutes to allow alcohol to evaporate. Pour into a small bowl and set aside to cool.

➤ In the meantime, pour 1½ cups of almond milk in a medium pot. Stir cornstarch into remaining ½ cup milk (still cold) until dissolved completely. Add to pot and whisk continuously on medium-high heat. Add sugar, vanilla and nutmeg and continue whisking for about 5 to 6 minutes or until mixture thickens and begins to bubble. (Be careful not to burn bottom — you may need to adjust the heat.) Keep warm.

➤ To assemble, you'll need a 9-inch pie plate or shallow bowl. Dunk cookies, one at a time, in marsala mixture for about 3 seconds. Shake off excess and place in pie plate. Repeat with other cookies until you've made one layer and filled in all gaps with cookies. Pour half the cream mixture over cookies. Add another layer of cookies, dunking one at a time. Pour remaining cream over top layer. Let cool 10 minutes. Add hemp seeds and sprinkles, if desired.

➤ Serve warm or refrigerate for up to 12 hours to set.

TIP Sweet marsala, not dry marsala, is ideal for desserts. I like the Sperone Cremovo brand for its smooth taste.

⌂ HIGH IN...CALCIUM

Not only is almond milk much lower in fat than the cream or whole milk typically used to prepare a cookies in cream recipe, but it also has an equal amount of calcium to regular milk. Almond milk is also boosted with the same amount of vitamin D as milk.

5 SERVINGS   30 MIN OR LESS   DAIRY-FREE* CHECK LABEL

PER SERVING 180 CALORIES | 4 G TOTAL FAT (2 G SATURATED FAT) | 0 MG CHOLESTEROL | 129 MG SODIUM | 26 G CARBOHYDRATE | 1 G FIBER | 2 G PROTEIN

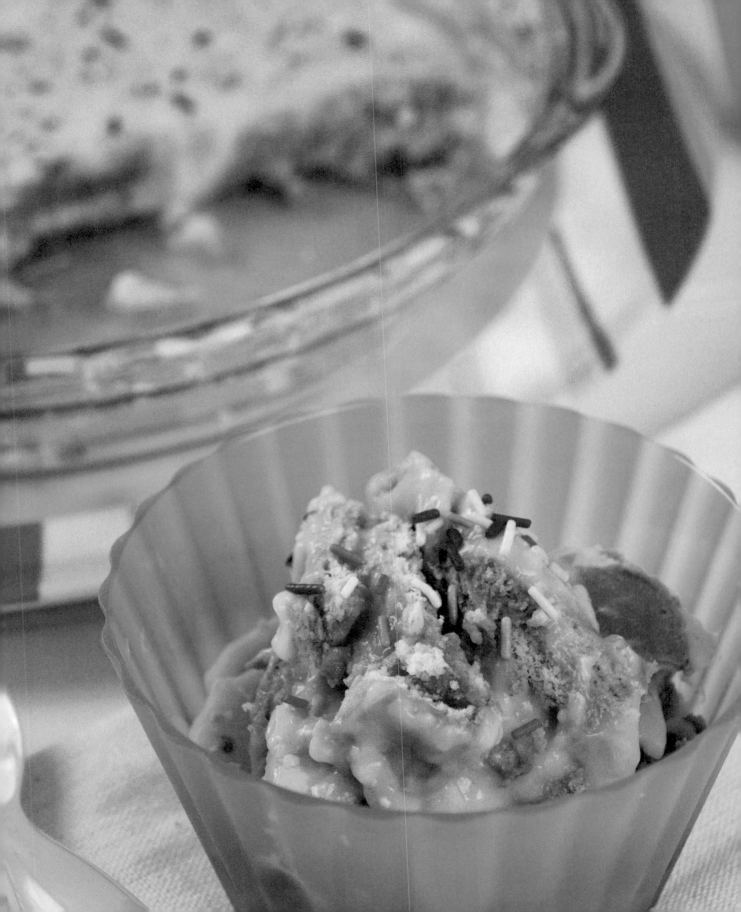

Pistachio Granita

Granita di pistacchio

I HAD MY FIRST TASTE OF LEMON GRANITA, stuffed into a brioche (a sweet bun like a croissant), for breakfast while visiting Italy the summer I was eight years old. I was still in bed in the early morning hours when my nonna ran after the granita truck — a sort of equivalent of the ice cream truck — and delivered what I thought was surely a forbidden treat. I learned that the decadent meal was a traditional Sicilian breakfast. Well, I don't have to tell you what I had for breakfast every single day while I was there! What was more incredibly lip-smacking was that granitas weren't limited to only lemon — other refreshing flavors included thirst-quenching watermelon and creamy pistachio. I was hooked!

1 cup	large unsalted dry-roasted pistachios, shelled
3 cups	water
⅓ cup	honey
½ cup	almond milk
¼ tsp	pure vanilla extract
Pinch	salt

➤ Grind pistachios in a food processor until they're extremely fine. Set aside.

➤ In a large pot, bring water to a boil. Whisk in honey until fully dissolved and remove from burner to cool. Stir in almond milk, vanilla, salt and ground pistachios. Whisk gently to ensure the pistachios are well incorporated. Let mixture cool completely.

➤ Pour mixture into a non-reactive, freezer-safe pan or bowl. (I use a 9 x 13-inch glass baking pan.) Cool down for 10 minutes, whisk mixture gently and carefully place in freezer on a flat surface to chill for about 2 hours, when mixture will start to form ice crystals. Use a fork to scrape icy bits from sides and mix well. Place back in freezer and repeat scraping every 30 minutes to an hour. Scoop into glass cup or bowl and serve immediately.

MAKE AHEAD Prepare ingredients the night before and freeze. Pulse granita in the bowl of a food processor until smooth just before serving.

⌂ HIGH IN...FIBER

Like other nuts, pistachios offer a great deal of fiber in just a small amount, about 3 grams per 1-ounce serving. The phytosterols and good fats in pistachios also make them a healthy snack in small quantities.

8 SERVINGS · **GLUTEN-FREE** · **DAIRY-FREE** · **MAKE AHEAD**

PER SERVING 155 CALORIES | 7 G TOTAL FAT (1 G SATURATED FAT) | 0 MG CHOLESTEROL | 9 MG SODIUM | 22 G CARBOHYDRATE | 1 G FIBER | 3 G PROTEIN

Tartufo Cake

Torta di tartufo

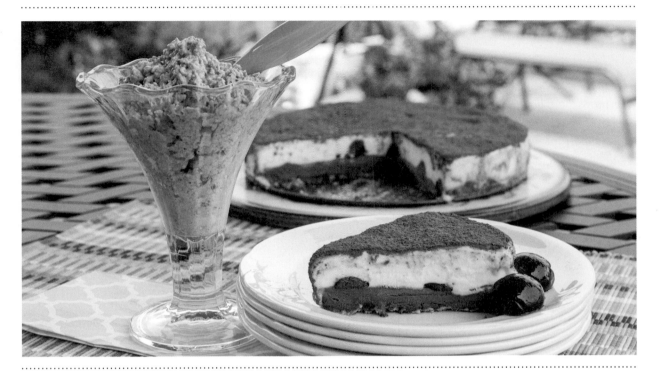

¾ cup	toasted unsalted whole almonds
4 cups	(1 L) chocolate frozen yogurt
4 cups	(1 L) vanilla frozen yogurt
1 cup	pitted frozen or fresh cherries, halved
2 tbsp	unsweetened cocoa powder
Your favorite liqueur for serving (optional)	

MAKE AHEAD Prepare this cake two to three days before you're ready to serve it. Freeze completely, then cover it completely with foil paper or seal in an air-tight container.

➤ Place almonds in the bowl of a food processor and pulse until small pieces form. Set aside.

➤ Cover the bottom of a 10-inch springform pan evenly with almond pieces. Now, you'll need to work quickly so be sure you have all your ingredients at hand. Scoop out chocolate frozen yogurt and place evenly over almonds.

➤ Use the back of a spoon, then your hands, to press down and fill the layer evenly. Scatter cherries evenly over chocolate frozen yogurt. Scoop out vanilla frozen yogurt and place evenly over cherries. Use the back of a spoon, then your hands, to press down and fill layer evenly. Be sure that top is smooth — wet your hands if you need to.

➤ Place cocoa powder into a sifter and sift evenly over vanilla layer. Freeze overnight. Cut into equal slices and serve with a drizzle of liqueur, if desired.

 16-20 SERVINGS 30 MIN OR LESS GLUTEN-FREE   MAKE AHEAD

PER SERVING(20) 99 CALORIES | 3 G TOTAL FAT (1 G SATURATED FAT) | 10 MG CHOLESTEROL | 62 MG SODIUM | 15 G CARBOHYDRATE | 1 G FIBER | 2 G PROTEIN

Christmas Fig Cookies
Purciddati di Natale

EVEN BEFORE OUR FAMILY PLANS THE CHRISTMAS MENU, we set a date to make these heavenly cookies, a long-standing tradition in our house. My parents, my niece, my kids — we all get in on the action, if not to get our hands into the dough or to pulse the chunky filling, then it's to be the first ones in line to taste them as they come out of the oven piping hot. With a sensory-awakening mix of ingredients like figs, oranges, almonds, cloves and chocolate, can you blame us for wanting to hold onto this ritual forever?

Fig Filling

3 tbsp	granulated sugar
½ cup	water
10.5 oz	(300 g) Turkish dried figs, stems removed and chopped
½ cup	toasted unsalted whole almonds
Peel of 1 mandarin, finely chopped	
1 tsp	Amaretto liqueur
2 tsp	unsweetened cocoa powder
1 tsp	pure vanilla extract
1 tsp	ground cinnamon
¼ tsp	ground cloves
2 tbsp	reduced-sugar apricot jam

Cookie Dough

2 cups	cake & pastry flour
1 cup	whole wheat flour
1 pkg	(0.6 oz/16 g) Bertolini Lievito Vaniglinato
1 pkg	(0.3 oz/8 g) vanillin sugar
2 tsp	ground flaxseed
½ cup	trans-fat-free shortening (see tip)
½ cup	granulated sugar
2	large eggs
Zest and juice of ½ lemon	
1 tsp	Amaretto liqueur
2 to 3 tbsp cold water	
Egg white for brushing	

➤ To make filling, combine sugar and water in a medium pot and whisk until sugar is fully dissolved; bring to a gentle boil. Set aside.

➤ In the bowl of a food processor, add figs, almonds, mandarin peel, Amaretto, cocoa powder, vanilla, cinnamon and cloves. Pulse a few times, then slowly pour in half the sugar-water and whisk until it forms a chunky paste, about 2 to 3 minutes. Scrape down sides in between. Add fig mixture and apricot jam into pot with remaining sugar-water and stir on low heat until sugar-water is fully absorbed, about 8 to 10 minutes. Let cool for 1 hour or refrigerate overnight.

➤ To make the cookie dough, combine flours, Lievito Vaniglinato, vanillin sugar and flaxseed in a large bowl and mix well.

➤ Cream shortening and sugar in the bowl of a food processor fitted with pastry/dough blade. Add eggs, one at a time, and beat briefly after each addition. Add lemon zest and juice and Amaretto. Stream in flour mixture and 1 tbsp of cold water at a time if dough seems dry; process just until blended. Don't over-process or dough will be tough. Place dough in a greased glass or ceramic bowl, cover with plastic wrap and let rise for 1 hour.

➤ Preheat oven to 350°F. Working in batches, take a handful of dough, knead and roll out as thinly as possible to form a disk shape. Invert an 8-inch (20-cm) side plate and press into dough. Cut around plate; remove dough around it. Cut circle into 8 triangles. Add 1½ tsp of filling at wide edge, flatten slightly and roll into a crescent. Place crescents 1 inch (2.5 cm) apart on a baking sheet lined with parchment paper. Brush tops with egg white. Bake in preheated oven for 15 to 20 minutes, or until bottoms are golden brown and tops are lightly golden.

MAKE AHEAD Make fig filling one to two days before and refrigerate.

TIP I use Earth Balance natural shortening, a plant-based shortening that is trans-fat free, dairy-free and gluten-free.

60 COOKIES

DAIRY-FREE

MAKE AHEAD

PER COOKIE 69 CALORIES | 2 G TOTAL FAT (1 G SATURATED FAT) | 6 MG CHOLESTEROL | 21 MG SODIUM | 11 G CARBOHYDRATE | 1 G FIBER | 1 G PROTEIN

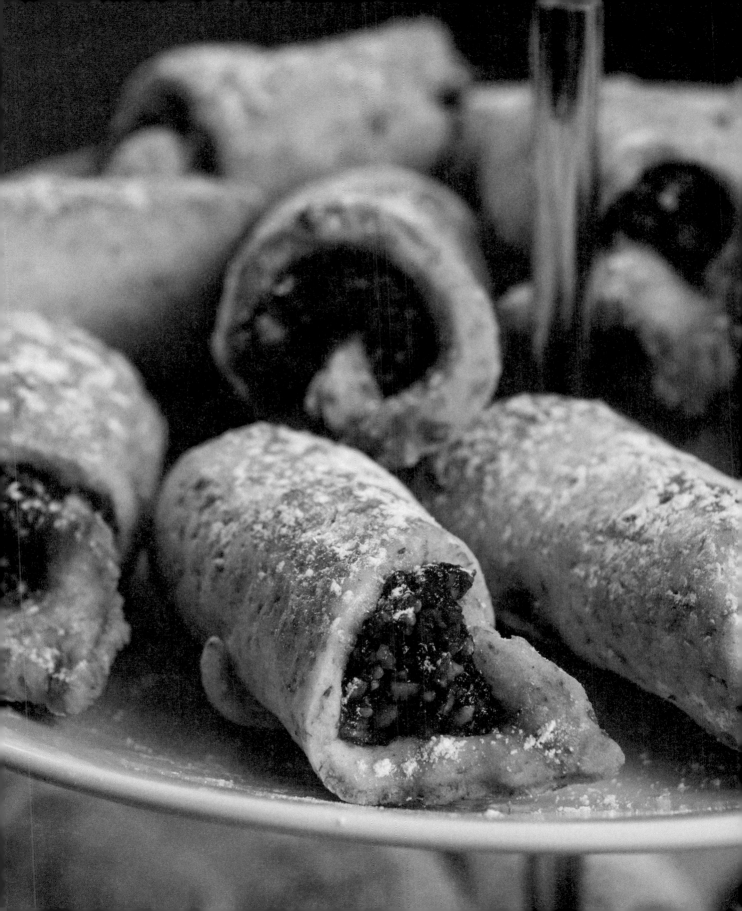

Dark Chocolate Almond Torrone

Torrone di mandorle al cioccolato fondente

AROUND THE HOLIDAYS, mom was always tussling with some sticky concoction involving almonds and sugar. Her traditional *torrone* took fragrant roasted almonds, coated them in a honey mixture and left them to dry like peanut brittle. Delish! But if I have to choose, it's the Italian nougat torrone with an irresistibly chewy center that I love even more, for obvious reasons. To make the divine confectionary, however, requires a more finicky process much like candy-making, and I never had the patience for it. Luckily for you (OK, for me!), my sister learned a "secret" shortcut recipe for torrone from a relative and agreed to share it. We often make it together — I recommend the extra pair of hands to hold the pot while you stir the extra tacky mixture before it sets and is cut into decadent morsels.

17.5 oz	(500 g) good-quality unsalted whole almonds (about 3½ cups)
17.5 oz	(500 g) dark baking chocolate (wafers)*
17.5 oz	(500 g) mini marshmallows
½ tsp	light butter
½ tsp	pure vanilla extract
2	sheets (about 8 x 11 inches/ 20 x 28 cm each) edible rice paper (see tip)

TIP Edible rice paper or wafer paper can be found in bulk food stores. Don't confuse this paper with rice wrappers.

MAKE AHEAD Roast the almonds up to a day or two ahead.

⇆VARIATIONS Try different nuts like hazelnuts or pistachios.
➤ For for a more decadent version, use a white chocolate instead of a dark chocolate.

➤ Preheat oven to 350°F. Place almonds on a baking sheet and roast until fragrant and lightly browned, about 10 minutes. Let cool.

➤ In a large pot set on medium-low heat, add chocolate wafers and stir continuously until about half melted. Add marshmallows and butter and continue stirring until fully combined. Be careful that the bottom doesn't brown (or reduce heat). Add vanilla and almonds and remove from heat. Stir almonds until evenly coated.

➤ Line a glass, ceramic or plastic 8 x 11-inch (20 x 28-cm) container with one long sheet of plastic wrap that extends beyond the handles (you'll later need to use the wrap to coerce the torrone out). Layer lined bottom with 1 sheet of rice paper that fills in most of the bottom of pan. Pour mixture onto rice paper, spread it out leaving ½ inch (1 cm) perimeter around rice paper. Place second sheet of rice paper on top, pressing it into mixture and smooth out evenly. Take another glass dish (slightly smaller) and place it on top to flatten out gently. Don't press too hard or mixture will ooze out from sides and stick on top of paper.

➤ Remove dish and let torrone sit overnight, uncovered.

➤ Once set, pull up plastic wrap and wiggle out whole piece of torrone. (It'll feel like a hard piece of brick.) Place on a large cutting board. With a wide, sharp knife (a chef's knife will do), cut torrone vertically to form 4 long pieces, almost 2 inches (5 cm) wide for each. You may need to trim outside edges. Take each vertical piece and cut pieces horizontally on a slight angle about ¾ inch (2 cm) thick.

➤ Store in a tight, sealed container in a dry place for up to three to four weeks.

50-55 PIECES   GLUTEN-FREE*   MAKE AHEAD
                       CHECK LABEL

PER PIECE(55) 137 CALORIES | 9 G TOTAL FAT (3 G SATURATED FAT) | 0 MG CHOLESTEROL | 11 MG SODIUM | 13 G CARBOHYDRATE | 2 G FIBER | 3 G PROTEIN

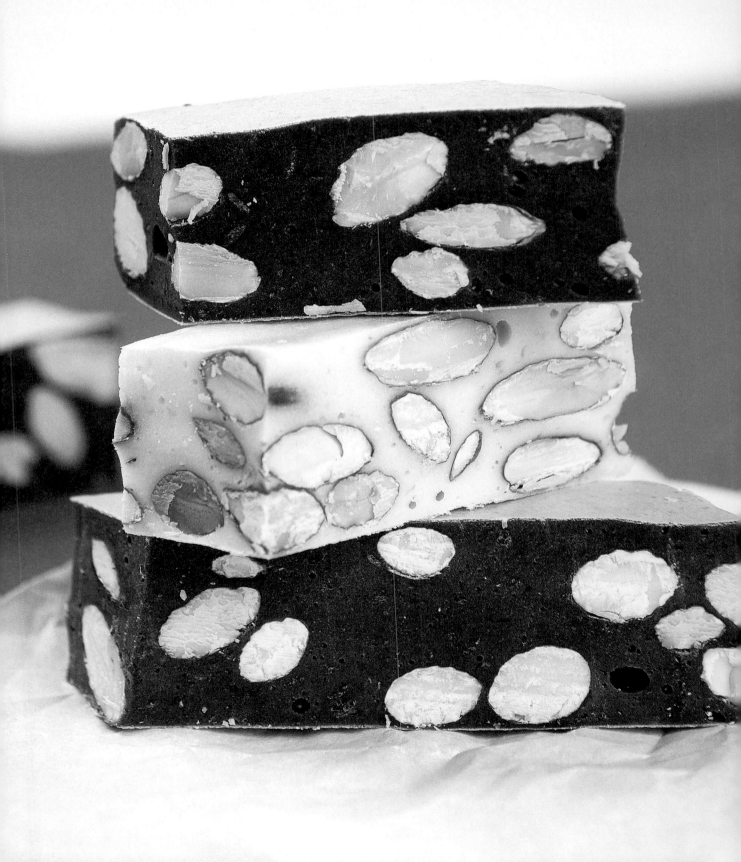

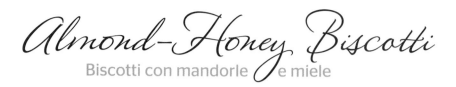

Almond-Honey Biscotti

Biscotti con mandorle e miele

WHEN MY PARENTS BABYSAT MY KIDS and their other grandkids as toddlers, the highlight was Nonno's afternoon coffee break, which can be equated to the English teatime. That's because my dad's coffee mug became a dunking pot for biscotti like these ones. The kids would climb onto his lap, and once he set down the mug, the dunking frenzy began. Even today, while most of the kids are now too big to sit on his lap, they sometimes sneak in a dunk or two.

1 cup	unsalted whole almonds
3	large eggs
½ cup	honey
1 tbsp	brown sugar
1 tbsp	anise-flavored or sambuca liqueur
1 tsp	pure vanilla extract
1 tsp	pure almond extract
1 tsp	grated orange zest
2¾ cups	whole wheat flour (see variation)
2 tsp	ground flaxseed
1 tsp	baking powder
¼ tsp	salt
⅓ cup	dark (at least 60% cocoa) chocolate chips
1 tbsp	egg white

⇆ VARIATION For a slightly nutty flavor and more protein, substitute ½ cup quinoa flour for the same amount of whole wheat flour. For more chocolatey oomph, dip bottoms of biscotti into melted dark chocolate and let dry.

MAKE AHEAD Roast almonds up to a day or two ahead of making these biscotti.

➤ Preheat oven to 350°F. Place almonds in a single layer on a baking sheet and bake until fragrant and lightly browned, about 10 to 12 minutes. Let cool.

➤ In a large bowl, whisk together eggs, honey, brown sugar, liqueur, vanilla extract, almond extract and orange zest.

➤ In a medium bowl, combine flour, flaxseed, baking powder and salt. Mix well and gradually stir into egg mixture until a soft dough forms. Fold in almonds and chocolate chips.

➤ Divide dough in half and shape sticky dough into 2 logs on a floured surface. Transfer logs onto a baking sheet lined with parchment paper. Flatten logs to form a rectangle, about 9 inches (23 cm) long and 3 inches (7.5 cm) wide and no more than ½ inch (1 cm) high (dough will rise while baking). Lightly brush tops and sides of logs with egg white.

➤ Place baking sheet on *middle* rack and bake in preheated oven for 25 minutes or until loaves are golden brown and firm. Remove loaves from oven and let cool for about 15 minutes. Reduce oven temperature to 325°F.

➤ Transfer loaves to a cutting board and, using a long serrated knife, cut diagonally into ½-inch (1-cm) slices. Place slices back on lined baking sheet, cut side down, and bake for 7 to 8 minutes. Turn slices over and bake on other side for 7 to 8 minutes, until lightly browned. They'll get hard and crispy as they cool down. For extra crunch, increase baking time to 12 to 15 minutes each side.

➤ Let cool completely and store biscotti upright in an airtight container for up to a month.

36-40 BISCOTTI   40 MIN OR LESS   DAIRY-FREE   MAKE AHEAD

PER BISCOTTI(40) 79 CALORIES | 3 G TOTAL FAT (1 G SATURATED FAT) | 14 MG CHOLESTEROL | 8 MG SODIUM | 11 G CARBOHYDRATE | 1 G FIBER | 3 G PROTEIN

Almond Cookies

Biscotti con pasta di mandorle

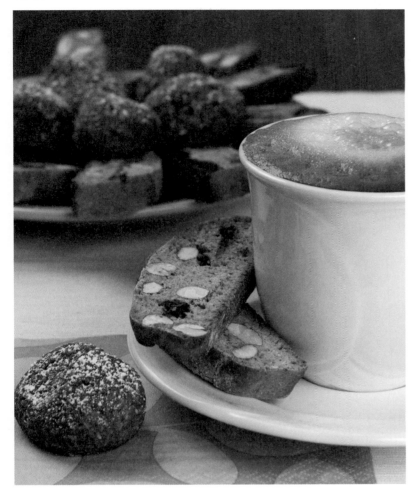

> ➤ Preheat oven 325°F.

> ➤ Combine almond meal and coconut palm sugar in a large bowl. Slowly add egg whites, mixing to incorporate well. Stir in lemon zest, vanilla and baking powder.

> ➤ Line a 9 x 12-inch cookie sheet with parchment paper. Roll dough by the tablespoons into balls. Pinch sides and place on cookie sheet about 1 inch (2.5 cm) apart.

> ➤ Bake for 15 minutes or until golden on bottom and cracked on top. Reposition cookie sheet on the *middle* oven rack and cook for 5 more minutes. Remove from oven and let cool for 10 minutes. Dust with icing sugar.

TIP Almond meal can also go by the name ground almonds or almond flour. The ingredient list should include only ground almonds (with no fillers), which have been ground to the consistency of a coarse flour.

3 cups	almond meal (see tip)
1 cup	coconut palm sugar
3	egg whites
Zest of 1 lemon	
½ tsp	pure vanilla extract
½ tsp	baking powder
Icing (confectioner's) sugar	

↻ LOW ON...THE GLYCEMIC INDEX

Coconut palm sugar, which replaces granulated sugar in this recipe, is believed to be lower on the Glycemic Index, and better able to stabilize blood sugar when compared to other sweeteners. Its taste is closer to brown sugar. You'll find coconut palm sugar in the baking section or the organics section of your grocery store.

  22-25 COOKIES   **30 MIN OR LESS**   **GLUTEN-FREE**   **DAIRY-FREE**

PER COOKIE(25) 64 CALORIES | 1 G TOTAL FAT (0 G SATURATED FAT) | 0 MG CHOLESTEROL | 64 MG SODIUM | 10 G CARBOHYDRATE | 0 G FIBER | 3 G PROTEIN

Vanilla Latte Panna Cotta

Panna cotta al caffé latte con vaniglia

FOR AS LONG AS I'VE KNOWN MY BROTHER-IN-LAW, he caps off his dinners with an espresso, a ritual played out by many Italians. Others in my family prefer a latte, and so when we host dinners, we have several brewing machines fixing the perfect elixirs. It's fitting, then, that one of my desserts honors the much-loved espresso bean in this popular dessert that's almost as easy to make as pressing the button on the coffee machine.

3 tbsp	almond slices
1½ cups	2% evaporated milk
1½ cups	almond milk
½ cup	strongly brewed coffee
1½ tbsp	agave syrup or 2 tbsp honey
1 tsp	pure vanilla extract
Pinch	ground espresso or coffee beans
Pinch	ground cinnamon
1½ tbsp	unflavored gelatin
¼ cup	low-fat 2% vanilla Greek yogurt
1	square (1 oz/28 g) dark baking chocolate, chopped

➤ Preheat oven to 350°F. Place almond slices in a single layer and roast until lightly browned, about 8 minutes; set aside.

➤ Combine evaporated and almond milks and coffee in a medium saucepan and heat over medium heat until hot but not boiling. Stir in agave syrup, vanilla, ground espresso and cinnamon. Heat another 1 to 2 minutes. Remove from heat.

➤ In the meantime, sprinkle gelatin over 4 tbsp of boiling water in a small bowl. Let stand for 2 to 3 minutes to let it bloom (powder is fully dissolved and absorbed by liquid). Give it a quick stir if not fully absorbed; whisk gelatin into milk mixture until dissolved. Pour into a large, heat-proof bowl and whisk in yogurt until fully incorporated.

➤ Pour equal amounts of mixture into 8 ceramic ramekins or custard cups (3 inch/125 mL each). Let cool for 15 minutes.

➤ Place ramekins on a baking sheet and transfer to refrigerator to set for at least 3 hours or preferably overnight.

➤ Serve panna cotta in ramekins or place ramekins halfway into a basin of hot water for 5 seconds, run a knife around perimeter to loosen edges and invert onto individual dessert plates or bowls. Garnish with about 1 tsp toasted almond slices and some chopped chocolate.

♡ LOW IN...FAT

The name "panna cotta," meaning "cooked cream," already reveals that the traditional concoction has its foundation in rich full cream. But this blend of creamy Greek yogurt, lower-fat milk and flavorful almond milk doesn't let on that there's no cream to be found on this ingredient list.

8 SERVINGS   30 MIN OR LESS   GLUTEN-FREE

PER SERVING 111 CALORIES | 4 G TOTAL FAT (2 G SATURATED FAT) | 4 MG CHOLESTEROL | 78 MG SODIUM | 14 G CARBOHYDRATE | 1 G FIBER | 5 G PROTEIN

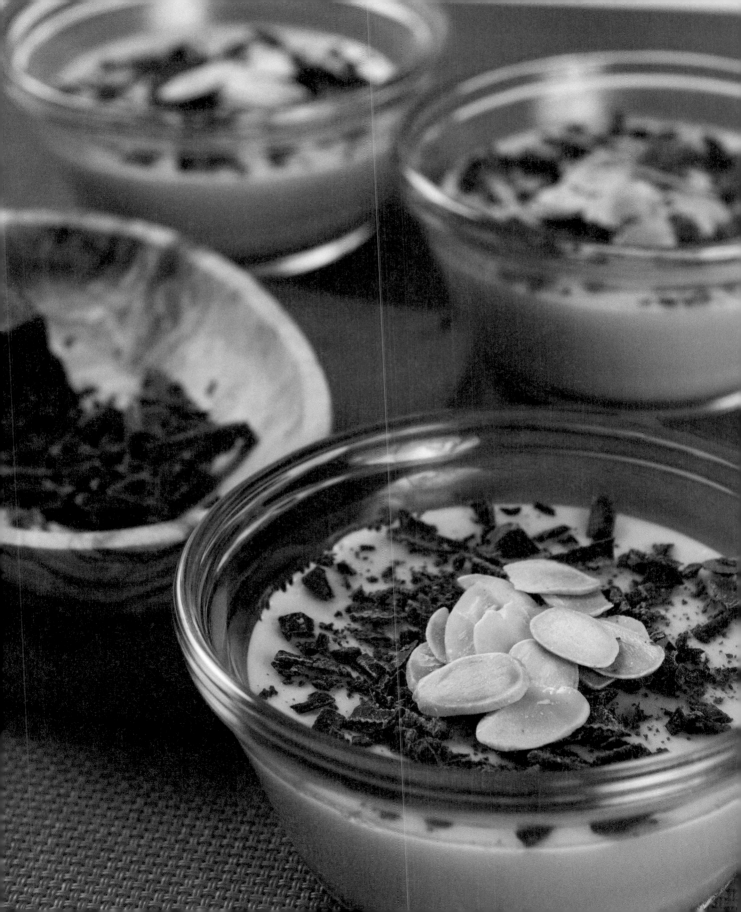

Rosa's Gluten-Free Super Sponge Cake

Pan di spagna di Rosa sensa glutine

AFTER YEARS OF TINKERING WITH THE RIGHT COMBINATION OF GLUTEN-FREE FLOURS, my mom has perfected this super-moist cake recipe, an adaptation from her dear late friend Rosa's much-loved dessert. While the cake always (I mean, *always*) gets rave reviews, it's even more special to us because it reminds us of Rosa's generous spirit and passion for life. Rosa, who lived down the street, never stopped in without bearing gifts of fresh fruit from the market, freshly baked cookies and this cake that exemplifies the legacy she's left behind.

¾ cup	brown rice flour
½ cup	tapioca flour/starch
½ cup	potato starch
7	large eggs, separated
¼ tsp	cream of tartar
¾ cup	granulated sugar
⅓ cup	high-oleic canola oil
3 tbsp	low-fat 2% vanilla Greek yogurt
⅓ cup	water
1 tsp	pure almond extract
1 pkg	(0.6 oz/16 g) Bertolini Lievito Vaniglinato (*see tip, page 258*)

TIP Use this cake in place of lady finger cookies to make a gluten-free tiramisu (*see recipe, page 260*).

➤ Combine rice flour, tapioca flour and potato starch in a medium bowl and set aside.

➤ In a stand mixer fitted with a whisk attachment, beat egg whites with cream of tartar on high speed until very stiff peaks form. Gently transfer egg-white mixture to another bowl. Set aside and keep cool.

➤ Preheat oven to 350°F.

➤ In stand mixer fitted with a whisk attachment, beat egg yolks with sugar on medium speed until well blended and pale in color. Gradually add oil, yogurt, water and almond extract and beat until well blended.

➤ Stream in reserved flour mixture; beat batter on medium-high for at least 10 minutes, scraping down sides halfway through. Don't cut this time down — you want to create as many air pockets in the batter as possible for a super spongy cake. Gently stir in Lievito Vaniglinato just until combined. Fold egg whites into batter with a spatula until well blended.

➤ Pour batter into a large greased 10-inch tube cake pan (preferably with feet) that's been dusted with flour. Bake in preheated oven for 40 minutes or until a pick inserted in the center comes out clean. Let cool and invert cake for at least 20 minutes to ensure it has fully detached from pan. You may need to run a knife around the edges of pan and tube to fully release cake.

➤ Invert onto a serving platter and serve with a dusting of icing sugar and/or fresh strawberries or raspberries and a dollop of vanilla-flavored Greek yogurt.

14-16 SERVINGS　　　　**GLUTEN-FREE**

PER SERVING(16) 150 CALORIES | 5 G TOTAL FAT (0 G SATURATED FAT) | 0 MG CHOLESTEROL | 37 MG SODIUM | 24 G CARBOHYDRATE | 1 G FIBER | 3 G PROTEIN

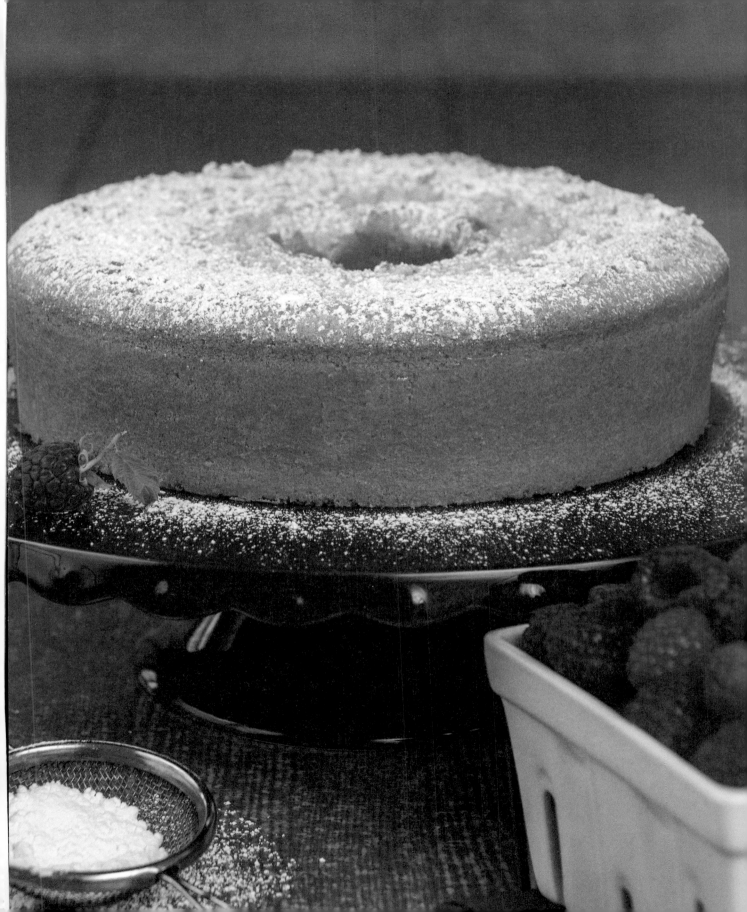

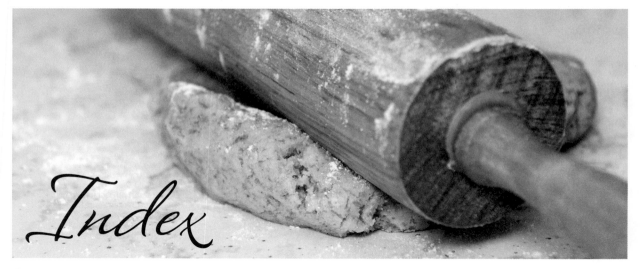

Index